High-Intensity 300

Dan Trink

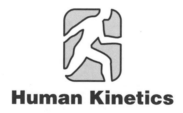

Human Kinetics

Library of Congress Cataloging-in-Publication Data

Trink, Dan, 1972-
  High-Intensity 300 / Dan Trink.
    pages cm
  Includes index.
1. Bodybuilding. 2. Physical fitness. I. Title. II. Title: High-Intensity Three hundred.
  GV546.5.T74 2014
  613.7'13--dc23

                              2014007402

ISBN: 978-1-4504-5527-5 (print)

This publication is written and published to provide accurate and authoritative information relevant to the subject matter presented. It is published and sold with the understanding that the author and publisher are not engaged in rendering legal, medical, or other professional services by reason of their authorship or publication of this work. If medical or other expert assistance is required, the services of a competent professional person should be sought.

The web addresses cited in this text were current as of March 2014, unless otherwise noted.

Acquisitions Editor: Tom Heine; **Developmental Editor:** Anne Hall; **Managing Editor:** Tyler M. Wolpert; **Copyeditor:** Patricia MacDonald; **Graphic Designer:** Joe Buck; **Graphic Artist:** Tara Welsch; **Cover Designer:** Keith Blomberg; **Photograph (cover):** © Corey Jerkins/age fotostock; **Photographs (interior):** Neil Bernstein; **Photo Asset Manager:** Laura Fitch; **Visual Production Assistant:** Joyce Brumfield; **Photo Production Manager:** Jason Allen; **Printer:** United Graphics

We thank the Stephens Family YMCA in Champaign, Illinois, for assistance in providing the location for the photo shoot for this book.

Human Kinetics books are available at special discounts for bulk purchase. Special editions or book excerpts can also be created to specification. For details, contact the Special Sales Manager at Human Kinetics.

Printed in the United States of America   10 9 8 7 6 5 4 3 2 1

The paper in this book is certified under a sustainable forestry program.

Human Kinetics
Website: www.HumanKinetics.com

United States: Human Kinetics
P.O. Box 5076
Champaign, IL 61825-5076
800-747-4457
e-mail: humank@hkusa.com

Canada: Human Kinetics
475 Devonshire Road Unit 100
Windsor, ON N8Y 2L5
800-465-7301 (in Canada only)
e-mail: info@hkcanada.com

Europe: Human Kinetics
107 Bradford Road
Stanningley
Leeds LS28 6AT, United Kingdom
+44 (0) 113 255 5665
e-mail: hk@hkeurope.com

Australia: Human Kinetics
57A Price Avenue
Lower Mitcham, South Australia 5062
08 8372 0999
e-mail: info@hkaustralia.com

New Zealand: Human Kinetics
P.O. Box 80
Torrens Park, South Australia 5062
0800 222 062
e-mail: info@hknewzealand.com

E5962

For Ricki Jean and Henry

Contents

Acknowledgments

I've never created an exercise. I've simply taken things I've learned from others and put them together in a way that made sense to me. Therefore, I'd like to thank all the great teachers, coaches, trainers and people who have taken the time and put in the effort to teach me what they thought was important about exercise, nutrition, and fitness--most notably, Joe Dowdell and Edward Williams from Peak Performance in New York City, who have served as my mentors for the past five years. I could probably fill half this book with the names of trainers, coaches, doctors, athletes, and educators who have influenced me and to whom I owe a huge debt of gratitude. I do not want to name a few and risk leaving out the names of others so I will simply say that if we spent time together in the classroom, on the gym floor, on the phone, in your seminar series, or even just exchanged a few passing words in the hallway during a fitness summit or expo, thank you for taking the time to share your knowledge, ideas, and passion with me.

I've learned as much (if not more) from spending time on the training floor as I have reading books, taking classes, or attending seminars. With that in mind, I'd also like to thank all the great training partners I've had over the years including Kyle Fields, Ed Williams, Adam Copeland, Antonio Valverde, Sam Denis, and the countless other people I've come across in gyms who were willing to trade tips, provide motivation, or simply give me a spot. You've all influenced this book as much as anyone has.

Thank you to the entire crew at Human Kinetics, particularly Tom, Anne, Tyler, and Neil, who've worked tirelessly and graciously to turn my enormous manuscript into the structured, sane and digestible book that you now hold in your hands.

Finally, I would truly be nowhere without my family. So, I'd like to thank my parents, Alex and Judy, for always being loving and supportive. And to Ricki Jean and Henry, my wife and son, whose belief in me allows me to have belief in myself. You both have taught me the true meaning of strength.

Introduction

There may be no more controversial topic in the world of fitness right now than high-intensity training (HIT). Fans of HIT rave about the constant variety and lack of boredom characteristic of these types of workouts. They revel in the fact that most training sessions last 30 minutes or less, so they are easily incorporated into their busy day. And, most important, they are blown away by the results these programs deliver. Devotees can experience dramatic changes in both body composition (especially fat loss) and performance, changes they never gained with more traditional weight or cardio programs.

Of course, high-intensity training has its detractors—those who claim these programs push beginning trainees too hard too fast, resulting in serious injury. Or, that by not following a more tried and true training progression, these enthusiasts become the gym-floor equivalent of a "jack of all trades, master of none." Detractors may say that HIT enthusiasts won't excel at any specific aspect of the strength training continuum, whether it be the ability to move massive weights or develop sport-specific skills that transfer to the track, court, or field.

But what if there were an exercise program that delivered on the strengths of the traditional approach while also exploiting the benefits of high-intensity training? Workouts that were quick, exciting, and constantly varied but also safe, effective, and grounded in a science-based approach that ensured you were progressing through the most important qualities you would want out of a solid training program?

What you currently hold in your hands is exactly that training program.

High-Intensity 300 delivers 300 unique workouts designed to make you leaner, make you stronger, and help you improve performance. And each workout is designed to be completed in 30 minutes or less. It's truly the best of both worlds.

And though you will be training hard right from the get-go, I want you training as safely as possible. For this reason, I am including a dynamic warm-up sequence for you to complete before each workout, making sure your muscles are primed and ready to go.

I am also including a ramp-up chapter to teach you how to perform the basic movement patterns that are the foundation of every workout in the book. I'll give you general tips on nutrition so you are properly fueled for each training session as well as warning signs of overtraining. If you are an experienced trainee, you may be able to skip over this chapter and jump right into the more demanding workouts. But I guarantee, even gym veterans can improve form and technique by going through the fundamentals in this chapter.

After you ramp up, you'll notice that every chapter of *High-Intensity 300* is focused on achieving a specific goal. In Ultimate Fat Loss (chapter 2), you'll be working with higher reps and lighter weights (or even body weight) at a quicker pace in order to get used to many of the movement patterns that reoccur throughout the book. Getting Stronger (chapter 3) requires that you add some weight to the bar in an effort to increase your strength levels. We then move on to Targeted Muscle Builders (chapter 4), where the workouts focus on developing one or two muscle groups per workout. This approach allows you to build more lean muscle mass and focus on any specific body parts you want to improve.

To bring up your work capacity and overall conditioning, the workouts in Last (Wo)Man Standing (chapter 5) will challenge your ability to effectively perform coordinated movements while trying to manage fatigue. The Core of the Matter (chapter 6) delivers some extra work to develop your midsection for aesthetic, performance, and strength benefits. Let's Push!, Let's Pull! (chapter 7) is built around a tried and true training approach of working noncompeting muscle groups in a superset fashion, allowing you to get a lot of work in very efficiently.

And, finally, we put it all together with 40 Toughest Workouts (chapter 8), a series of workout challenges that require you to use all the skills you've developed in the previous chapters, with a focus on maximizing performance. Working on developing different strength qualities over a set period of time is one of the key aspects that make this program superior to the more typical haphazard approach. Even though we maintain the intensity and variety that keep these workouts exciting, you'll ultimately reap greater benefits by focusing on one given strength quality (whether getting stronger, bigger, or leaner) for a given training block. This allows you to approach your training in one of two ways. You can either immediately focus on a specific goal by jumping to that section (e.g., the fat-loss chapter) or perform the workouts in the order given and become a fitness machine, training all the various fitness qualities by the time you make it to the end of the book. The choice is yours.

If you are fairly new to training, you may be wondering if you are ready for high-intensity work. Luckily, all the workouts in this book can be performed by anyone who is currently involved in a fitness program. You'll notice that each workout has an easy option, which gives novice trainees a way of scaling down the workouts to make them more appropriate to their fitness levels. And each exercise is described in detail so you'll never be left wondering how to perform a given movement. You will also find an option for stepping it up that challenges advanced trainees to push the intensity to an even higher level. So whether you've been training for only a short while or have spent countless hours sweating it out on the gym floor, these workouts are expertly designed for you.

All the greatest training programs have one thing in common: They deliver progress and results. The workouts in *High-Intensity 300* are no different. At the onset of this program, you will complete a few fitness tests. These may test how much weight you can move in a particular lift or how many reps you can perform in a specific amount of time. Then, every two months as the program progresses, we'll retest. It's a surefire way to see, feel, and experience your progress. There is nothing more exhilarating than outperforming a personal best in a specific lift or timed workout, and I guarantee you will experience that feeling.

Finally, I want you to spend your time training, not reading. After the initial ramp-up chapter, you'll notice that the remaining workouts are short on text but high on intensity. In each workout I will highlight a specific exercise in order to give you tips on form and how to maximize the effects of the movement. But, other than that, once you are into the workouts, you will be into the workouts.

OK, time to get at it. I'm about to give you tons of great information and 300 different workouts that will challenge you, excite you, and push you to your limits. The desire to crush these workouts, to bring your best every time, and to achieve more than you thought you could—that is up to you!

Let's get to work.

CHAPTER 1

Ramping Up

As I mentioned in the introduction, this book is not meant to be a review of research studies on the benefits of high-intensity training (HIT). I want you to jump in, start training, and get the results you are looking for. However, it's always good to understand the thinking and mechanisms behind any training plan you engage in. First, getting insight into the thought process behind the workout plan is a great way to gauge whether this is the right training program for your goals.

Second, when you are in the middle of a tough set, your lungs burning, sweat pouring off your forehead, and having that occasional *what have I gotten myself into* moment of self-doubt, you will, in the back of your mind, have an understanding of why you are doing what you are doing and why it is so effective. This should serve as motivation to keep on going. Now let's get into the three big concepts that make up the rationale behind high-intensity workouts.

What Is Intensity?

Most people think of intensity in the gym setting as the amount of effort you are putting into a workout. A slow walk on the treadmill while reading the morning paper is a low-intensity workout, while an all-out, sweat-pouring-off-your-forehead, heart-about-to-jump-out-of-your-chest circuit is high intensity. This is intensity of effort, the type of intensity you should be focusing on when completing chapters such as 40 Toughest Workouts, Last (Wo)Man Standing, and Ultimate Fat Loss. But intensity of effort is only one of the definitions of intensity that will be used in this book.

When it comes to official training lingo, intensity represents a specific percentage of your 1-repetition maximum (the maximum amount of weight you can lift for exactly 1 rep, or 1RM), or how much weight is on the bar relative to how much weight you can actually use if you were going all out. This becomes critical when trying to

build strength during the workouts in the chapter Getting Stronger. Finally, there is muscular intensity, or how much localized muscle fatigue you are incurring during your workout. A workout that blasts your biceps with several back-to-back exercises as you might find in Targeted Muscle Builders would fall into this category.

So, let's review. Intensity of effort is how hard you perceive yourself to be working, intensity of load is how much weight you are lifting relative to the maximum you are capable of lifting (e.g., 85 percent of your 1RM), and muscular intensity involves repeatedly working a specific muscle to a level of exhaustion. It is important to get a grasp of what type of intensity you are trying to focus on during any given workout.

The Science Behind High-Intensity Training

Along with the performance and aesthetic benefits that people gain from high-intensity training come the scientifically researched mechanisms that cause these desired adaptations. And although the science can get complicated and expansive, it is worth understanding some key concepts and mechanisms behind why HIT is so effective. Following are three key principles as to why HIT is an efficient and results-driven approach to training.

Concept 1: EPOC

The biggest concept to wrap your head around when it comes to the benefits of high-intensity training is something called excessive postexercise oxygen consumption (EPOC). After either resistance training or cardiorespiratory training (or a combination of both), the body continues to need oxygen at a higher rate than before exercise began. This occurs so the body can get back to homeostasis, or its typical resting metabolic rate. Repaying the oxygen debt caused by training requires additional energy expenditure. What this means, in a nutshell, is that you will continue to utilize energy (in the form of burning calories) well after your exercise session is over. High-intensity workouts drive up the effect of EPOC even more because you create a larger oxygen deficiency during the intensified effort of this type of training.

The bottom line? The greater the intensity of the workout, the greater the EPOC and, therefore, the greater the energy expenditure (calories burned) both during and after the workout. This afterburn can last for 36 hours postworkout, so don't underestimate just how powerful it is. Now, not every workout here tries to cash in on the EPOC effect. Many workouts focus more on building strength or gaining muscle mass—which leads perfectly into our next concept.

Concept 2: Building and Maintaining Lean Mass

In all the workouts that follow, there is a component of resistance—whether it's barbells, kettlebells, dumbbells, machines, or even body weight. The prevailing thought used to be that if you wanted fat loss, the majority of your training had to be centered around traditional long, slow cardiorespiratory activities such as jogging or cycling. And although those activities still have some value when looking for fat loss, they pale in comparison to resistance training. Why? Because resistance training builds lean muscle tissue. Lean muscle helps you gain strength, of course, but it is also metabolically active, and it takes a lot of energy to maintain muscle and keep it functioning. So, essentially, the more muscle mass you have, the more calories you can consume without gaining additional body fat.

Concept 3: Exercise Density

Density is simply the amount of work you perform in a given amount of time—in this case, 30 minutes or less in each workout. By packing more work into a shorter amount of time you drive up your work capacity, which is critical for cardiorespiratory health and sports performance. (Ever notice that it is the athlete who can give the greatest effort in the fourth quarter or final round that is usually the most successful?) These workouts are truly the ultimate in exercise efficiency, getting the most work done, in the least amount of time, while delivering optimal body composition and performance results.

Assessing Your Fitness

It's difficult to know where you are going if you have no idea where you have been. Yet so many people begin training programs without any type of self-assessment (maybe with the exception of jumping on the scale) as a baseline by which to judge future progress. You are not going to make that mistake. Following are two basic benchmark workouts. One will measure the total number of reps you can perform of several movements. The other will test the time it takes to get through an exercise circuit. Be sure to record your results so you can reassess these in the future.

Benchmark Workout 1

Complete one set of the maximum number of repetitions for each movement. Rest 3 to 5 minutes between each movement. The number after each exercise indicates the workout number where the exercise is featured with detailed instructions.

1. Barbell back squat (#63) with 50 percent of your body weight.
2. Kneeling lat pull-down (beginner) (#120) with 50 percent of your body weight/chin-up (intermediate or advanced) (#73)
3. Incline push-up (beginner) (#115)/push-up (intermediate or advanced) (#12)
4. Plank (figure 1.8) to be held for the maximum amount of time

Table 1.1 should be used as a guide to evaluate your appropriate difficulty levels for workouts. If you can only perform fewer than 10 reps of the barbell back squat, fewer than 5 reps of the chin-ups or pull-downs, fewer than 15 reps of the push-ups, and less than 45 seconds of the plank, you should opt for the easy variation found at the end of each workout. There is no shame in having to start with

Table 1.1   Difficulty Level Based on Number of Repetitions Completed

Exercise	Easy	Standard	Step it up
Barbell back squat	<10	10-20	>20
Chin-up / pull-down	<5	5-10	>10
Push-up	<15	15-25	>25
Plank	<45 sec	60-120 sec	>120 sec

the easy variation, and with some consistent training you will be able to move to the standard workouts in no time.

If you can perform between 10 and 20 reps of the squat, 5 and 10 reps of the chin-ups or pull-downs, 15 and 25 reps of the push-ups, and 46 seconds and 2 minutes of the plank, you should be attempting the standard versions of the workouts.

If you are exceeding all the rep ranges (20+ squats, 10+ chins-ups or pull-downs, 25+ push-ups, 2 minute+ plank), then feel free to attempt the suggestions for stepping it up to make the workouts more challenging and intense.

What happens if you can do certain exercises at one level and other exercises at a different level? The goal of *High-Intensity 300* is to provide workouts that are customizable to your fitness levels and goals while giving you a training challenge. So use the highest intensity you can manage for any exercise. Just note which level you were able to achieve, and when a comparable exercise comes up in the training program, use the intensity that is appropriate. However, if you are on the fence about which intensity to use, start with something a bit easier. You will get more benefit out of performing your workouts with great technique and a lighter load than adding more weight to the bar and using bad form. Remember, training is a lifelong endeavor. There is no need to rush into adding more load than you can handle.

Benchmark Workout 2

Complete all repetitions of all three exercises in the shortest amount of time possible. Like before, the number after the exercise indicates the workout where it's featured.

1. 30 prisoner squats (#188)

2. 20 incline push-ups (beginner) (#115)/20 push-ups (intermediate or advanced) (#12)

3. 20 kneeling lat pull-downs (beginner) (#120) with 50 percent of body weight/10 pull-ups (intermediate or advanced) (#231)

Use table 1.2 as a guide to determine the appropriate difficulty level. If your total time is under 2:30 for all three exercises, you can consider utilizing the step-it-up option. If your time is between 2:30 and 5 minutes, the standard workouts should be appropriate for you. If your time is more than 5 minutes or you cannot complete the workout, I would recommend sticking with the easy option for now.

Table 1.2 Difficulty Level Based on Time Taken (Min) per Set

Easy	Standard	Step it up
>5:00	2:30-5:00	<2:30
>5:00	2:30-5:00	<2:30
>5:00	2:30-5:00	<2:30

Retest both benchmark workouts every two months and record your results. If your results shift from one category to the next (e.g., you performed the second benchmark workout in 5:25 two months ago and you finished in 4:45 upon retesting), feel free to attempt the more challenging workout for the remainder of the program.

Finally, several of the workouts recommend using loads that are a percentage of your 1RM of a specific movement. Therefore, it would be beneficial to test or at least have a solid idea of your 1RM in the conventional deadlift, barbell bench press, barbell front squat, barbell back squat, and weighted chin-up before you start tackling these workouts. Table 1.3 can be used to keep track of your 1RM for these exercises.

Table 1.3 Chart to record 1RM

Exercise	Personal 1RM
Conventional deadlift	
Barbell bench press	
Barbell front squat	
Barbell back squat	
Weighted chin-up	

Ramping Up to Daily Workouts

Here's the thing about high-intensity training—it's intense. Many trainees are susceptible to injury because although they have a lot of motivation and energy to begin a really challenging training program, their bodies just aren't ready for that type of effort. What follows are some basic rules and parameters you should remember when performing HIT (or, frankly, any workout program).

We also discuss the basic movement patterns—what they are and how to perform them correctly—as well as the thought process behind the easy and step-it-up options you will find at the end of each workout.

Rules to Train By

In my years as a strength and conditioning specialist, five big-picture rules have allowed my clients to continue to make progress and, most important, remain injury free. Although I do want you to train with intensity, my number one priority is to make sure you stay safe. Those who can stay healthiest can train the most and, in the long run, make the most progress—so, please, take these rules seriously. Your long-term success depends on it.

Always, Always, Always Put Safety First

I completely understand the desire to train hard and push your limits in an effort to challenge yourself and get the best possible results. In truth, this attitude is needed if you want to optimally progress your training. However, intensity and effort should never be a substitute for common sense, technique, and safety. Always err on the side of caution so you are certain to lift weights you can handle without injury, and always strive to use technically acceptable form during every movement. I realize that, in the middle of a great session, with adrenaline coursing through your veins, you may want to push the weights you choose beyond the limits of your capabilities. However, make sure your increases are reasonable (5 percent or less from the maximum weight you lifted last time you performed the movement), and do not make choices based on your ego or your desire to show off. Your results will never be optimal if you repeatedly can't train due to injury.

When attempting maximal or near-maximal weights, always have experienced spotters on hand when appropriate who can make sure you are safe and get you out of any failed lifts. Finally, you will notice an icon next to particularly complicated or difficult exercises that require technical efficiency to be performed safely or correctly. Please be sure you are comfortable with the techniques required for those exercises before attempting the workouts or utilizing them at higher intensities.

Don't Skip the Dynamic Warm-Up

Dynamic warm-ups (described in detail later in the chapter) activate and prepare your entire body, as well as specific muscle groups, for the workout ahead by increasing core and muscle temperature and by laying down the foundations of the movement patterns you will be going through during your training. It is very easy, especially when pressed for time, to discard this portion of the training program and get right to "the good stuff." I urge you not to do that. Your overall movement as well as performance during the rest of the training session will be enhanced if you put the appropriate effort into your dynamic warm-up. It will also help safeguard you against potential injuries. So don't skip it.

Choose Your Loads Wisely

As you might imagine, in a book of this nature it is very difficult to make blanket recommendations on specific loads because everyone is a different size and has a different degree of strength and different levels of training experience. Some of you will have a pretty good idea of your 1RM for all the major lifts (remember, 1RM stands for 1-repetition maximum, or the largest load you can handle for exactly 1 repetition of a specific exercise). A basic rule to follow when choosing appropriate weight is to select a load that allows you to complete the prescribed number of repetitions with perfect form. For beginners, choose a load that allows you to complete one or two more repetitions than the prescribed number (so if the program calls for 12 reps of a dumbbell overhead press, choose a weight with which you could complete 14 reps). This will take some trial and error in the early going, but you will learn to assess your limitations and abilities fairly quickly.

Make a Great Effort

Of course, safety is critical, but you do want to put in a great effort every time you train. Remember, these are high-intensity workouts. If you are tempted to pick up the latest gossip magazine between sets, you're probably not working hard enough. One of the benefits of these workouts is that they are all relatively short. Therefore you should be able to completely focus your mind on the task at hand and put in maximal effort.

Have Your Mind on Recovery

What you do outside the gym is just as critical to your results as what you do inside it. To get the most out of your training, you must take specific measures toward recovery. Getting 7 to 9 hours of sleep each night is ideal. And even though the length of these workouts should allow for recovery and increased training frequency, a day or two of rest per week is essential to stave off fatigue and allow for maximal effort and performance. (It's the reason there are 300 workouts in this book and not 365—be sure to take some days off!) Try to manage lifestyle and additional stress through various relaxation techniques. Be sure your nutrition is on point (more on this later). Burning the candle at both ends by training hard and living hard will not yield optimal results. Remember, the workouts are 30 minutes or less, but health and fitness are truly 24/7 priorities.

Training Terms and Specifics

A few terms and concepts that appear throughout the book may be familiar to you if you've been following or reading training programs for a while, or they may be completely new to you if you are a beginner. A *superset* is any group of two or more exercises done in succession with either no rest or a specific amount of rest between movements. They are indicated by assigning a letter in front of the exercise name followed by ascending numbers. Here's an example:

A1. Trap bar deadlift
- 3 sets × 8 reps, 60 seconds of rest

A2. Lying hamstring curl
- 3 sets × 10 reps, 45 seconds of rest

A3. Seated calf raise
- 3 sets × 12 reps, 45 seconds of rest

This sequence would have you performing 8 reps of the trap bar deadlift, followed by 60 seconds of rest. You would then perform 10 reps of the lying hamstring curl followed by 45 seconds of rest, then finish the superset with 12 reps of the seated calf raise. After another

45 seconds of rest, you would go back to the trap bar deadlift and repeat the entire sequence until all 3 sets are complete.

A *complex* is a specific type of superset in which several exercises are strung together using one implement (such as a dumbbell, kettlebell, or barbell), with no rest between movements. The goal is to seamlessly transition from one movement to the next until all repetitions are complete, rest the assigned amount of time, and then repeat for a total number of sets. For example a barbell complex may look like this

Hang power clean
- 4 sets × 6 reps

Push press
- 4 sets × 6 reps

Bent-over row
- 4 sets × 6 reps
- 60 seconds of rest

In this case you would grab the barbell and perform 6 reps of the hang power clean, transition directly into the 6 reps of push press, and then finish the complex with 6 reps of the bent-over row. You would then rest for 60 seconds and repeat the process for a total of 4 sets.

Other concepts such as timed circuits, tonnage sets, ladders, and never-ending sets all appear throughout the book and are explained in detail before those workouts.

Fundamental Movement Patterns

Although there are hundreds (maybe thousands) of exercises, the majority are mainly variations on eight fundamental movement patterns: hip hinge, squat, overhead press, chest press, chin-up, row, crunch, and plank. By following these guidelines and tips for performing these patterns correctly and effectively, you'll be successful no matter what twist, variation, or implement (dumbbell, barbell, body weight) is being utilized.

Hip Hinge

Found in movements such as the conventional deadlift (#5) and the double-arm kettlebell swing (#13)

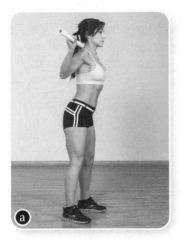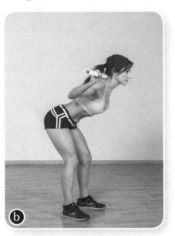

The hip hinge may be the most difficult fundamental movement pattern for trainees to perform correctly, which is why I chose to place it first on the list. The hip hinge relies on good spinal posture and the ability to activate the posterior chain (i.e., all the muscles in the back of your body—namely the hamstrings, glutes, spinal erectors, and muscles of the upper back). Since people cannot see these muscle groups in the mirror, they can have a hard time visualizing how they work.

A great way to practice the hip hinge is to utilize a PVC pipe or broomstick across your traps as in a back squat (a). Keep your chest tall and maintain a straight, flat back throughout the entire movement (b). Unlock your knees, but do not let them bend. Drive your butt back by hinging at your hips (standing a few inches away from a wall and reaching your butt back until it touches is a great feedback mechanism). If you are doing this correctly, you should begin to feel a stretch in your hamstrings. If you are doing this incorrectly, you will begin to feel it in your lower back. The mental key to this entire movement is to think about driving your hips back, not bringing your chest closer to the ground.

Common mistakes: rounding the lower back, utilizing knee bend to gain additional range of motion, assuming a forward-rounded shoulder posture, initiating movement by bringing the chest forward as opposed to driving the hips back.

Squat

Found in movements such as the barbell back squat (#63) and the barbell front squat (#44)

Perhaps no other movement has been scrutinized and is as polarizing as the squat. Although everyone agrees this is a critical movement pattern, how to teach it and what the end product should look like are topics of much debate. I recommend practicing your squat form two ways. The first is a goblet squat in which

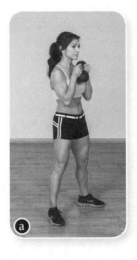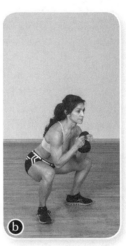

you hold either a light dumbbell or kettlebell directly in front of your chest (a). The other is using an unloaded barbell across your traps in order to work on your back squat technique. Each of these loading parameters will put you in a different posture (you will be more upright throughout the movement in a goblet squat, which mimics the front squat position, while your torso will be more forward leaning in the back squat).

Initiate both movements by unlocking your hips and driving them back (as in the hip hinge) while unlocking your knees and allowing them to bend. Utilize this combination of hip hinging and knee bending to lower your hips toward the ground. Be sure to keep a flat back and a tall chest throughout the entire movement. Once you get as low as your range of motion will allow (b), reverse the motion and return to the starting position. Two things to remember during your ascent: When in the back squat position, drive your elbows forward to help your torso stay tall as you return to the top position. And, in both movements, be sure to keep your entire foot down by driving your heels into the ground.

The split squat and lunge utilize a position where one foot is forward and the other foot is back. Keep the stance between the feet long from front to back, with a tall chest. Full range of motion is achieved when the back knee is anywhere from touching to 2 inches (5 cm) above the floor.

Common mistakes: jamming the knees forward, not keeping the torso tall and folding forward, allowing the knees to cave inward when initiating the lifting phase of the movement.

Overhead Press

Found in movements such as the push press (#16) and the push jerk (#81)

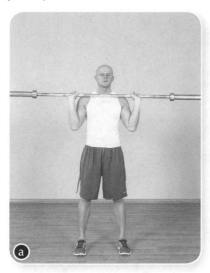

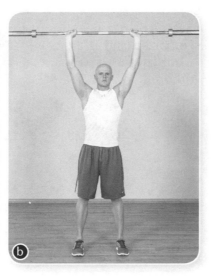

Any overhead pressing movement should be performed only by those who have no shoulder pain or impingement and have sufficient range of motion with arms overhead. For many people, overhead presses are more safely and effectively performed by keeping the grip narrow (directly outside shoulder width) and the elbows tucked in toward the rib cage (*a*). This is true when using any implement including dumbbells and kettlebells. From a performance standpoint, it is critical to keep the bar from getting out in front of the toes as it is being pressed overhead (*b*). Keep the bar over the middle of the foot by retracting the head back (as if making a double chin). Finally, although it is a completely valid method and makes its way into a few workouts, overhead pressing from behind the head is not possible for many people who lack the shoulder and trunk flexibility to perform this motion correctly. If you fall into that category, substitute with a front-loaded variation.

Common mistakes: using too wide a grip, leaning back during the lifting phase in order to gain leverage, using only partial range of motion by not bringing the bar under the chin at the bottom.

Chest Press

Found in movements such as the barbell bench press (#54) and the incline dumbbell chest press (#210)

Similar to the overhead press, for most people the chest press will be most safely and effectively performed with a fairly narrow grip (powerlifters notwithstanding). As you descend into the bottom position of the movement, keep your elbows tucked toward your sides (as opposed to allowing them to flare out). On barbell chest press movements such as the bench press, start with your eyes directly under the bar (this will prevent you from pressing into the barbell catches when pressing back up) (*a*). Full range of motion is achieved when the bar touches your chest between the collarbones

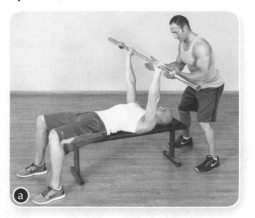

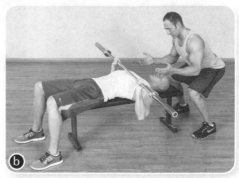

and the bottom of the sternum (*b*). When chest pressing from a bench, be sure to keep your head and the area between your shoulder blades and butt in contact with the bench at all times and your feet flat on the floor. As with the majority of movements, use a spotter when attempting challenging loads.

Common mistakes: flaring the elbows outward during the lowering phase, not achieving full range of motion, bringing the butt or head off the bench during the lifting phase.

Chin Up

Found in movements such as the pull-up (#231), chin-up (#73) and the lat pull-down (#120)

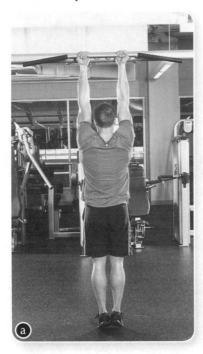
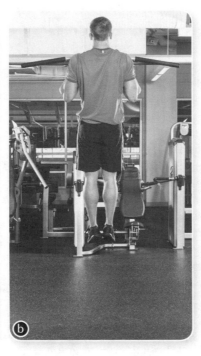

Regardless of which grip you are using, perform a chin-up by beginning at the bottom position, with arms fully extended (a). Drive your body up to the bar by retracting your shoulder blades first and pulling your chest up toward the bar, keeping your knees back. A rep is achieved by getting your chin over the bar (b). Return to the starting position (arms fully extended).

Common mistakes: not fully extending at the bottom position, bringing the knees forward to gain leverage, "arming" it up by not retracting the shoulder blades and utilizing the muscles of the back, swinging to gain momentum (sometimes known as kipping).

Row

Found in movements such as the seated cable row with hip flexion (#174) and the underhand-grip seated cable row (#69)

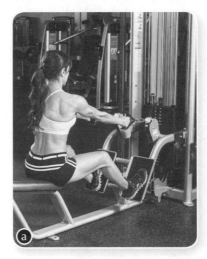
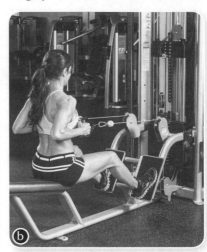

Rows have several variations, all utilizing different stances and postures. For bent-over rows, it is critical to keep a neutral spine and flat back. Shoulder blades should be retracted, and your torso should be just short of parallel to the floor. For the barbell and bilateral dumbbell versions, several different hand positions and grips can be utilized, and those will be detailed in the individual workouts. For the single-arm dumbbell work, utilize the same back position but support your knee and nonworking hand on a bench. For seated cable versions of the row, make sure your chest is tall and you are sitting upright (a). Keep a fixed torso, and resist the urge to flex your trunk forward or backward to accommodate the weight as you pull the cable toward your body (b).

Common mistakes: rounding the upper back during bent-over variations, not keeping the torso parallel to the ground during bent-over variations, using torso rotation during single-arm movements, flexing at the trunk during unsupported seated variations.

Crunch

Found in movements such as the sit-up (#251) and the hanging leg raise (#217)

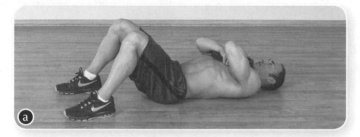

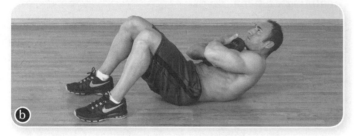

A crunch (for our purposes) is defined as any movement where the abdominals are flexed, bringing the rib cage closer to the hip bones. The key to success in the ground-based versions of this movement pattern is to make sure the back is flat and the chest is lifted up toward the ceiling. Arms can be placed behind the head or crossed in front of the chest, or you can hold a weighted implement (a) or an anchor point overhead (on movements such as the reverse crunch). Be sure to keep a neutral spine as you lift toward the ceiling (b), and never pull forward when your hands are behind your head.

Common mistakes: rounding the upper back, moving the torso forward rather than upward, pulling the head forward, utilizing the hip flexors by overextending the range of motion.

Plank

Found in movements such as the push-up (#12) and the side plank (#175)

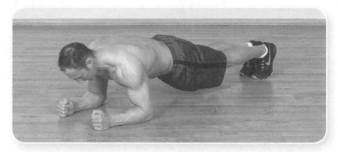

The plank involves an isometric contraction, meaning the muscles have tension but are not changing length. Being able to brace and activate your core muscles in this manner are critical components of so many movements including deadlifts, squats, and military presses. Maintaining a neutral spine, flat back, engaged hips, and active abdominal musculature is critical for achieving good posture. Thinking of the phrase *head to heel, strong as steel* will reinforce the rigidity this position requires.

Common mistakes: sagging at the hips, poking the head and chin forward, rounding the mid- and upper back, bringing the hands together rather than keeping them shoulder-width apart.

Taking It Easy Versus Stepping It Up

I was determined to make *High-Intensity 300* an exercise program that everyone, regardless of training experience, could benefit from. The challenge lies in the fact that everyone has different strength levels, familiarity with the lifts, and overall training experience. With that in mind, each workout has two additional versions to the standard workout: easy and step it up. The easy option regresses the workout by either recommending movements that are simpler to perform or reducing the recommended reps, sets, or weight used in the standard version. Step it up does the opposite, adding intensity to the workout by increasing one or more of the variables. Since most of the standard workouts are to be completed in 30 minutes or less, they should be quite challenging, so be sure you are really confident in your abilities before attempting the stepped-up versions of the programs. You can't say I didn't warn you.

KNOWING WHEN YOU'VE OVERDONE IT

Given that these programs are well designed, follow specific training phases, can be scaled up or down based on your abilities, and are of short duration, the chances of overuse injuries and overtraining are minimized. However, even the best athletes working with great coaches on smart training programs can overdo it. If you injure yourself during a lift, be sure to get checked out by a health care professional and give the injury time to properly heal and be rehabilitated. If your desire to train decreases, your heart rate is constantly elevated, you have a hard time sleeping, or you find yourself consistently moody or depressed, you may be suffering from overtraining. Try taking a few days off and see if the symptoms subside. If they do, great. If not, consider taking some extended time off of training to let your metabolism, nervous system, and mental energy return to normal. Just because there are hundreds of workouts in this book does not mean you are required to train every day. Learn to listen to your body and know when it needs to rest. Without proper recovery and a good mental frame of mind, you will never realize the gains you should be making from this training program.

Eating to Build Muscle

Just as recovery is critical for positively adapting to this training program, so is proper nutrition. And although I don't like to assign specific percentages to the importance of the components of a fitness program (e.g., 80 percent of progress is nutrition), rest assured that properly fueling your workouts before and after training will play an enormous role in how you progress over time. It is not the intention of this book to lay out a specific diet plan for optimizing body composition through diet (there are plenty out there to choose from), but here are some general recommendations that will have you on your way to reaping the most benefits from your training.

Eat a protein-rich breakfast.

Starting your day with a protein-rich breakfast has been shown to help improve body composition by optimizing hormonal production and providing a feeling of satiety (fullness), which leads to better portion control throughout the rest of the day.

Shoot for a total of 1.4 to 1.8 grams of protein per kilogram of body weight per day.

Protein is the key component for building and maintaining lean muscle tissue, especially in people who are engaging in resistance training programs. If the metric system isn't your thing, this translates into .7 to .9 grams of protein per pound of body weight per day. You can always check on the foods labels or on websites such as www.calorieking.com or www.nutritiondata.com to find out how much protein is in the food you eat.

Include protein and slow-digesting carbohydrate in your preworkout meal.

A preworkout meal of protein and slow-acting carbohydrate will give you energy for the training session and prime your muscular system for protein synthesis. How long before a training session you should eat this meal is based on individual tolerance (some people can eat 15 minutes before a training session, while others find it difficult to train with 2 hours of eating). A very broad recommendation is to have your preworkout meal 90 minutes to 2 hours before training. Good slow-digesting carbohydrate sources include brown rice, sweet potatoes, and quinoa.

Consume a carbohydrate and protein drink immediately after finishing your workout.

Glycogen is, simply put, the most efficient energy source within a muscle. During a workout, glycogen is depleted by working muscles. You want to restore glycogen as soon as possible after weight training to begin the rebuilding and repair process, and the quickest way to do this is by ingesting fast-digesting liquid carbohydrates. Glycogen also works as a facilitator, allowing cell-building protein to enter the muscles. A good general recommendation is to drink a postworkout shake that has a ratio of 2:1 carbohydrates to protein.

Limit the amount of processed foods you consume each day.

Restricting the amount of highly processed foods you consume will improve the health of your entire digestive system as well as other systems in the body. A healthy digestive system is critical for getting the most out of the nutrients you do consume. So fewer processed foods means a healthier digestive system, which, in turn, means more nutrients getting to your muscles.

Be sure to keep vegetable intake high.

Vegetables contain high levels of micronutrients, which are the vitamins, minerals, and phytochemicals responsible for making sure your cells are functioning properly. So get in more veggies. Your mom and your muscles will be happy you did. And, while we are on the topic, one or two servings of fruit per day can also help deliver vitamins and additional energy during tough workouts.

Dynamic Warm-Up Exercises

Dynamic warm-up movements increase core temperature, prepare the nervous system for the workout ahead, and fire the major muscle groups in preparation for training. These exercises should be held for 1 or 2 seconds in each position and have repeatedly been proven more effective than static stretching before resistance training. Each workout lists several (usually three or four) of these movements that you should complete before your training session, chosen based on the movements and muscle groups you'll be focusing on that day. The dynamic warm-up sequence should be included in the 30 minutes of training. I cannot emphasis enough how important it is to not skip this aspect of the training program. Your ability to move well, stay injury free, and get the most out of your workout hinges on completing the dynamic warm-up sequence assigned to these workouts.

World's Greatest Stretch

This warm-up earns its not-so-modest name by efficiently activating several key muscle groups in one movement.

1. Start by stepping out into a long lunge with your left leg forward. Keep your back leg as straight as possible in order to get a stretch in your hip flexors.

2. Reach down and place your hands on either side of your front foot (a). Now take your left elbow and reach it down toward the instep of your sneaker by rotating at your thoracic spine (midback) (b).

3. Take that same arm (the left) and rotate around until it is straight and reaches toward the ceiling (c).

4. Now return to the long lunge position, with both hands on either side of your foot (your right hand has not moved since you first placed it there) (d). Bring your hips back and up, and straighten your front leg as much as possible in order to stretch the hamstring on your right leg. Bend the back knee until it reaches the floor, and lift your chest (e).

5. Stand up and move your left foot forward toward your right.

6. Repeat the sequence on the other side by lunging the right foot forward. Completing the sequence on each side constitutes 1 rep.

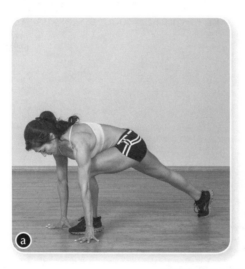
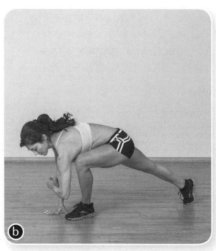
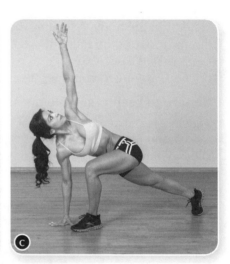
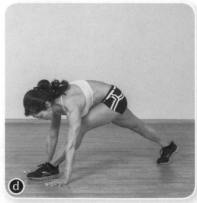
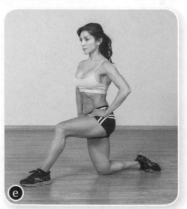

Quadruped T-Spine Rotation

1. Start in a quadruped position by getting on the floor with your hands directly under your shoulders and your knees under your hips (as if you were about to begin crawling).

2. Place your left hand behind your head.

3. Reach your left elbow to your right wrist by twisting at your thoracic spine (midback) (a). Keep your hips square to the ground to ensure you are not utilizing your lower back.

4. Rotate to the left and reach your elbow to the ceiling (b). Repeat all the reps on the right side before switching to the left.

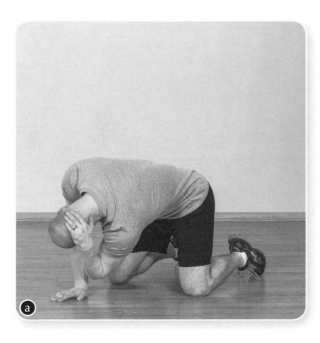

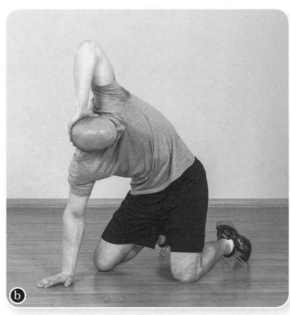

Cat–Cow

1. Begin in a quadruped position by getting on the floor with your hands directly under your shoulders and your knees under your hips (as if you were about to begin crawling).

2. Press your hands into the floor and lift your midback up toward the ceiling, tucking your chin toward your chest (a).

3. Hold for 2 seconds and then reverse the motion, bringing your rib cage down toward the floor and retracting your shoulder blades (b).

4. Hold the bottom position for 2 seconds. Repeat for prescribed number of reps.

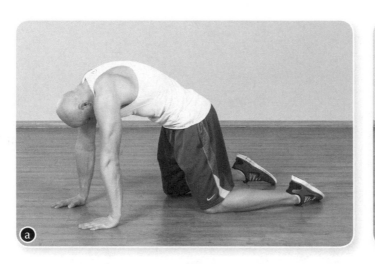

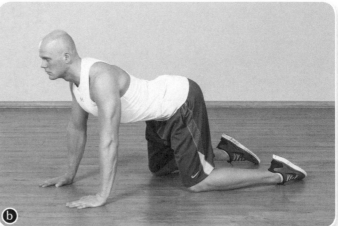

Shoulder Sweeps

1. Lie on the floor, facing up with your legs straight. Bring your left knee up, bending it 90 degrees and laying it over your right leg. Place an object (such as a foam roller, yoga block, small medicine ball, or folded towels) under your knee for support. Place your right hand on your left knee, ensuring that it maintains contact with the object throughout the entire movement. Place your left hand directly overhead, with your palm up (a).

2. Keeping as much of your arm in contact with the floor as possible throughout the entire movement, sweep your arm downward toward your legs (b).

3. As your arm begins to go past your shoulder, your hand will flip over to a downward-facing position. As you keep rotating downward, bend your arm in an effort to get your thumb to touch your middle back (c).

4. Reverse the movement (your arm will straighten and your palm will rotate over to a palm-up position). Once your arm reaches the starting position, allow your elbow to bend and reach your thumb to your left ear. Remember that the goal is to keep as much of your arm and hand in contact with the floor at all times. Repeat all reps on one side before switching to the other.

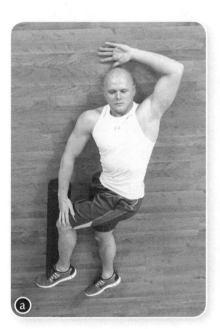
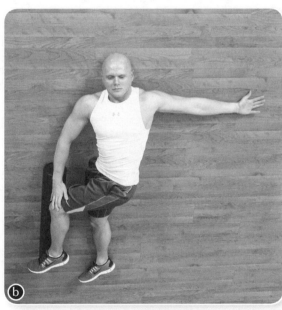
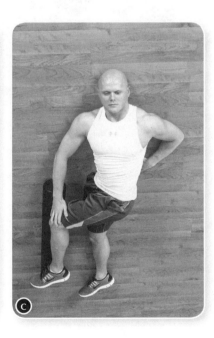

Inchworm

1. From a standing position, bend at the waist, keeping your knees locked out, and reach your hands to the floor (a).

2. Slowly begin to walk your hands out as far as possible in an alternating fashion (b) until your entire body is parallel to the floor (c).

3. Once you've reached your limit, begin to walk your feet toward your hands, keeping your legs straight and raising your hips toward the ceiling (d).

4. Once you get your feet as close to your hands as possible, walk your hands out again, and repeat the entire sequence for the recommended number of repetitions.

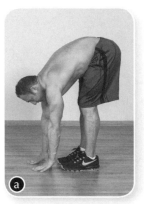
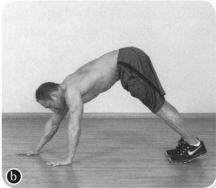
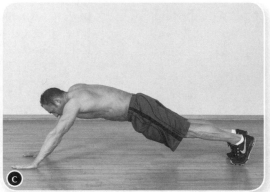
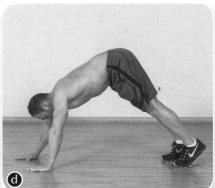

Hip Rocker

1. Begin in the bottom position of a lunge, with your right leg forward, left leg back, and both knees at 90 degrees (you may want to place a pad or towel behind your back knee for comfort). Bring your left foot up toward your glutes. Using your left hand, grab the left ankle and bring that foot as close to the left glute as possible (a).

2. Rock forward, creating a good stretch in the left hip flexor and quad (b). At the same time you are creating mobility in the right ankle by driving the front knee forward and out (toward the small toe). Hold for 2 seconds and rock back to the starting position. You may want to hold onto a bench for stability throughout the movement. Complete all the recommended repetitions for one side before switching.

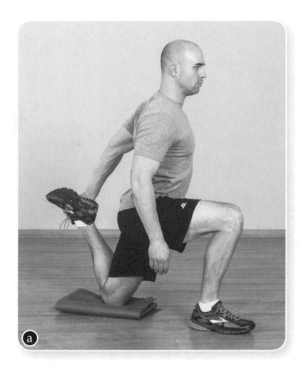
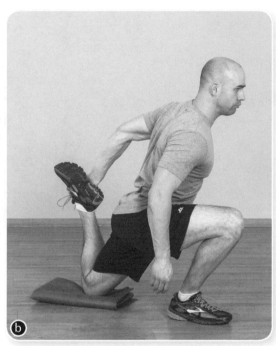

Kneeling Adductor Stretch

1. Start in a tall kneeling position (meaning both knees on the floor and bent to 90 degrees, with your feet behind you).

2. Lift your leg and bring it out directly to the side so your knee and foot are perpendicular to your torso.

3. Gently lean to your right, stretching your adductor (groin muscle) on your left leg. Hold for 2 seconds before returning to the start. Repeat for the recommended number of reps before switching to the left side.

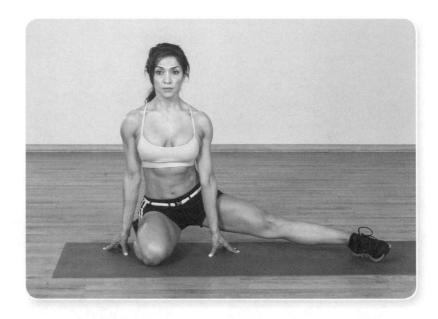

Inverted Hamstring Stretch

1. From a standing position, extend your arms out toward your sides, with your palms facing up.

2. Maintaining a tall chest and flat back, bring your left foot behind you, with the left heel reaching behind you and arcing up toward the ceiling (a). Be sure to keep both legs straight. Your chest will lower until it is parallel to the ground (b). Note: Focus on bringing the back heel up toward the ceiling rather than lowering your chest to the ground to get the most out of this movement. Complete all reps on one side before switching to the other.

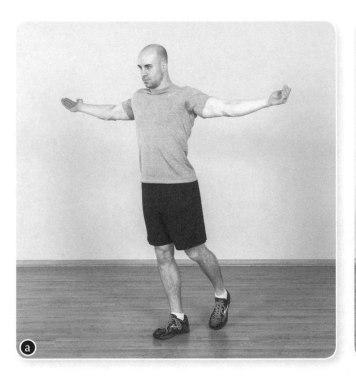

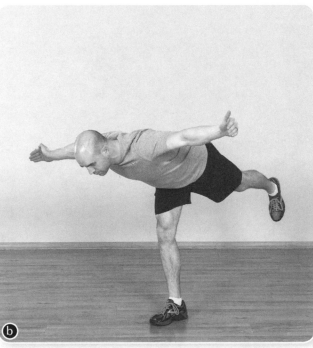

Squat to Stand

1. With feet greater than hip-width apart, bend forward and grab under the toes of both feet with your hands.

2. Pull your hips downward, lifting your chest until you are in the bottom of a deep squat position (a).

3. Release your right hand, and reach overhead and back as far as possible before bringing it back under your right toes (b).

4. Repeat on the left side (c).

5. Release both hands, extend them overhead, and stand straight up (d).

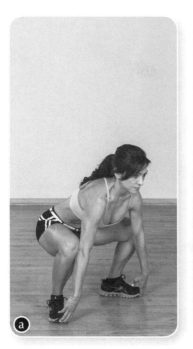 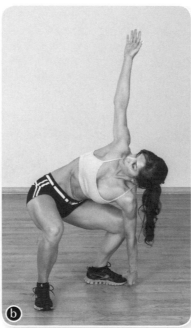 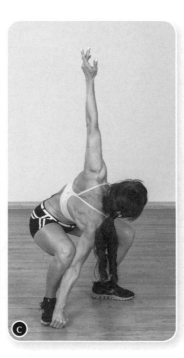 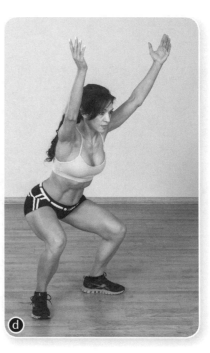

Glute Bridge

1. Lie on your back with your knees bent 90 degrees and your feet flat on the floor (a).

2. Lift your hips until you have created a straight line from your knees to your shoulders (your head, upper back, arms, and feet should be the only body parts in contact with the floor) (b).

3. Flex your glutes at the top for 2 seconds before returning your hips back to the floor. Repeat for the recommended number of reps.

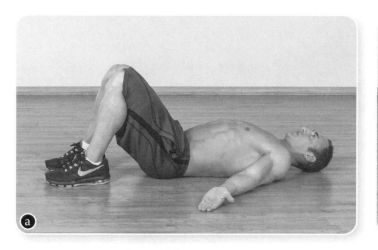

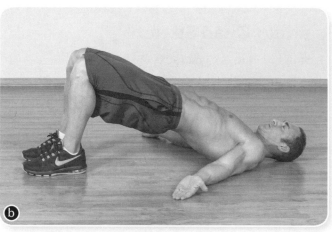

Essential Static-Stretch Cool-Downs

There is much debate as to how effective static stretching is for improving flexibility (and if it is actually effective at all). However, I do recommend static stretching postworkout simply because it's a guaranteed way to cool down and calm the nervous system after an intense bout of training. As with the dynamic warm-up exercises, each workout will focus on a few static stretching exercises that work on the muscle groups used during the workout.

Standing Quad Stretch

1. Stand next to a squat rack.
2. While holding on to one of the supports with your right hand, reach back with your left hand and grab your left ankle, bringing your heel up to your butt.
3. Keep your knees together, drive your hip slightly forward, and squeeze your right glute.
4. Hold the stretch for 20 seconds and then repeat on the other side.

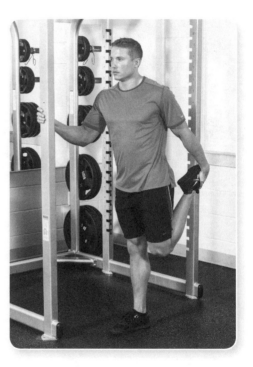

Double Lat Stretch

1. Grab a pole or the support on a squat rack with both hands, interlocking your fingers.
2. Sit back into your hips and allow your torso to bend forward (at the end position your eyes should be facing the ground and your arms should be directly overhead).
3. Allow your weight to shift onto your heels in order to get a stretch in your lats.
4. Hold for 20 seconds.

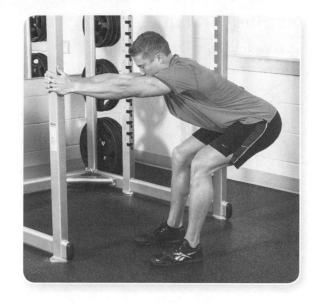

Pec Stretch

1. Grab the support on a squat rack with your right hand.
2. Slowly turn yourself away from the support, creating a stretch in the front of your shoulder and chest.
3. Hold the stretch for 20 seconds and then repeat on the other side.

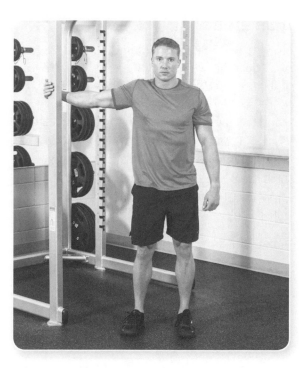

Hamstring Stretch

1. Stand with your feet at hip-width.
2. Bring your fingertips toward your toes by reaching your hips back (avoid rounding your upper back).
3. Once you can no longer push your hips back any more, you have reached the end of your range of motion.

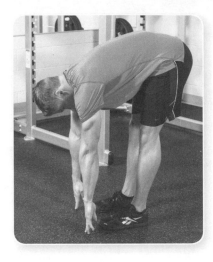

Calf Stretch

1. Using a calf-stretching board, low step, or part of a squat rack, place the ball of your right foot at the edge of the step while keeping your heel on the ground (a).
2. Stand tall and step forward with your right leg so your right foot is in front of your left.
3. You should feel a strong stretch in the right calf muscle (b).
4. Hold for 20 seconds and then repeat on the other side.

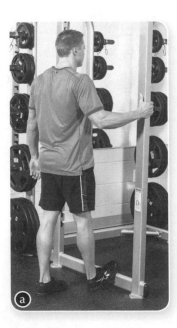 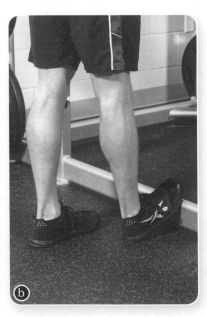

90-Degree Stretch

1. Place your right leg on a bench or stretching table so that the lateral (outside) of your foot, lower leg, and upper leg all rest on the table. The goal is to keep your lower leg at a 90-degree angle to your upper leg.

2. Keep your entire right leg in contact with the table or bench.

3. Your left leg should be directly under your hip and either straight (if using a high table) or with a bent knee (if stretching on a lower bench). You should feel a stretch in your right hip.

4. Hold for 20 seconds and then switch sides.

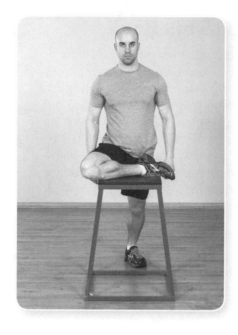

Cross-Body Stretch

1. Standing tall, bring your right arm directly across your body, keeping it straight and parallel to the ground.

2. Using your left hand, bring the right arm closer to your body by pressing the upper right arm with the palm of your left hand. Be careful not to push at the elbow joint.

3. Hold for 20 seconds and then repeat on the other side.

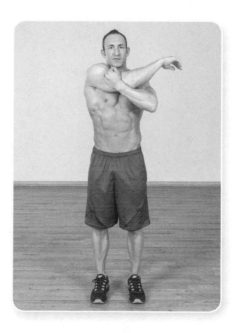

How to Best Use This Book

Certainly you can look at this book as a series of randomized individual workouts, but in truth, it is laid out as a series of training phases (strength, hypertrophy, strength-endurance, metabolic, hybrid). If followed in sequence, this program can get you fitter, stronger, and leaner than you have likely ever been in your life. However, everyone has different goals and training priorities. If you are looking to put on size, you can certainly skip directly to the chapter Targeted Muscle Builders and get started there. Need to lose fat for a photo shoot or wedding? Then Ultimate Fat Loss may be a good beginning. You can also think of this book as a source of ideas and randomly pick workouts to fill a void between your own training phases, use a few of the fat-loss workouts as metabolic finishers, or simply learn a new variation of a presented exercise. At the end of the day, I want this book and your fitness program to suit your needs.

Finally, you may have some hesitation about training with such high frequency. But plenty of research shows how training often, even high-intensity training, can be very beneficial for body composition, performance, and health. On top of this, the fact that all these sessions are designed to be completed in 30 minutes or less makes the risk of overtraining extremely minimal. With that being said, it's very likely that you won't make every training session every day. And it's always a smart idea to listen to your body. If it is telling you to take a day off, you should definitely do so. Just pick it back up where you left off. The key is to not only train consistently but to also give your full effort every time you step into the gym.

CHAPTER 2

Ultimate Fat Loss

In addition to helping you shed fat, the goal of this chapter is to introduce you to many of the exercises and get you familiar with the effort you will need to put forth throughout the book. Most of these workouts utilize supersets (exercises performed back to back, with little or no rest between movements). It is important to choose your loads wisely because using great technique and adhering to the rest periods are critical for keeping you injury free and helping you drop any unwanted body weight. Prepare for your heart rate to go up and your pants size to go down.

Short Circuit

Circuit training is a great way to burn fat while maintaining a resistance element in your training program (meaning you reduce the risk of losing muscle while dropping body weight). The key to circuits is to keep moving—so reduce the rest intervals to 30 seconds or less. Your muscles will be burning, you'll be gasping for air, and you'll be sweating as if you just crossed the Sahara, but these sacrifices will be worth it. There's simply no better way to torch fat inside the gym.

Warm-Up

5 reps of inchworm, 6 reps per side of quadruped T-spine rotation, 10 reps of cat–cow

● Featured Exercise

Narrow-Grip Chin-Up

1. Grab a pull-up bar with a double underhand grip (palms facing you). Your pinkies should be touching each other.
2. Begin from a dead hang with your arms straight (a). Initiate the pull from your back, depressing your shoulder blades and pulling your chest up toward the bar. Then drive your elbows back and down, lifting your torso toward the bar.
3. Once you have reached the top of your range of motion (b), lower under control until your arms are completely straight. Repeat for reps.

Complete Workout

Complete 5 rounds of the following circuit.

Narrow-grip chin-up
- 6 reps
- 10 seconds of rest

Goblet squat (#2)
- 8 reps
- 10 seconds of rest

Push-up (#12)
- 10 reps
- 10 seconds of rest

Burpee (#7)
- 12 reps
- 60 seconds of rest

OPTIONS

Easy Option Perform 3 rounds of the circuit. Use an assistance band or lat pull-down machine as a substitution for the narrow-grip chin-up.

Step It Up Add 2 reps per set to each exercise in the circuit.

Cool-Down Double lat stretch, cross-body stretch, hamstring stretch.

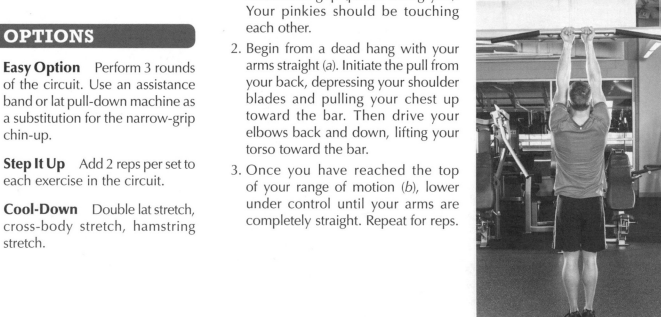
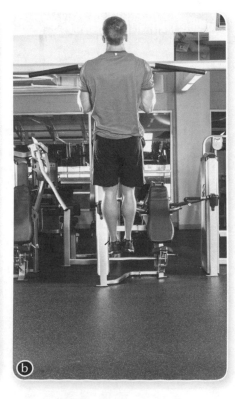

The Holy Grail

Goblet squats are an excellent squat variation for beginners and even advanced lifters as they put your torso in the ideal upright position for great technique and proper depth. They are also taxing on the musculature of the upper back and the core, making this a true total-body movement. If you are having problems maintaining posture in the front squat or back squat, master the goblet squat first.

Warm-Up

6 reps of squat to stand, 6 reps per side of quadruped T-spine rotation, 8 reps of glute bridge, 10 reps of cat–cow

● Featured Exercise

Goblet Squat

1. Grab a kettlebell by placing your hands in a V and wrapping them around the handle (*a*).
2. Keeping your feet slightly turned out at shoulder width, your chest tall and the weight directly in front of your collarbones, unlock your hips and knees and lower your body toward the floor.
3. In a controlled manner, sit as low as possible while maintaining an upright torso (*b*). Once depth is achieved, reverse the movement back to the starting position. Repeat for reps.

Complete Workout

Perform 4 rounds of the following circuit.

Goblet squat
- 10 reps
- 30 seconds of rest

Alternating dumbbell row (#246)
- 10 reps/side
- 30 seconds of rest

100-yard (100 m) sprint* (#41)
- 2 minutes of rest

*Can be performed on a track, field, or treadmill.

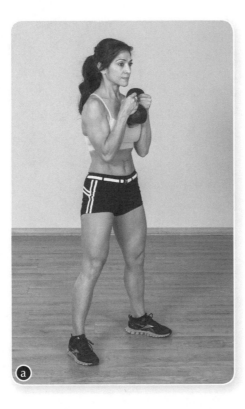
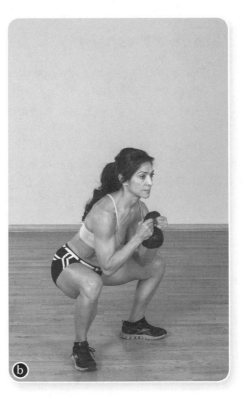

OPTIONS

Easy Option   Complete 3 rounds of the circuit.

Step It Up   Complete 5 rounds of the circuit.

Cool-Down   Hamstring stretch, calf stretch, pec stretch.

3

Band of Brothers

Utilizing bands allows you to overload specific aspects of an exercise, a technique often used by powerlifters during their training. For example, when you pull against bands during a deadlift, you are increasing the resistance as the bands stretch, making the lockout at the top more difficult than it ordinarily would be. In this workout, you'll be placing a band around your back to make the push-up more challenging. This will make the top half of the movement more difficult, overloading your triceps.

Warm-Up

4 reps per side of the world's greatest stretch, 6 reps per side of hip rocker and inverted hamstring stretch, 8 reps per side of shoulder sweeps

● Featured Exercise

Banded Push-Up

1. Place one end of a resistance band in each hand, and loop the rest of the band around your back.
2. Assume a push-up position with your hands just outside shoulder width, arms straight and your body in a straight line from shoulders to heels (a).
3. Lower your body to the ground, keeping your elbows tucked toward your sides (b). Do not let your hips sag or rise as you perform the movement.
4. Once you reach the bottom position, forcefully drive up until your arms reach lockout. Repeat for reps.

Complete Workout

Perform as many rounds of this circuit as possible in 12 minutes, resting only when needed.

Single-arm farmer's walk (#29)
- 40 yards (40 m)

Banded push-up
- 12 reps

Double-arm kettlebell swing (#13)
- 20 reps

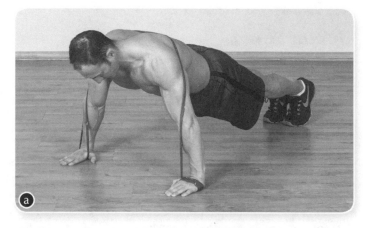

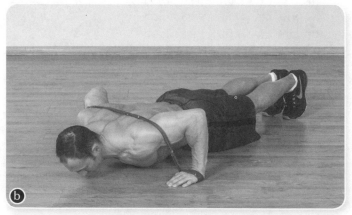

OPTIONS

Easy Option   Perform as many rounds as possible for 7 minutes.

Step It Up   Perform as many rounds as possible for 15 minutes.

Cool-Down   Standing quad stretch, 90-degree stretch, double lat stretch.

Code Red

Your heart rate monitor may just read *code red* in the middle of this training session. The metabolic demands of both the jump squat and the pull-up make this an unbelievably efficient fat-burning workout. A simple but brutal circuit, this one is certainly not for the faint of heart.

Warm-Up

6 reps of squat to stand, 6 reps per side of quadruped T-spine rotation, 8 reps of glute bridge, 10 reps of cat–cow

Featured Exercise

Prisoner Jump Squat

1. Place your hands behind your head with your fingers intertwined. Do not pull down on your neck (*a*).
2. Bring your hips back and bend your knees until you are in a full squat position (*b*).

3. Reverse motion and jump off the ground (*c*). Land with knees slightly flexed, and proceed directly to the next rep. Repeat for reps.

Complete Workout

Perform 10 rounds of the following circuit, resting as little as possible between exercises and between rounds.

Prisoner jump squat
- 10 reps

Neutral-grip pull-up (#237)
- 10 reps

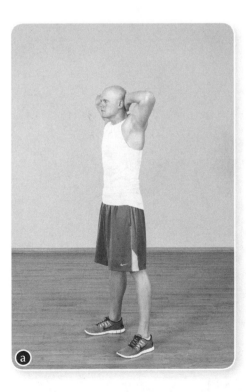
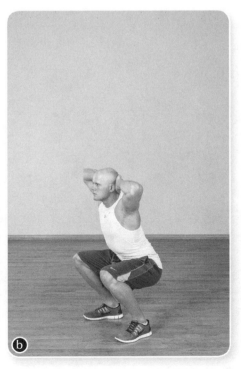
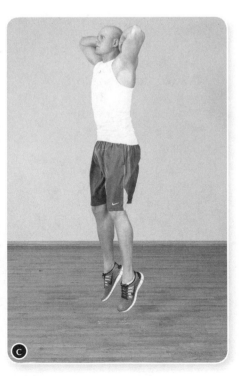

OPTIONS

Easy Option   Perform only 5 reps of the pull-up.

Step It Up   Perform 15 reps of the prisoner jump squat.

Cool-Down   Hamstring stretch, calf stretch, pec stretch.

Dead Man Jumping

If there is any movement where proper form is essential to reduce the risk of injury, it might just be the deadlift. The most common mistake? Rounding the lower back. Avoid this costly error by squeezing your shoulder blades down and back (get a mental image of sticking your shoulder blades in your back pockets) and sticking your chest out in the bottom position. This will help ensure you have a flat back and neutral spine throughout the entire movement.

Warm-Up

4 reps per side of the world's greatest stretch, 5 reps each of inchworm and inverted hamstring stretch, 10 reps of glute bridge

● Featured Exercise

Conventional Deadlift

1. Utilize a hip-width stance, hinge at your hips (see chapter 1, Ramping Up, for a full description of the hip hinge), bend your knees slightly, and grab the bar with either a double overhand or mixed grip (a).

2. Keeping the bar close to your shins, pull it off the ground by extending at the knees and driving your hips forward.

3. Lock out fully at the hips, and maintain a neutral spine at the top of the movement (b).

4. Return the bar to the ground by first hinging at your hips and then slightly bending your knees as the bar gets closer to the ground. Repeat for reps.

Complete Workout

Complete 4 rounds of this circuit in as little time as possible. Load the bar with your body weight for the conventional deadlift, and utilize a 24-inch (60 cm) box for the box jump.

Box jump (#198)
- 5 reps

Conventional deadlift
- 10 reps

OPTIONS

Easy Option   Use 75 percent of your body weight for the deadlifts.

Step It Up   Use 125 percent of your body weight for the deadlifts.

Cool-Down   Double lat stretch, hamstring stretch, calf stretch.

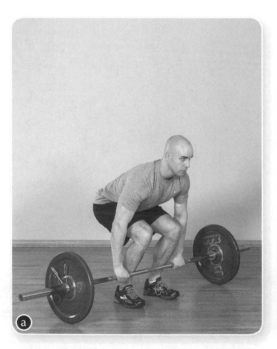
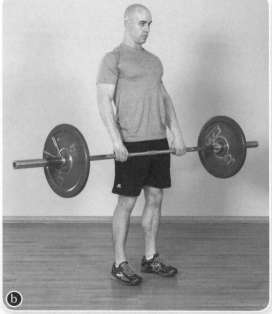

Clean, Press, Thrust

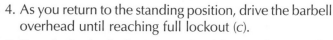
Weightlifting movements (particularly the snatch and its variations) can be done with specifically designed straps. These straps sit on the hands rather than the wrists and are designed to release from the bar quickly. Do not get these confused with deadlifting straps that wrap around your wrists and give you extra support with the grip. Performing snatches with the wrong straps can prove to be disastrous if you miss the lift, particularly behind you. So, if you do choose to use straps in your weightlifting, make sure you are using the correct ones.

Warm-Up

5 reps of squat to stand; 6 reps per side of kneeling adductor stretch, hip rocker, and quadruped T-spine rotation

● Featured Exercise

Barbell Thruster

1. Rack a barbell on your shoulders with a double overhand grip. Your elbows should be forward of the bar.

2. Unlock your hips and squat down toward the floor, keeping your chest tall and eyes forward throughout the entire movement (*a*).

3. Once you've reached the bottom of your range of motion (your upper leg should be at or below parallel to the floor), reverse your motion, driving your hips forward (*b*).

4. As you return to the standing position, drive the barbell overhead until reaching full lockout (*c*).

5. Rerack the barbell at your shoulders and repeat for reps.

Complete Workout

Complete 5 rounds of the following circuit in as little time as possible, resting as much as needed between reps, sets, and rounds. Use the same loaded barbell for all movements (put the barbell down only as needed).

Barbell clean and push press (#79)
- 3 reps

Push press (#16)
- 6 reps

Barbell thruster
- 9 reps

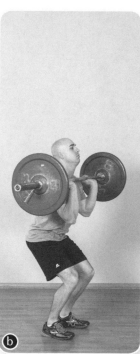
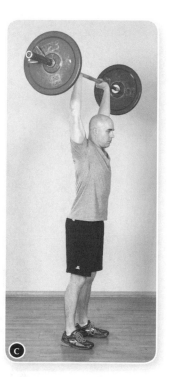

OPTIONS

Easy Option   Perform 3 rounds of the circuit.

Step It Up   Add 2 reps to each of the exercises.

Cool-Down   Standing quad stretch, 90-degree stretch, cross-body stretch.

Unlucky 7s

If three 7s come up on a slot machine, you've hit the jackpot. Completing 7 rounds of 7 reps for each movement in this workout, however, will leave you feeling anything but lucky. Do not let the fact that this workout includes only body-weight movement fool you into believing it's easy. The combination of pulling, pushing, squatting, and jumping will have your entire body feeling like the spinning reels of that slot machine.

Warm-Up

6 reps of squat to stand, 6 reps per side of quadruped T-spine rotation, 8 reps of glute bridge, 10 reps of cat–cow

● **Featured Exercise**

Burpee

1. Begin in a tall standing position (a). Place your hands on the floor, and jump your feet back into push-up plank position (b).

2. Keeping your elbows closely tucked to your sides, perform one push-up.

3. Simultaneously bring both knees into your chest and rock back so the soles of your feet are on the floor.

4. Jump up (you are attempting to jump at least 6 inches [15 cm] in the air with every rep) (c) and land with soft knees. Come to a full standing position and repeat for reps.

Complete Workout

Complete 7 rounds of the following circuit, resting as little as possible.

Prisoner jump squat (#4)
- 7 reps

Chin-up (#73)
- 7 reps

Burpee
- 7 reps

OPTIONS

Easy Option   Perform the circuit for 5 rounds.

Step It Up   Add a weighted vest for the entire workout.

Cool-Down   Standing quad stretch, 90-degree stretch, double lat stretch.

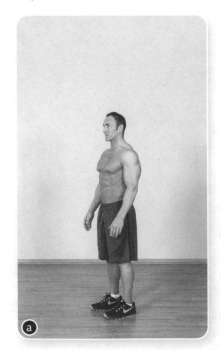
(a)

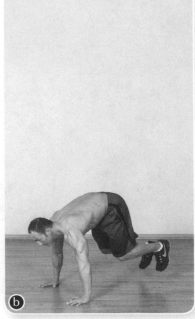
(b)

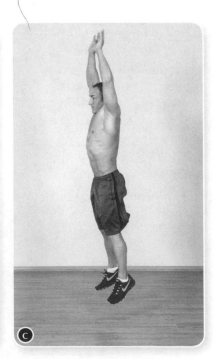
(c)

Circuit Maximus

Most circuses have so much going on it's hard to know where to look at first. This workout uses so many major muscle groups in one workout, you'll have a hard time figuring out which one is being challenged the most. By alternating between upper and lower body exercises using major compound movements, this metabolic challenge could just be "the greatest workout on earth."

Warm-Up

4 reps per side of the world's greatest stretch, 6 reps per side of hip rocker and inverted hamstring stretch, 8 reps per side of shoulder sweeps

● Featured Exercise

Trap Bar Deadlift

1. Load up a trap bar and step inside, assuming a shoulder-width stance.
2. Grab the handles directly in the center, bend your knees, bring your hips back, and keep your chest tall (a).
3. Lift the bar by driving your hips forward and bringing your knees to lockout (b). This movement is best thought of as a combination of a squat and deadlift.
4. Maintain a neutral spine while lowering the bar back to the starting position by hinging your hips back.

Complete Workout

Complete 4 rounds of the following circuit.

Trap bar deadlift
- 10 reps
- 60 seconds of rest

Barbell bench press (#54)
- 10 reps
- 60 seconds of rest

Alternating step-back lunge (#24)
- 10 reps/leg
- 60 seconds of rest

Alternating dumbbell row (#246)
- 10 reps/side
- 2 minutes of rest

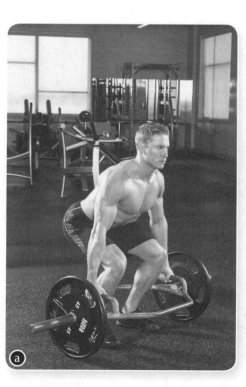

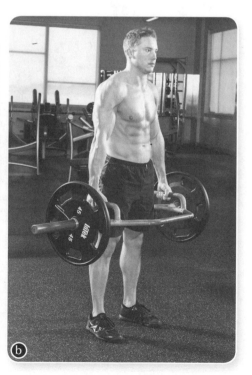

OPTIONS

Easy Option Complete 3 rounds of the circuit.

Step It Up Reduce the rest to 45 seconds between movements.

Cool-Down Standing quad stretch, 90-degree stretch, double lat stretch.

The Purple Heart

Named after an award given to those military personnel who are wounded or killed while serving, the Purple Heart definitely takes a lot of guts to get through. By combining a tough upper body movement (chin-up), a tough unilateral lower body movement (step-up), and an all-out sprint on the bike, this workout will prepare you for any battle.

Warm-Up

4 reps per side of the world's greatest stretch, 6 reps per side of hip rocker and inverted hamstring stretch, 8 reps per side of shoulder sweeps

● **Featured Exercise**

Russian Step-Up

1. Load up a barbell on the outside of a squat rack. Unrack the barbell so it is sitting on your upper traps.

2. Using a box or bench that allows your leg to be bent at a 90-degree angle, place your left leg on top of the box (*a*).

3. Drive off your left foot down into the box, driving up until your left leg achieves complete lockout. Your right foot should trail behind but not be placed on top of the box (*b*).

4. Lower yourself with control back to the starting position, and complete all reps on the left side before starting the right.

Complete Workout

Perform 4 rounds of the following circuit.

Chin-up (#73)
- 10 reps
- 30 seconds of rest

Russian step-up
- 10 reps/leg
- 30 seconds of rest

Bike sprint
- 30 seconds
- 2 minutes of rest

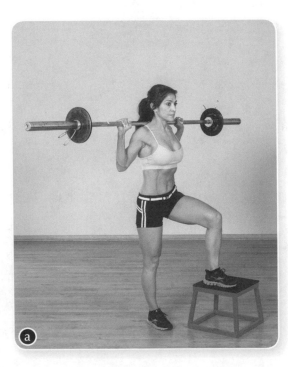
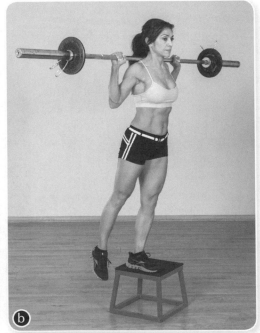

OPTIONS

Easy Option   Perform 3 rounds of the circuit.

Step It Up   Perform 5 rounds of the circuit.

Cool-Down   Hamstring stretch, calf stretch, pec stretch.

Over the Rainbow

The over-the-shoulder medicine ball toss (featured in this workout) mimics the movement required by strongmen when competing in an Atlas stones event, which requires placing increasingly heavy boulders onto a tall platform. But rather than placing a cement stone onto a podium, you are going to flip a relatively heavy medicine ball over your shoulder. Although you should always strive to keep your back in a safe position, you should be a lot less concerned with specific form in this exercise. There are many ways to get a heavy, odd object up to your shoulder, and as long as you are not promoting injury and the ball gets up and over, you're going about it the correct way.

Warm-Up

5 reps of inchworm, 6 reps per side of quadruped T-spine rotation, 10 reps of cat–cow

● Featured Exercise

Over-the-Shoulder Medicine Ball Toss

1. Place a relatively heavy medicine ball between your feet. Bend down, and with your arms between your knees, place your fingers under the ball (a).

2. Keeping your arms straight, deadlift the ball up to your hips. Walk your feet together and sit into a deep squat, placing the ball in your lap.

3. Wrap your arms around the ball and stand up, driving your hips forward explosively, using that momentum to allow the ball to travel up your body and to your shoulder (b).

4. Allow the ball to roll directly over your shoulder to the floor (c). Repeat for reps.

Complete Workout

Complete 5 rounds of the following workout as quickly as possible, resting as little as needed within or between sets.

Barbell thruster (#6)
- 12 reps

Over-the-shoulder medicine ball toss
- 12 reps

OPTIONS

Easy Option Reduce the number of rounds to 3.

Step It Up Increase the number of reps per set to 15.

Cool-Down Double lat stretch, cross-body stretch, hamstring stretch.

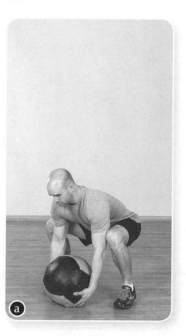
(a)

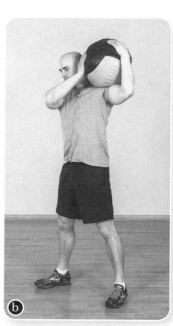
(b)

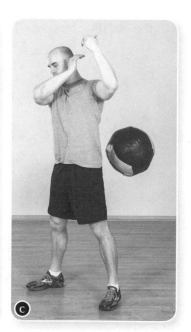
(c)

Go Heavy

You don't need a gym full of equipment or even a set of weights to get in a great workout. If you find yourself traveling or wanting to train when your gym is closed, just find yourself a heavy object such as a firewood log or cinder block and lift it overhead, lunge while holding it, and walk with it for long distances. You will quickly see that fatiguing your muscles and jacking your heart rate through the roof does not require anything fancy.

Warm-Up

4 reps per side of the world's greatest stretch, 6 reps per side of hip rocker and inverted hamstring stretch, 8 reps per side of shoulder sweeps

● Featured Exercise

Heavy Object Front Carry

1. Grab a heavy object (e.g., a weight plate, sandbag, cinder block, tree log, Atlas stone, medicine ball), and hold it directly in front of your chest.
2. With your chest tall and head up, walk with the object the distance prescribed.

OPTIONS

Easy Option   Reduce the number of reps per set to 6 (push press), 8 (pull-up), and 8 (burpee).

Step It Up   Add 2 more rounds of the circuit (5 rounds total).

Cool-Down   Standing quad stretch, 90-degree stretch, double lat stretch.

Complete Workout

Perform 3 rounds of the following circuit with as little rest as needed between movements within sets. The goal is to complete the 3 rounds as quickly as possible.

Push press (#16)
- 8 reps

Pull-up (#231)
- 12 reps

Heavy object front carry
- 100 feet (30 m)

Burpee (#7)
- 10 reps

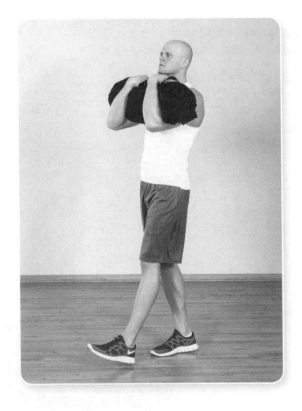

All Out

It's become common knowledge that sugar is bad for your health and body composition. However, sugar (when combined with protein) can be beneficial directly after your workout. Drinking a postworkout drink that has 2 to 3 grams of simple carbohydrate (such as sugar) for every gram of protein can help replenish muscle glycogen and begin muscle protein synthesis. Both these processes support muscle growth and faster repair, allowing you to more easily adapt and recover from your training session.

Warm-Up

6 reps of squat to stand, 6 reps per side of quadruped T-spine rotation, 8 reps of glute bridge, 10 reps of cat–cow

● Featured Exercise

Push-Up

1. Start with hands directly under shoulders and your body in a push-up position, creating a straight line from shoulder to heel (a).
2. Keeping your elbows tucked toward your rib cage and maintaining a neutral spine, slowly lower your body until your chest touches the ground (b).
3. Drive your hands into the floor and reverse the motion until your elbows reach lockout and you have returned to the starting position. Repeat for reps.

Complete Workout

Perform as many rounds as possible of the following workout in 8 minutes.

Push-up
- 15 reps

Frog sit-up (#27)
- 25 reps

Single-contact mountain climber (#281)
- 35 reps

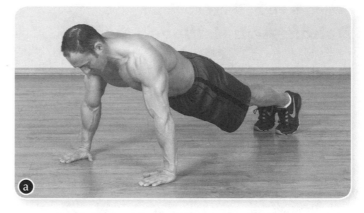

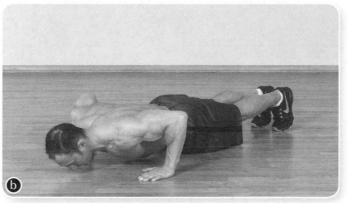

OPTIONS

Easy Option   Perform as many rounds as possible in 6 minutes.

Step It Up   Increase the number of reps per exercise by 5 (20, 30, 40).

Cool-Down   Hamstring stretch, calf stretch, pec stretch.

Bell of the Ball

The kettlebell swing is an excellent exercise for training explosive power through your hips while developing strength in your glutes, hamstrings, lower back, and grip. This will transfer to other explosive strength moves such as hip thrusters, good mornings, deadlifts, and back extensions.

Warm-Up

4 reps per side of the world's greatest stretch, 5 reps each of inchworm and inverted hamstring stretch, 10 reps of glute bridge

● Featured Exercise

Double-Arm Kettlebell Swing

1. Grab a kettlebell with a double overhand grip (*a*).

2. Begin gaining momentum by forcefully swinging the kettlebell between your legs, making sure to keep it high (directly below your crotch).

3. As the kettlebell is traveling through your legs, perform a hip hinge (described in chapter 1, Ramping Up), keeping your arms straight and chest tall (*b*).

4. Reverse motion by driving your hips forward, keeping your arms straight, and propelling the kettlebell forward. All the power should be generated by your hips—do not use your arms to lift the kettlebell.

5. Once the kettlebell reaches its pinnacle (*c*), reverse the motion and drive it back through your legs. Repeat for reps.

Complete Workout

Set a timer for 20 minutes. In the first minute, you must complete 20 kettlebell swings. In the second minute, aim to complete 19 swings. In the third minute, try for 18 reps. Continue this pattern until you complete a single swing in the 20th minute. You can strategize and plan your rest in any way you see fit, either completing all reps as close to the top of the minute as possible or breaking up the reps throughout each minute.

Double-arm kettlebell swing
- 20 sets (20, 19, 18, 17, 16, 15, 14, 13, 12, 11, 10, 9, 8, 7, 6, 5, 4, 3, 2, 1 reps)

OPTIONS

Easy Option   Set the timer for 12 minutes and start with 12 reps.

Step It Up   Set the timer for 25 minutes and begin with 25 reps.

Cool-Down   Double lat stretch, hamstring stretch, calf stretch.

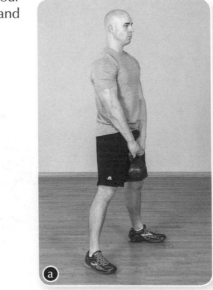
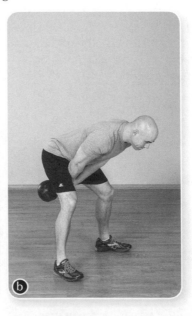
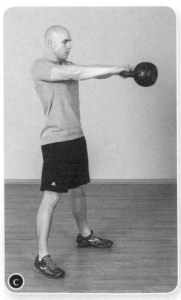

The Big Bang

Plyometric exercises are an excellent way of utilizing the stretch–shortening cycle to develop athletic performance. The stretch–shortening cycle is defined as an active stretch of a muscle followed by an immediate shortening of that same muscle; it is a key component in explosive movements, ranging from jumps to bounds to clapping push-ups. This workout utilizes several plyometric movements to challenge your conditioning and ability to repeat explosive efforts.

Warm-Up

5 reps of squat to stand; 6 reps per side of kneeling adductor stretch, hip rocker, and quadruped T-spine rotation

● Featured Exercise

Split Jump

1. Begin in a long split stance, with your left foot forward, right foot back.

2. Lower yourself by bending your knees until your back (right) knee is just above the floor (a).

3. Explosively drive off the floor, propelling your body straight up.

4. While airborne, quickly switch legs so your right is forward and your left is back (b).

5. Land with soft knees and immediately lower your body into the next jump (c). Repeat for reps.

Complete Workout

Perform 6 rounds of the following circuit.

Box jump (#198)
- 6 reps
- 30 seconds of rest

Split jump
- 8 reps/side
- 30 seconds of rest

Burpee (#7)
- 10 reps
- 30 seconds of rest

Prisoner squat (#188)
- 12 reps
- 2 minutes of rest

OPTIONS

Easy Option   Perform 4 rounds of the circuit.

Step It Up   Increase the number of reps to 10 per side of the split jump, 12 of the burpee, and 15 of the prisoner squat.

Cool-Down   Double lat stretch, hamstring stretch, calf stretch.

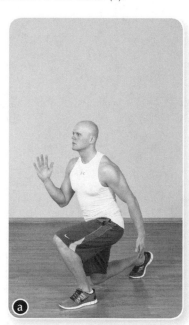
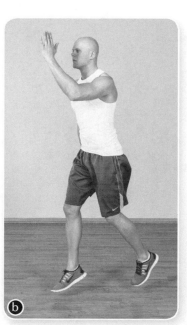
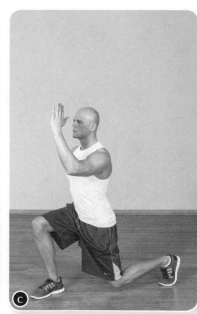

666 Barbell Beast

According to the Bible, 666 is the number of the Beast, better known as the devil. For a devilishly challenging short workout, try loading a barbell with one-third of your body weight, and do the following 6 moves for 6 rounds, 6 reps each—hence the 666. Once you pick up the bar, don't put it down until the entire sequence is over. Performing a circuit in this manner (one implement, one way, all exercises back to back) is called a complex and is one of the most effective schemes for fat loss.

Warm-Up

4 reps per side of the world's greatest stretch, 6 reps per side of hip rocker and inverted hamstring stretch, 8 reps per side of shoulder sweeps

● Featured Exercise

Hang Clean

1. Start by holding the barbell with an overhand grip, placing hands and feet slightly wider than shoulder-width apart. The bar should rest just below your knees (a).

2. Explosively jump upward, extending your body into triple extension—extending at the ankles, knees, and hips (b).

3. Aggressively pull your body under the bar, rotating your elbows around the bar. Catch the bar on your shoulders while moving into a squat position (c).

4. Upon hitting the bottom of your squat, stand up immediately (d).

5. Flex your knees slightly, and return the barbell to the starting position against your thighs. Repeat for reps.

Complete Workout

Perform 6 reps of each movement for rounds of the following complex, resting 60 seconds between rounds.

Hang clean

Barbell front squat (#44)

Barbell overhead press (#36)

Barbell back squat (#63)

Barbell Romanian deadlift (#295)

OPTIONS

Easy Option   Perform 4 rounds of the complex, resting 75 seconds between rounds.

Step It Up   Load the bar with 50 percent of your body weight, and reduce the rest to 45 seconds between sets.

Cool-Down   Standing quad stretch, 90-degree stretch, double lat stretch.

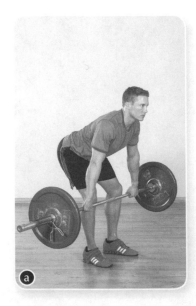
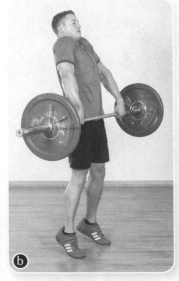
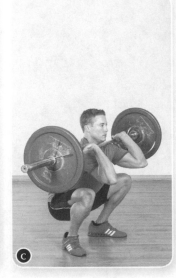
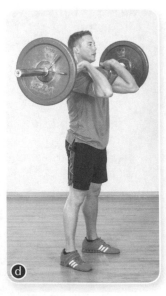

The Hero

You'll need nothing less than a heroic effort to complete this brutal complex. A great way to remember the order of the exercises (because, clearly you don't want to be looking at this book in the middle of the set) is to keep in mind that all the movements follow a top-down order. You start overhead with the push press, and then the rack position is at the shoulders for the front squat, at your hips for the Romanian deadlift, just above your knees for the bent-over row, and on the ground for the deadlift.

Warm-Up

4 reps per side of the world's greatest stretch, 6 reps per side of hip rocker and inverted hamstring stretch, 8 reps per side of shoulder sweeps

Complete Workout

Complete 4 rounds of the following complex, resting 90 seconds between rounds.

Push press
- 6 reps

Barbell front squat (#44)
- 6 reps

Barbell Romanian deadlift (#295)
- 6 reps

Conventional deadlift (#5)
- 6 reps

● Featured Exercise

Push Press

1. Begin with a barbell in the rack position, sitting across your anterior (front) deltoids, your hands in a clean grip and your upper arms parallel to the ground.
2. Keeping your back straight, bend your knees until you have reached a quarter-squat position (*a*).
3. In one explosive motion, straighten your legs and drive the bar overhead (*b*).
4. Return the barbell to the starting position and repeat for reps.

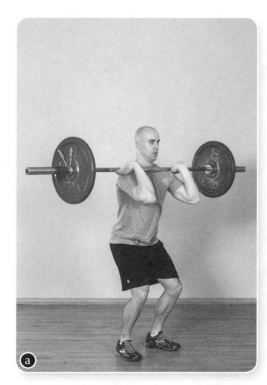

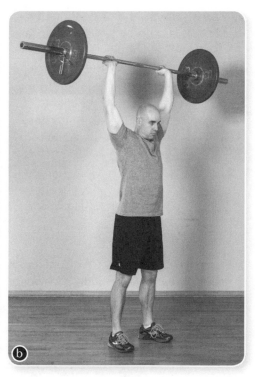

OPTIONS

Easy Option Complete 3 rounds of the complex.

Step It Up Add an additional round of the complex, and reduce the rest between rounds to 60 seconds.

Cool-Down Standing quad stretch, 90-degree stretch, double lat stretch.

Triple Five Clean

One of the simplest and most effective tools you can use to ensure you are moving well and training hard is a foam roller. Rolling around on a foam roller can help ease knots and fascial adhesions as well as make your muscles more supple and pliable. This will not only make you feel better but also allow the joints surrounding those muscle groups to move more freely, which will pay big dividends in helping you get stronger and stay injury free. It's truly one of the greatest investments you can make in your training.

Warm-Up

5 reps of inchworm, 6 reps per side of quadruped T-spine rotation, 10 reps of cat–cow

Complete Workout

Perform 5 rounds of the following complex, with no rest between movements. Rest 2 minutes between rounds.

Power clean (#52)
- 5 reps

Barbell front squat (#44)
- 5 reps

Split jerk
- 5 reps

● Featured Exercise

Split Jerk

1. Begin with the barbell resting across the front of your shoulders. Hands should be grasping the bar just outside shoulder width. Your elbows should be in front of you (a).

2. Dip down into a quarter-squat position by driving your knees forward (do not bring your hips back as you would at the beginning of a traditional squat).

3. Forcefully reverse the motion, splitting your legs so one foot lands in front of you and the other behind (as if in the middle of a lunge) as the bar locks out overhead (b).

4. Recover by bringing your front foot back to a neutral position, followed by your back foot. Lower the bar back to your shoulders.

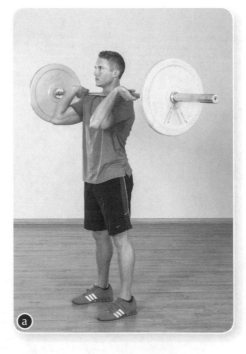
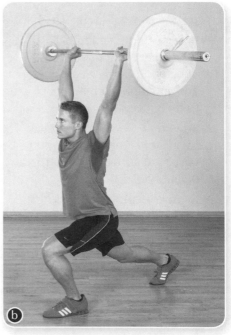

OPTIONS

Easy Option   Perform 3 reps of each exercise per round.

Step It Up   Add another round to the complex (6 rounds total).

Cool-Down   Double lat stretch, cross-body stretch, hamstring stretch.

250 × 25

A kettlebell swing is one of the greatest exercises you can use to train the hip-hinge pattern (see chapter 1, Ramping Up). It also teaches explosiveness, challenges grip strength, and, when done for high reps or combined with other exercises, is very metabolically challenging. For these very reasons, you'll see the swing pop up in many workouts throughout this book. Master this critical movement, and watch your athletic ability and work capacity improve.

Warm-Up

4 reps per side of the world's greatest stretch, 5 reps each of inchworm and inverted hamstring stretch, 10 reps of glute bridge

● Featured Exercise

Single-Arm Kettlebell Swing

1. Grab a kettlebell with a single-arm overhand grip.
2. Keeping your arm straight, forcefully drive the kettlebell back between your legs (be sure to keep it high, just under your crotch) by hinging at your hips (*a*).
3. Forcefully drive your hips forward, forcing the kettlebell up and out in front of your body (*b*). Do not use your arms to lift the kettlebell—allow the power to come from your lower body.
4. Once the kettlebell reaches its apex, forcefully bring the bell down between your legs. Repeat for reps.

Complete Workout

Complete 4 rounds of the following workout, resting as little as possible between movements.

Rower (#212)
- 250 meters

Single-arm kettlebell swing
- 25 reps

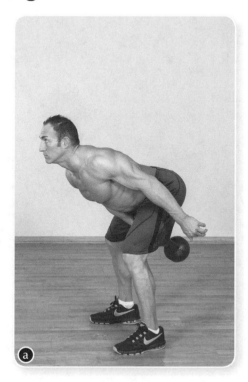

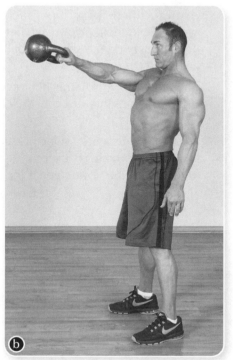

OPTIONS

Easy Option Reduce the number of kettlebell swings to 15 reps, and reduce the row to 200 meters.

Step It Up Add an additional round, bringing the total up to 5.

Cool-Down Double lat stretch, hamstring stretch, calf stretch.

Circuit Breaker

The circuit breaker workout utilizes multijoint compound movements with short rest periods. This combination of factors drives up metabolic and cardiorespiratory demand to a level that may just break your mind, spirit, and soul. Complete this workout and prove to yourself that you can rise to any challenge.

Warm-Up

6 reps of squat to stand, 6 reps per side of quadruped T-spine rotation, 8 reps of glute bridge, 10 reps of cat–cow

● Featured Exercise

Kettlebell Sumo Deadlift

1. Place a kettlebell directly between your feet. Utilize a shoulder-width stance.
2. Keeping your chest tall and your spine neutral, hinge your hips back (see chapter 1, Ramping Up), reach between your legs, and grab the kettlebell with a double overhand grip (a).
3. Keeping your arms straight, forcefully drive your hips forward until they reach lockout (b).
4. Maintain your neutral spine position as you hinge your hips back, returning the kettlebell to the floor. Repeat for reps.

Complete Workout

Complete the following circuit five times.

Kettlebell sumo deadlift
- 10 reps
- 30 seconds of rest

Barbell front-foot elevated split squat (#140)
- 10 reps/side
- 30 seconds of rest

Farmer's walk (#187)
- 4 sets × 40 yards (40 m)
- 2 minutes of rest

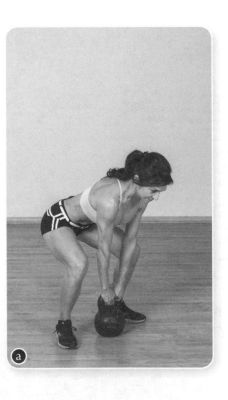

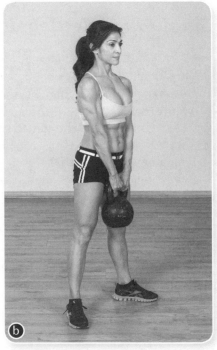

OPTIONS

Easy Option   Increase the rest period to 60 seconds between sets.

Step It Up   Replace the kettlebell sumo deadlift with a sumo deadlift (#82).

Cool-Down   Standing quad stretch, 90-degree stretch, double lat stretch.

Wham Bam Slam

In addition to being a fantastic way to get out aggression, the medicine ball slam (featured in this workout) is a great tool for dynamically training hip extension and core flexion. Since you are using gravity instead of overcoming it as you do with most medicine ball exercises, you should use a relatively heavy ball. However, you do want to maintain a component of speed with this exercise. Finally, the medicine ball slam can be a great way to drive up metabolic demand, particularly when added to a low-rest circuit and done for higher reps.

Warm-Up

5 reps of inchworm, 6 reps per side of quadruped T-spine rotation, 10 reps of cat–cow

● Featured Exercise

Medicine Ball Slam

1. Grab a relatively heavy medicine ball, and hold it above your head with your feet just outside shoulder width (*a*).
2. Reach back with your hips and forcefully slam the ball on the floor or a pad directly in front of you (*b*).
3. Pick up the ball and repeat for reps. Make sure the ball is directly overhead at the start of every rep. Make sure the ball is directly overhead at the start of every rep.

Complete Workout

Complete 4 rounds of the following workout as quickly as possible, resting as little as needed between exercises and rounds.

TRX jumping split squat (#201)
- 8 reps/side

Pull-up (#231)
- 12 reps

Over-the-shoulder medicine ball toss (#10)
- 15 reps

Medicine ball slam
- 20 reps

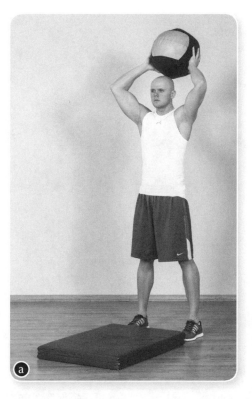

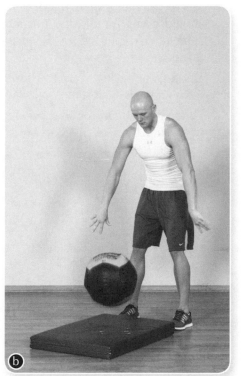

OPTIONS

Easy Option Perform 3 rounds of the circuit.

Step It Up Add 2 reps per set to the TRX jumping split squat and 3 reps per set to the pull-up.

Cool-Down Double lat stretch, cross-body stretch, hamstring stretch.

Bottoms Up

Handstands and handstand push-ups are extremely challenging yet beneficial movements because they train upper body strength, shoulder and core stability, and balance. They also have carryover to several other fitness modalities including yoga, gymnastics, and acrobatics. However, unlike simpler exercises that have a low learning curve, handstand push-ups are a skill that takes time and practice to develop.

Warm-Up

4 reps per side of the world's greatest stretch, 6 reps per side of hip rocker and inverted hamstring stretch, 8 reps per side of shoulder sweeps

 Featured Exercise

Handstand Push-Up

1. Place your hands on the floor wider than shoulder width, and with a staggered foot stance, kick your feet up against a wall. Be sure to keep your arms locked out (a).
2. Lower your body toward the floor, keeping your heels against the wall at all times.
3. When your head touches the floor (b), press back up until your arms reach lockout. Repeat for reps.

OPTIONS

Easy Option   Perform 3 rounds of the circuit, and replace the handstand push-up with the banded push-up (#3).

Step It Up   Perform 5 rounds of the circuit.

Cool-Down   Standing quad stretch, 90-degree stretch, double lat stretch.

Complete Workout

Perform 4 rounds of the following three exercises, resting as little as possible.

Handstand push-up
- 5 reps

Sumo deadlift (#82)
- 5 reps

Pull-up (#231)
- 10 reps

Warning: Handstand push-ups are an advanced exercise that requires a considerable amount of strength, stability, and coordination to perform without injury. It is highly recommended that you practice and perfect this technique before attempting it in a fatigued state.

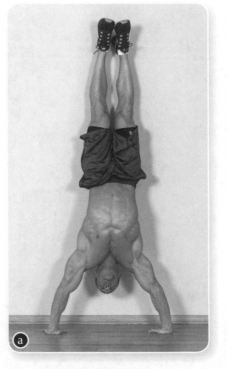
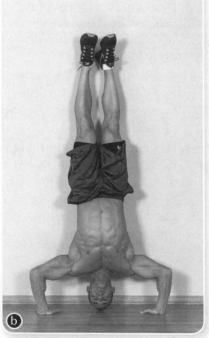

The Sentinel

Barbells, dumbbells, kettlebells, TRX, sleds, machines, and every other piece of equipment in your gym should be seen as tools that get specific jobs done. Knowing that every piece of equipment has its benefits and can be used to your advantage is a much better way of approaching your training than simply falling in love with one tool and using it exclusively.

Warm-Up

4 reps per side of the world's greatest stretch, 5 reps each of inchworm and inverted hamstring stretch, 10 reps of glute bridge

● Featured Exercise

Alternating Single-Arm Kettlebell Swing

1. Begin with a kettlebell on the floor directly in front of you. Hinge your hips back, reach down, and grab the handle with your right hand.

2. Swing the kettlebell back between your legs, making sure to keep the kettlebell high, your back flat, and your knees slightly bent (a).

3. Drive your hips forward, straighten your legs, and allow the kettlebell to "pop" off your hips until it reaches a height between your navel and sternum.

4. When the kettlebell reaches its pinnacle, release the handle with your right hand and immediately grab it with your left (b).

5. Repeat the movement (c), alternating from one hand to the other until all reps are complete.

Complete Workout

Complete 10 circuits of the following exercises every minute on the minute (begin the circuit at the top of the minute, complete all reps, rest the remainder of that minute, begin again at the top of the next minute).

Alternating single-arm kettlebell swing
- 10 reps (5 per side)

Burpee (#7)
- 10 reps

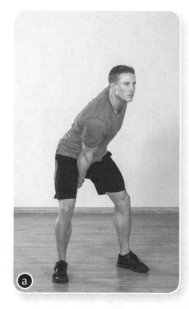
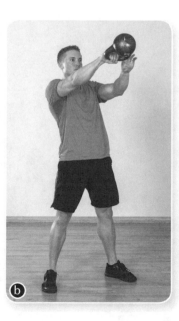
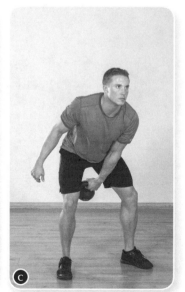

OPTIONS

Easy Option Perform the circuit 6 times.

Step It Up Perform 20 reps (10 reps per side) of the alternating single-arm kettlebell swing.

Cool-Down Double lat stretch, hamstring stretch, calf stretch.

Pain and Gain

There is an old gym adage that states *no pain, no gain.* And although it's true that you will have to push yourself to the point of some discomfort to make progress, there is a difference between working hard and getting out of your comfort zone and putting yourself at risk for injury by using poor form or too much load on any given exercise. Training does not have to be painful to be effective. As long as you are challenging yourself while maintaining good technique, you'll make progress. Remember, it's hard to improve when you are constantly sidelined by injury.

Warm-Up

6 reps of squat to stand, 6 reps per side of quadruped T-spine rotation, 8 reps of glute bridge, 10 reps of cat–cow

● Featured Exercise

Overhead Walking Lunge

1. Grab a barbell with a slightly outside shoulder-width grip and press it straight overhead (*a*). It should remain there until all reps are completed.

2. Step forward with your left leg, and bend both knees until your back knee either touches or is 1 inch (2.5 cm) above the floor (*b*). Your torso should remain tall, and your front shin (lower leg) should be perpendicular to the floor.

3. Drive off the front foot to return to a tall standing position, bringing the back foot in line with the front.

4. Step forward with the right foot and repeat the sequence (*c*). Continue to alternate in this fashion until all reps are completed.

Complete Workout

Perform 5 rounds of the following circuit, resting as little as possible.

Box jump (#198)
- 6 reps

Barbell thruster (#6)
- 8 reps

Overhead walking lunge
- 10 reps

Toes to bar (#28)
- 12 reps

OPTIONS

Easy Option Complete 3 rounds total.

Step It Up Complete 6 rounds total.

Cool-Down Standing quad stretch, 90-degree stretch, double lat stretch.

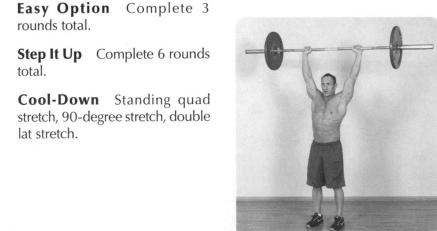

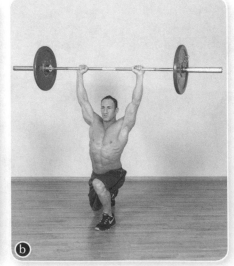

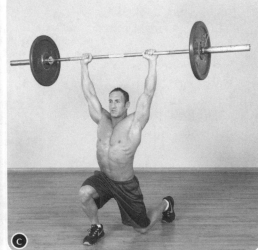

Row a Go Go

The rower is an excellent piece of equipment requiring strength and coordination of the quads, hamstrings, glutes, lats, forearms, and biceps as well as high cardiac capabilities to keep up with the metabolic demand. Too often overlooked, the rower is an efficient choice for driving up work capacity and is an especially effective tool for interval training.

Warm-Up

4 reps per side of the world's greatest stretch, 6 reps per side of hip rocker and inverted hamstring stretch, 8 reps per side of shoulder sweeps

● Featured Exercise

Alternating Step-Back Lunge

1. Holding a barbell across your upper back (a), step back with your left foot, lowering until your left knee just touches the ground. Your front (right) knee should be at a 90-degree angle at this bottom position (b).

2. Drive off your front (right) foot to bring your back (left) foot to the original starting position.

3. Repeat this movement with the right foot reaching back (c). Continue to alternate until all repetitions are achieved.

Complete Workout

Perform 4 rounds of the following circuit.

Dumbbell push press (#51)
- 10 reps
- 30 seconds of rest

Alternating step-back lunge
- 10 reps/leg
- 30 seconds of rest

Rower (#212)
- 250 meters
- 2 minutes of rest

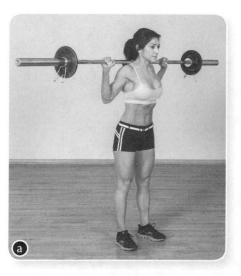
(a)

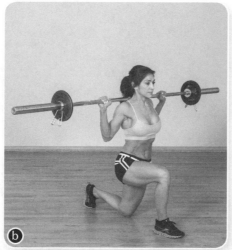
(b)

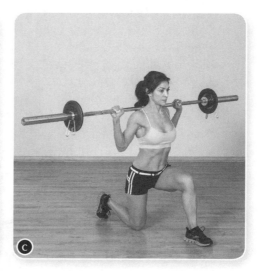
(c)

OPTIONS

Easy Option Reduce the number of rounds to 3.

Step It Up Increase the number of rounds to 5.

Cool-Down Hamstring stretch, calf stretch, pec stretch.

50-40-30-20-10

Don't end up being the most hated guy or girl in the gym. Make sure you mind your gym etiquette and wipe down your area after use, allow people to work on equipment, and offer to spot when someone is going for a max lift. Remember, the gym is not just another place of business, it's a community of people trying to improve themselves. Do your best to be a valuable part of that community, and you'll always get a spot when you need it.

Warm-Up

4 reps per side of the world's greatest stretch, 6 reps per side of hip rocker and inverted hamstring stretch, 8 reps per side of shoulder sweeps

● Featured Exercise

Wall Ball

1. Begin with a medicine ball in front of your chest and your hands on either side of it (a).

2. Squat down until your hip creases are below your knees (you can put a medicine ball behind you and touch the ball with your glutes as a reference) (b). Be sure to keep your chest tall and a neutral spine position as you squat.

3. Once you reach the bottom position, stand up and throw the ball against a target 9 to 12 feet (3 to 4 m) above the floor (c). This should be done as one continuous motion.

4. Catch the ball and immediately descend into the squat. Repeat for reps.

Complete Workout

Perform 1 round of the following circuit, resting as little as possible between exercises.

Wall ball
- 50 reps

Over-the-shoulder medicine ball toss (#10)
- 40 reps

Push-up (#12)
- 30 reps

American kettlebell swing (#206)
- 20 reps

Pull-up (#231)
- 10 reps

OPTIONS

Easy Option   Cut all the reps by 50 percent (25, 20, 15, 10, 5).

Step It Up   Perform 2 rounds of the circuit.

Cool-Down   Standing quad stretch, 90-degree stretch, double lat stretch.

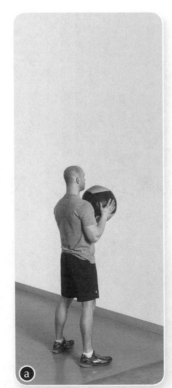
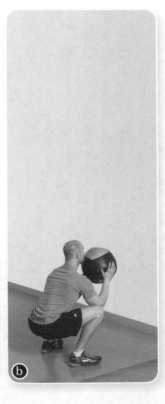
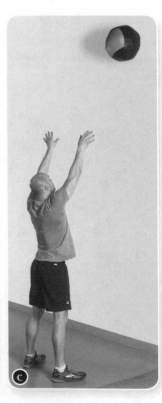

5-10-15

You should be able to complete this three-exercise circuit (the name 5-10-15 stands for the number of reps of each exercise) in less than 15 minutes. But don't let that short time frame fool you. This total body crusher puts the *work* in *workout*, hitting all the major muscle groups of the upper body as well as challenging your grip, glutes, and hamstrings. By the time it's over you'll feel as if you've just trained for hours on end.

Warm-Up

4 reps per side of the world's greatest stretch, 6 reps per side of hip rocker and inverted hamstring stretch, 8 reps per side of shoulder sweeps

● Featured Exercise

Double-Arm Kettlebell Swing

1. Grab a kettlebell with a double overhand grip (*a*).

2. Begin gaining momentum by forcefully swinging the kettlebell between your legs, making sure to keep it high (directly below your crotch).

3. As the kettlebell is traveling through your legs, perform a hip hinge (described in chapter 1, Ramping Up), keeping your arms straight and chest tall (*b*).

4. Reverse the motion by driving your hips forward, keeping your arms straight, and propelling the kettlebell forward. All the power should be generated by your hips—do not use your arms to lift the kettlebell.

5. Once the kettlebell reaches its pinnacle (*c*), reverse the motion and drive it back through your legs.

Complete Workout

Perform all reps in the following sequence as described. The goal is to complete 5 rounds in as little time as possible.

Pull-up (#231)
- 5 reps

Push-up (#12)
- 10 reps

Double-arm kettlebell swing
- 15 reps

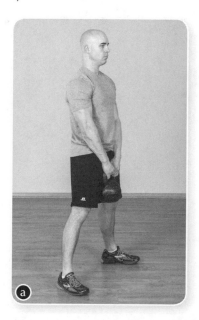
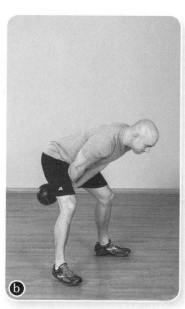
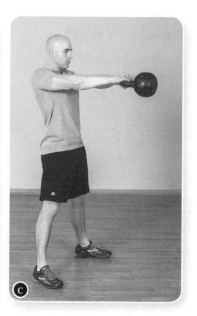

OPTIONS

Easy Option   Reduce to 3 rounds.

Step It Up   Increase the reps to 10 for pull-ups, 15 for push-ups, and 20 for kettlebell swings.

Cool-Down   Hamstring stretch, calf stretch, pec stretch.

The Farmer and the Frog

Although the name of this workout sounds like the setup to a joke, I promise you it's no laughing matter. The combination of metabolic demand from the dumbbell thrusters, total body strength from the farmer's walks, and core mobility from the frog sit-ups will have you wishing for the end of round 4 by the time you begin round 2.

Warm-Up

6 reps of squat to stand, 6 reps per side of quadruped T-spine rotation, 8 reps of glute bridge, 10 reps of cat–cow

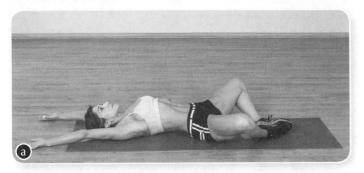

● Featured Exercise

Frog Sit-Up

1. Begin by lying on the ground with the soles of your sneakers touching each other and your heels close to your crotch (*a*).
2. Fully extend your arms overhead (*b*). Sit up until your hands touch the floor in front of your feet (*c*).
3. Return to the original position, making sure the backs of your hands touch the floor above your head. Repeat for reps.

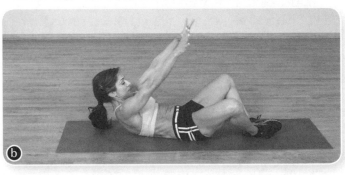

Complete Workout

Perform 4 rounds of the following circuit, resting as little as needed.

Dumbbell thruster (#208)
- 8 reps

Frog sit-up
- 15 reps

Farmer's walk (#187)
- 40 yards (40 m)

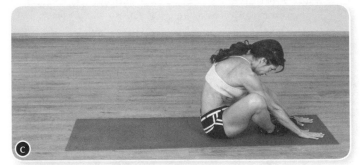

OPTIONS

Easy Option Perform 3 rounds of the circuit.

Step It Up Perform 5 rounds of the circuit.

Cool-Down Standing quad stretch, 90-degree stretch, double lat stretch.

Toes to Bar

Although training provides the stimulus for adaptation and growth, remember that actual muscle growth happens outside the gym—not during training. Take your recovery seriously by getting plenty of rest and an adequate amount of sleep (between 7 and 9 hours per night). You'll get much more out of your training if you pay attention to what you are doing away from the gym.

Warm-Up

6 reps of squat to stand, 6 reps per side of quadruped T-spine rotation, 8 reps of glute bridge, 10 reps of cat–cow

Complete Workout

Perform 6 rounds of the following circuit.

Power clean (#52)
- 4 reps

Barbell bench press (#54)
- 8 reps

Toes to bar
- 12 reps
- 2 minutes of rest

● Featured Exercise

Toes to Bar

1. Grab a pull-up bar with a double overhand grip at shoulder width (*a*).
2. Depress your shoulder blades (this will help you prevent swinging), and while keeping your legs straight, bring your toes up to the bar between your hands (*b*).
3. Lower your legs back to the starting position and repeat for reps.

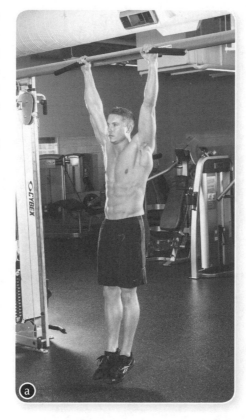

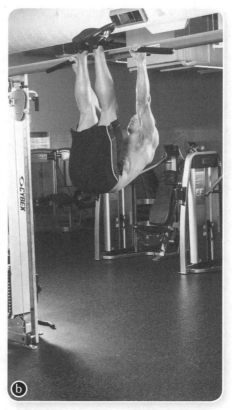

OPTIONS

Easy Option Perform 4 rounds of the circuit.

Step It Up Add 2 reps to each exercise (6 reps of the power clean, 10 reps of the barbell bench press, and 14 reps of the toes to bar).

Cool-Down Standing quad stretch, 90-degree stretch, double lat stretch.

American Eagle

Having a hard time not leaning to one side when doing single-arm farmer's walks, the single-arm kettlebell clean and press, or single-arm kettlebell snatches? Take your non-working hand, ball it up into a fist, and stick it out directly to the side. This simple move will improve your balance and stability and allow you to remain more upright on these unilateral movements.

Warm-Up

5 reps of inchworm, 6 reps per side of quadruped T-spine rotation, 10 reps of cat–cow

● Featured Exercise

Single-Arm Farmer's Walk

1. Grab a single kettlebell (or dumbbell) with one hand.
2. Stand tall with your shoulders down and back. Walk forward without leaning toward either side.
3. Walk the distance prescribed. Switch hands and repeat on the other side.

Complete Workout

Complete 8 rounds of this circuit as quickly as you can, putting the kettlebell on the ground as few times as possible. Suggested kettlebell weight: 53 lb (24 kg).

Goblet squat (#2)
- 8 reps

Single-arm farmer's walk
- 20 yards (20 m)/side

Double-arm kettlebell swing (#13)
- 25 reps

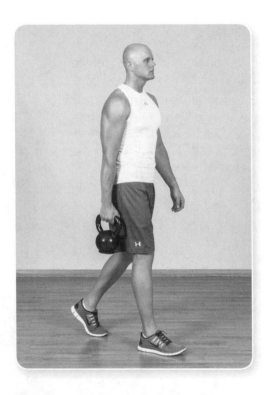

OPTIONS

Easy Option   Complete 5 rounds using a lighter kettlebell (44 lb [20 kg] or less).

Step It Up   Use a 62 lb (28 kg) or 70 lb (32 kg) kettlebell.

Cool-Down   Double lat stretch, cross-body stretch, hamstring stretch.

The Flame

Two things we don't do enough of at the gym are moving laterally (side to side) and training the core in disadvantageous positions (when not simply standing upright or lying on the ground). The side lunge and press (featured in this workout) remedies both of these neglected factors by requiring that you lunge laterally while pressing a dumbbell overhead, which is extremely demanding on your core. Add in the fact that this combo lift also uses a serious amount of energy per set, and you may consider this one of the most underrated exercises in the gym.

Warm-Up

5 reps of squat to stand; 6 reps per side of kneeling adductor stretch, hip rocker, and quadruped T-spine rotation

● Featured Exercise

Side Lunge and Press

1. Grab a pair of dumbbells and stand tall, with a hip-width stance.

2. Step directly to the left and bend at the knee in order to lower your body into a side lunge (*a*). Press both dumbbells overhead (*b*).

3. Lower the dumbbells to your shoulders and return to a standing position.

4. Repeat the movement for the other side. Continue to alternate until you have completed all reps.

Complete Workout

A1. Barbell thruster (#6)
- 3 sets × 8 reps
- 60 seconds of rest

A2. Wide-grip pull-up (#117)
- 3 sets × 8 reps
- 30 seconds of rest

B1. Side lunge and press
- 3 sets × 8 reps/side
- 30 seconds of rest

B2. Hanging knees to elbows (#205)
- 3 sets × 10 reps/side
- 30 seconds of rest

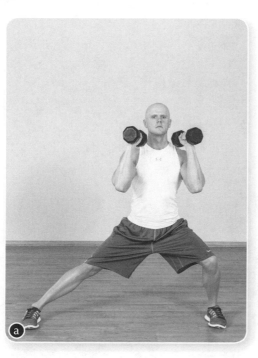

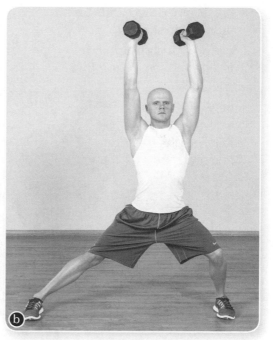

OPTIONS

Easy Option Complete 2 sets of each of the B exercises.

Step It Up Add 2 reps to each set of the B exercises.

Cool-Down Standing quad stretch, 90-degree stretch, cross-body stretch.

The Big Hurt

Sometimes a workout is all about gaining strength. Other times it's about feeling the muscle contraction and getting a pump. And sometimes it's just about survival. This workout falls into that last category. Although it's made up of only three movements, the full-body demand of each exercise combined with the lack of rest periods will challenge your work capacity in a big way because of the huge metabolic demand.

Warm-Up

4 reps per side of the world's greatest stretch, 6 reps per side of hip rocker and inverted hamstring stretch, 8 reps per side of shoulder sweeps

● Featured Exercise

Burpee

1. From a standing position (*a*), jump down into a push-up position (*b*).
2. Perform a push-up and, in one motion, return to your feet.
3. Jump, reaching your hands over your head (*c*).
4. Return to the starting position and repeat for reps.

Complete Workout

Complete 5 rounds of the following circuit in as little time as possible.

Box jump (#198)
- 5 reps

Pull-up (#231)
- 10 reps

Burpee
- 15 reps

OPTIONS

Easy Option   Reduce the total number of rounds to 3.

Step It Up   Add a set of 10 push-ups (#12) between the box jumps and pull-ups.

Cool-Down   Standing quad stretch, 90-degree stretch, double lat stretch.

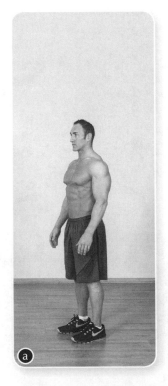

a

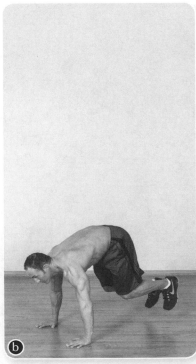

b

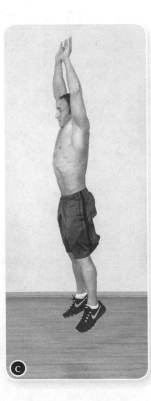

c

Hell's Bells

Although kettlebells are a fantastic strength and conditioning tool, the ballistic and somewhat technical nature of the lifts deserve respect. Be sure to refine your kettlebell technique with a certified instructor or review one of the many great kettlebell DVDs on the market to make sure you are using this equipment in a proper and effective manner. Your body will thank you.

Warm-Up

6 reps of squat to stand, 6 reps per side of quadruped T-spine rotation, 8 reps of glute bridge, 10 reps of cat–cow

● Featured Exercise

Kettlebell Clean and Press

1. Straddle a kettlebell with your feet slightly wider than shoulder width. Squat down with your arm between your legs, and grasp the kettlebell handle with an overhand grip (*a*).

2. Explosively pull the kettlebell up off the floor by extending your hips and knees (*b*). Keeping the kettlebell close to your body, shrug your shoulder and pull the kettlebell upward, allowing your elbow to bend out to the side.

3. Rotate your arm under the kettlebell, catching it on the outside of your arm, with your wrist locked and knees slightly bent (*c*).

4. Drive upward with your legs and arm until the kettlebell is overhead. Allow your body to dip slightly as you press the kettlebell until your arm is locked out and your wrist is straight (*d*).

5. Lower the kettlebell back to your shoulder and then down to the starting position on the floor. Repeat all reps for one side before switching to the other.

Complete Workout

Perform 5 rounds of the following circuit, attempting to use the same kettlebell for all movements.

Kettlebell clean and press
- 6 reps/side
- 30 seconds of rest

Kettlebell snatch (#34)
- 6 reps/side
- 30 seconds of rest

Kettlebell shoulder press (#298)
- 6 reps/side
- 30 seconds of rest

Double-arm kettlebell swing (#13)
- 25 reps
- 2 minutes of rest

OPTIONS

Easy Option Perform 4 total circuits.

Step It Up Complete 6 total circuits.

Cool-Down Standing quad stretch, 90-degree stretch, double lat stretch.

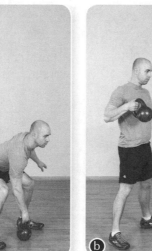
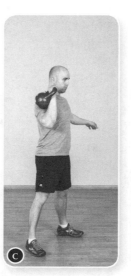
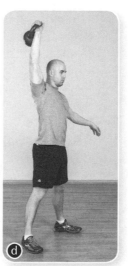

Grandmaster

Strength training can actually be more of a mental challenge than a physical one. Your body is capable of much more than you believe or give it credit for. The challenge lies in convincing yourself that you are able to add one more pound, add one more rep, or get through one more round. Obviously, you don't want to be reckless and do anything harmful, but next time you step into the gym, realize you are more than you think you are, and put that mindset into your workout.

Warm-Up

5 reps of squat to stand; 6 reps per side of kneeling adductor stretch, hip rocker, and quadruped T-spine rotation

Complete Workout

Complete 5 rounds of the following workout as quickly as possible, resting as little as needed within or between sets.

Jump squat (#92)
- 8 reps

Dumbbell thruster (#208)
- 10 reps

Over-the-shoulder medicine ball toss (#10)
- 12 reps

Air squat
- 15 reps

● Featured Exercise

Air Squat

1. Stand tall, with your feet between hip and shoulder width apart (experiment with the stance that is most comfortable for you) and turned slightly out (*a*).

2. Bring your hips back, bend your knees, and squat as deeply as possible. Keep your torso tall and bring your arms straight in front of you as you lower your body (*b*). Your hips should be between your heels in the bottom position.

3. Reverse the motion and stand up, bringing your arms back down to your sides. Repeat for reps.

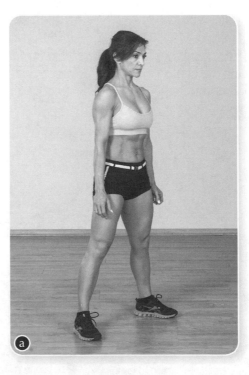

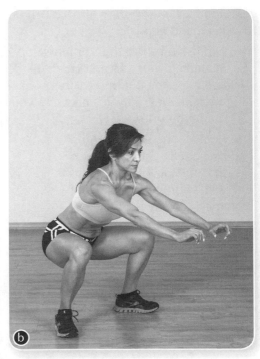

OPTIONS

Easy Option Reduce the number of rounds to 3.

Step It Up Add 2 reps per set to each exercise.

Cool-Down Standing quad stretch, 90-degree stretch, cross-body stretch.

Liberty Bells

Kettlebells are unique compared with other free-weight equipment (namely dumbbells and barbells) in that the weight is distributed directly below the handle as opposed to at the ends of it. This seemingly small difference completely alters the feel of the movement and requires you to manipulate your hand around the handle—a technique that takes a bit of time and *feel* to learn. This time spent is well worth it because the kettlebell will open you to a different style of training and be one more tool you can rely on to vary your workouts.

Warm-Up

4 reps per side of the world's greatest stretch, 6 reps per side of hip rocker and inverted hamstring stretch, 8 reps per side of shoulder sweeps

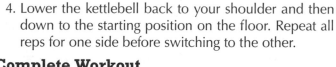

Kettlebell Snatch

1. Straddle a kettlebell, with feet slightly wider apart than shoulder width. Squat down with your arm between your legs, and grasp the kettlebell handle with an overhand grip (*a*).

2. Pull the kettlebell up off the floor by extending your hips, knees, and ankles. Keeping the kettlebell close to your body, shrug your shoulder and pull the kettlebell upward (*b*).

3. When the kettlebell reaches the top position overhead, rotate your hand around the handle of the kettlebell, catching it at its pinnacle directly over your shoulder (*c*).

4. Lower the kettlebell back to your shoulder and then down to the starting position on the floor. Repeat all reps for one side before switching to the other.

Complete Workout

Complete 5 rounds of the following circuit.

Kettlebell snatch
- 6 reps/side
- 30 seconds of rest

Single-arm kettlebell swing (#18)
- 8 reps/side
- 30 seconds of rest

Kettlebell shoulder press (#298)
- 6 reps/side
- 30 seconds of rest

Turkish get-up (#99)
- 4 reps/side
- 2 minutes of rest

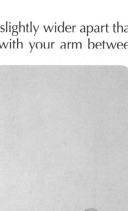
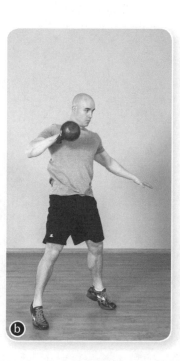
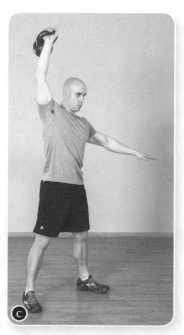

OPTIONS

Easy Option Complete 4 rounds of the circuit.

Step It Up Complete 6 rounds of the circuit.

Cool-Down Standing quad stretch, 90-degree stretch, double lat stretch.

Triple Five Snatch

Considering that most people sit at a desk and work on a computer all day and then go home and text on a smartphone all evening, you may be well served to do more pulling and back exercises during the week than pressing and chest exercises. Being in a forward shoulder position (as in typing) shortens the pectoral muscles while stretching and weakening the muscles in the upper back. By performing more pulling exercises, you can strengthen those back muscles and combat some of the damage you are doing during the rest of your day.

Warm-Up

5 reps of inchworm, 6 reps per side of quadruped T-spine rotation, 10 reps of cat–cow

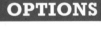 **Featured Exercise**

Power Snatch

1. Begin with the barbell on the floor. Grab the barbell with a double overhand snatch grip. Bring your hips down, and keep your chest tall and your shoulders in line with the bar (*a*).

2. Keeping your chest tall, push your knees back and lift your hips.

3. Once the bar has passed your knees and reached midthigh, begin dropping your hips.

4. As the bar continues to travel upward, explosively extend at your hips and knees, sending the bar directly overhead (*b*).

5. Receive the bar with arms locked out in the power position (do not squat below parallel) (*c*) before returning the bar back to the floor. Repeat for reps.

Complete Workout

Perform 5 rounds of the following complex with no rest between movements.

Power snatch
- 5 reps

Overhead squat (#167)
- 5 reps

Behind-the-neck jerk (#95)
- 5 reps
- 2 minutes of rest

OPTIONS

Easy Option   Perform 3 reps of each exercise per round.

Step It Up   Add an additional round of the complex (6 rounds total).

Cool-Down   Double lat stretch, cross-body stretch, hamstring stretch.

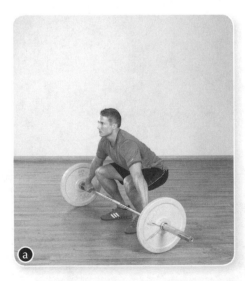

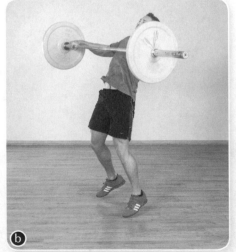

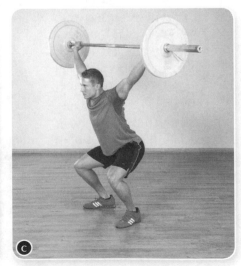

Body Armor

Many people discount the role of muscle mass in strength and athleticism. They often claim that too much mass will make you muscle-bound, inflexible, and unathletic—that big muscles are all show and no go. However, muscle mass is often responsible for increased strength because is beneficial for producing force on a joint. Muscle can also serve as body armor in sports that involve collisions such as football, lacrosse, and rugby. And as long as dynamic mobility is part of your overall training plan, you should not lose flexibility as you gain muscle.

Warm-Up

4 reps per side of the world's greatest stretch, 6 reps per side of hip rocker and inverted hamstring stretch, 8 reps per side of shoulder sweeps

● Featured Exercise

Barbell Overhead Press

1. Grab a loaded bar just outside shoulder width at collarbone height. The bar should be resting on top of your anterior deltoids (front of your shoulders) (*a*).

2. Take a deep breath in, brace your core, and begin driving the bar overhead.

3. As the bar passes over the top of your head, drive your body slightly forward so the bar is over the center of your foot (do not, however, jut your chin out or extend your neck).

4. Continue to press the bar overhead until you have achieved full lockout (*b*). Return the bar to the starting position and repeat for reps.

Complete Workout

Perform the following circuit in as little time as possible, resting only as needed. Place 50 percent of your body weight on the bar for the barbell overhead press.

Barbell overhead press
- 10 sets × 10, 9, 8, 7, 6, 5, 4, 3, 2, 1 reps

Wide-grip pull-up (#117)
- 10 sets × 10, 9, 8, 7, 6, 5, 4, 3, 2, 1 reps

Burpee (#7)
- 10 sets × 10, 9, 8, 7, 6, 5, 4, 3, 2, 1 reps

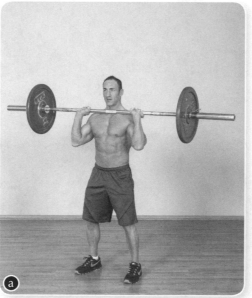
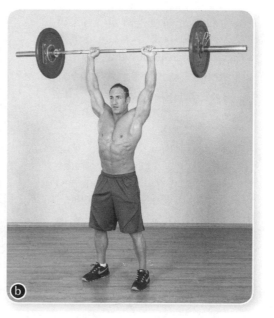

OPTIONS

Easy Option   Use one-third of your body weight for the barbell overhead press. Perform 7 sets total, starting with 7 reps per set and working down to 1 rep.

Step It Up   Use three-quarters of your body weight for the barbell overhead press.

Cool-Down   Standing quad stretch, 90-degree stretch, double lat stretch.

Going In for the Kill

Pay attention to how you move once you are already fatigued. Training in a fatigued state will often reveal your true movement weaknesses, which is knowledge you can exploit to improve your mobility or shore up weak muscle groups. Movement will almost never be ideal when you are in a fatigued state, so do not go for maximal lifts when you are gassed as this can open you up to injury. Even if a workout is being timed, taking an extra few moments to compose yourself, focus on form, and perform the exercise correctly will ultimately pay off.

Warm-Up

4 reps per side of the world's greatest stretch, 5 reps each of inchworm and inverted hamstring stretch, 10 reps of glute bridge

● Featured Exercise

Conventional Deadlift

Complete Workout

Complete the following circuit in as little time as possible, resting only as needed. Perform all three sets of the conventional deadlift, barbell push press, and wide-grip pull-up before moving on to the run, which can be performed outdoors or on a treadmill (the run is to be performed only once).

Conventional deadlift
- 6 reps

Barbell push press (#280)
- 9 reps

Wide-grip pull-up (#117)
- 12 reps

Run
- 1 mile (1.6 km)

OPTIONS

Easy Option   Perform 2 sets of the conventional deadlift, barbell push press, and wide-grip pull-up.

Step It Up   Perform 4 sets of the conventional deadlift, barbell push press, and wide-grip pull-up.

Cool-Down   Double lat stretch, hamstring stretch, calf stretch.

1. Approach a barbell set up on the floor by placing your feet under the bar until it is 2 to 3 inches (5 to 8 cm) in front of your shins. Your stance should be approximately hip width.

2. Bend down and grab the bar just outside your legs with either a double overhand or mixed grip.

3. Pull your hips down and bring your shins in contact with the bar. Keep your chest tall and maintain a neutral spine (a).

4. Stand up by raising simultaneously at your hips and shoulders, driving your hips forward until you reach lockout (b).

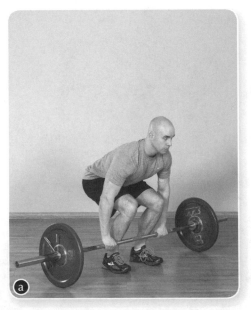 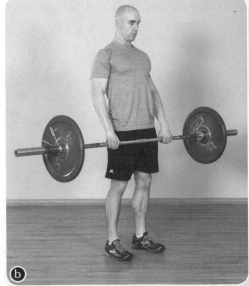

Balls to the Wall

If you are having problems achieving full range of motion in an exercise such as the squat or the deadlift, you may want to look at your ankle, hip, and thoracic spine mobility. Although these three areas are certainly not the cause of all mobility issues, they seem to be the main culprits for a lot of people. By doing some extra foam rolling and mobility work in these areas, you may free up some restrictions and be able to improve your range—making you a better, healthier athlete.

Warm-Up

6 reps of squat to stand, 6 reps per side of quadruped T-spine rotation, 8 reps of glute bridge, 10 reps of cat–cow

● Featured Exercise

3-for-1 Wall Ball

1. Stand tall, holding a medicine ball at chest height (*a*). Squat until the creases of your hips are below the height of your knees (your upper legs should be below parallel to the floor) (*b*).
2. In one motion, stand out of the squat and throw the ball at a 10- to 12-foot (3 to 4 m) target on a wall or beam in front of you (*c*).

3. Catch the ball and continue into three squats.
4. After the third squat, throw the ball at the target. Three squats and one throw are equal to 1 rep.

Complete Workout

Perform 3 rounds of the following circuit with as little rest as needed between movements within sets. The goal is to complete the 3 rounds as quickly as possible.

Barbell thruster (#6)
- 10 reps

3-for-1 wall ball
- 12 reps

Chin-up (#73)
- 15 reps

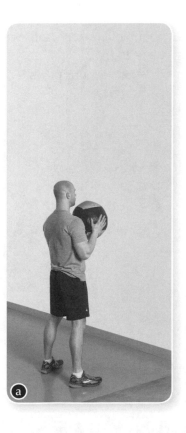
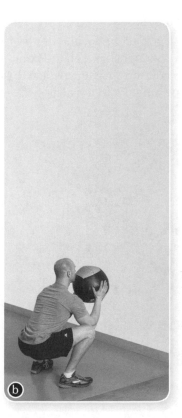
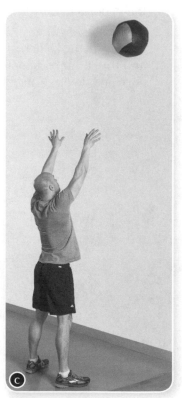

OPTIONS

Easy Option   Perform 2 total rounds of the circuit.

Step It Up   Add 2 more rounds of the circuit (5 rounds total).

Cool-Down   Hamstring stretch, calf stretch, pec stretch.

For Whom the Bells Toll

Developed in Russia in the 1700s, the kettlebell is a unique training tool. Unlike barbells or dumbbells, the kettlebell's center of mass is located directly below its handle as opposed to outside of it. This contributes to a unique "feel" you'll get while training with kettlebells, especially during ballistic exercises such as the clean, snatch, and swing

Warm-Up

4 reps per side of the world's greatest stretch, 6 reps per side of hip rocker and inverted hamstring stretch, 8 reps per side of shoulder sweeps

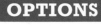 **Featured Exercise**

Kettlebell Renegade Row

1. Assume a push-up position, with your hands grasping the handles of a pair of kettlebells (a).
2. While pressing firmly into the kettlebell with your left hand, pick the kettlebell in your right hand off the floor and row it up by keeping your arm close to your rib cage and driving your elbow up toward the ceiling (b).

3. It is critical to keep your body (particularly your hips) parallel to the floor and not rotate during the movement.
4. Return the kettlebell to the floor and repeat, alternating sides.

Complete Workout

Perform 5 rounds of the following circuit.

Goblet squat (#2)
- 8 reps

Kettlebell clean and press (#32)
- 8 reps

Kettlebell sumo deadlift (#19)
- 8 reps

Kettlebell renegade row
- 8 reps

Double-arm kettlebell swing (#13)
- 20 reps
- 60 seconds of rest

OPTIONS

Easy Option   Complete 3 rounds of the circuit.

Step It Up   Increase the number of double-arm kettlebell swings to 30 reps.

Cool-Down   Standing quad stretch, 90-degree stretch, double lat stretch.

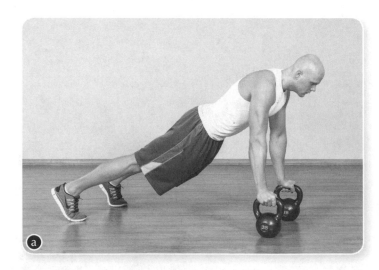

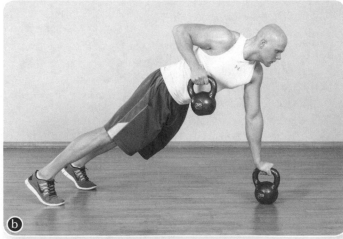

40 Reps of Hell

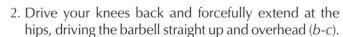

The phrase *floor to overhead*, which you will see used in this workout, is exactly what it sounds like—getting the bar from the floor to over your head any way you see fit, whether that is a clean and press, clean and split jerk, snatch, or any other movement you'd like. Similarly, *shoulder to overhead* means you can get the bar from the shoulder rack position to overhead using an overhead press, push press, push jerk, or split jerk. And feel free to mix these up during the workout, starting with the most challenging movements and progressing to the more mechanically efficient variations as you start to fatigue.

Warm-Up

4 reps per side of the world's greatest stretch, 5 reps of inchworm, 8 reps per side of shoulder sweeps

● Featured Exercise

Floor-to-Overhead Snatch

1. Grab a barbell with a snatch grip. Bend at the knees, lower your hips and keep your chest tall (*a*).

2. Drive your knees back and forcefully extend at the hips, driving the barbell straight up and overhead (*b-c*).

3. Catch the bar with knees slightly bent.

4. Stand tall and return the bar to the floor. Return to the start position and go directly into the next rep. Because the weight is light and you are prioritizing a high number of reps, you should be less concerned about making contact with the hips and pulling yourself under the bar as you would in a snatch/power snatch.

Complete Workout

Use a 95 lb (43 kg) barbell to complete the following workout in as little time as possible. Rest in between and within sets as needed, and set the bar on the floor at any time.

Floor-to-overhead snatch
- 20 reps

Shoulder-to-overhead snatch
- 20 reps

OPTIONS

Easy Option Reduce the weight of the barbell to 75 lb (34 kg) or less.

Step It Up Increase the weight of the barbell to 115 lb (52 kg) or more.

Cool-Down Pec stretch, double lat stretch, 90-degree stretch.

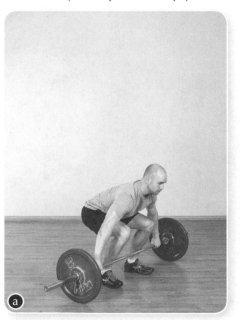

(a)

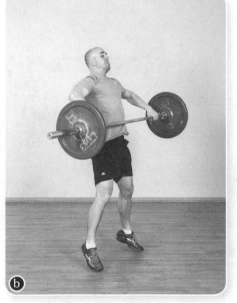

(b)

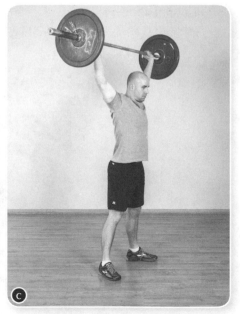

(c)

Born to Run

You learned to walk when you were about a year old. By the time you were two you probably knew how to run. How can something you've been doing for nearly your whole life feel so difficult? Whether you love to run or dread it, this repeat sprint workout will challenge your will and drive up your conditioning, making it the perfect aid for athletic performance or any fat-loss phase.

Warm-Up

4 reps per side of the world's greatest stretch, 6 reps per side of hip rocker and inverted hamstring stretch, 8 reps per side of shoulder sweeps

● Featured Exercise

Sprinting

1. Begin slowly running on a treadmill or a track.
2. Accumulate speed by striking your forefoot on the ground or treadmill and actively pulling your foot up toward your glutes (avoid striking your heel on the ground).
3. Prioritize longer strides and faster turnover to improve speed and performance during sprints.

Complete Workout

No specific rest periods are assigned to this workout. Rather, tackle the next set when you feel prepared to give an all-out effort.

100-yard (100 m) sprint*
- 10 sets
- Rest as needed

*Can be completed on a track, field, or treadmill

OPTIONS

Easy Option Reduce the number of sprints to 5. Sprint 75 yards (75 m).

Step It Up Keep all rest intervals under 1 minute for entire workout.

Cool-Down Standing quad stretch, 90-degree stretch, double lat stretch.

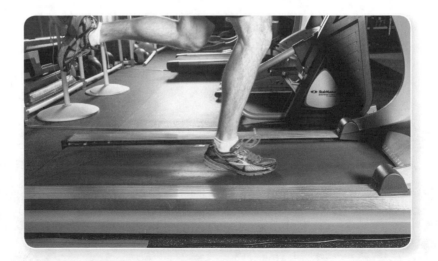

The Villain

Work capacity is a combination of muscular strength and aerobic endurance. The very definition of fitness may be the ability to maximize these two strength qualities for the longest time possible without a significant drop-off in performance. This workout tests work capacity by combining both strength and aerobic capabilities into one villainous circuit.

Warm-Up

4 reps per side of the world's greatest stretch, 6 reps per side of hip rocker and inverted hamstring stretch, 8 reps per side of shoulder sweeps

● Featured Exercise

Push-Up

1. Start with hands directly under shoulders and your body in a plank position, creating a straight line from shoulder to heel (a).

2. Keeping your elbows tucked toward your rib cage and maintaining a neutral spine, slowly lower your body until your chest nearly touches the ground (b).

3. Drive your hands into the floor and reverse the motion until your elbows reach lockout and you have returned to the starting position. Repeat for reps.

Complete Workout

Complete 4 rounds of the following circuit, resting as little as possible between exercises and rounds.

Rower (#212)
- 250 meters

Double-arm kettlebell swing (#13)
- 20 reps

Push-up
- 20 reps

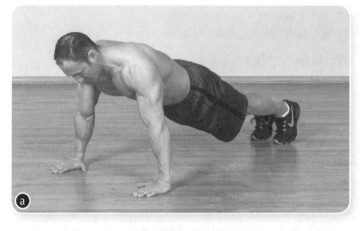

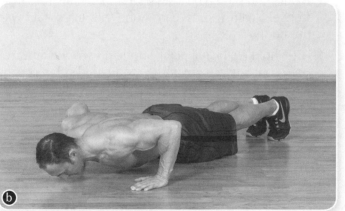

OPTIONS

Easy Option Decrease the number of reps for kettlebell swings and push-ups to 10 per set.

Step It Up Increase the row to 500 meters for each set.

Cool-Down Standing quad stretch, 90-degree stretch, double lat stretch.

Iron Giant

The term *giant set* refers to a circuit of different exercises (usually four or more) done back to back, with little to no rest between movements. Giant sets are a great method for fat loss in that they are very metabolically demanding (like traditional cardio) but utilize resistance, which promotes muscle gain or maintenance (unlike traditional cardio). So if you want your waist to shrink while keeping your strength high and muscle mass intact, give giant sets a try.

Warm-Up

4 reps per side of the world's greatest stretch, 6 reps per side of hip rocker and inverted hamstring stretch, 8 reps per side of shoulder sweeps

● Featured Exercise

Rolling Plank

1. Assume a side plank position, with your right elbow directly under your right shoulder, a straight line from your head to your heels, and your right foot directly in front of your left (your right heel should be just in front of your left toe). Your left arm should be extended toward the ceiling (a).

2. After holding the side plank for the prescribed time, roll your body onto both elbows into a full plank (b). Again, you should be holding a straight line from head to heels, with your forearms and toes in contact with the floor.

3. After holding the full plank for the prescribed time, roll onto your left forearm and perform a side plank on the left side, holding for the prescribed time (c).

4. Your hips should not sag during the entire movement, including the holds and the transitions from position to position.

Complete Workout

Complete 4 rounds of the following giant set, resting 20 seconds between movements and 2 minutes between rounds.

Goblet squat (#2)
- 12 reps

Incline dumbbell chest press (#210)
- 12 reps

Dumbbell Romanian deadlift (#267)
- 12 reps

TRX face pull (#270)
- 12 reps

Rolling plank
- 30 seconds per position

OPTIONS

Easy Option   Perform 3 rounds of the giant set. Rest 30 seconds between movements.

Step It Up   Reduce the rest to 15 seconds between movements.

Cool-Down   Standing quad stretch, 90-degree stretch, double lat stretch.

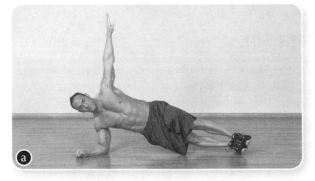

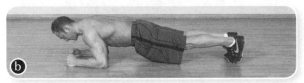

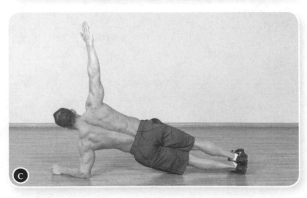

Aggressive

If one of your goals is improving body composition, you would be well served to take photos of yourself on a weekly basis. Photos are a great tool to help measure your progress. After all, if your goal is to look better, you may as well have an accurate account of how you look. Take four photos—one from the front, one from each side, and one from the back. And make sure you take any follow-up photos from the same angle and with the same camera and lighting. This way you'll be making a fair comparison from one set of photos to the next.

Warm-Up

4 reps per side of the world's greatest stretch, 6 reps per side of hip rocker and inverted hamstring stretch, 8 reps per side of shoulder sweeps

● Featured Exercise

Barbell Front Squat

1. Set up a barbell just below collarbone height in a squat rack.
2. Step under the bar so it sits on your front deltoids (shoulders), and grab the bar with a clean grip, with your elbows high and your upper arms parallel to the ground. Unrack the bar and take one step back with each foot (a).

3. Tighten up your upper body, unlock your hips, bend your knees, and lower your body toward the ground, trying to sit as low as possible while keeping the bar over the center of your foot (for more on proper squat technique, see chapter 1, Ramping Up) (b).
4. Once you reach the bottom of your range, reverse the motion and stand up. Repeat for reps.

Complete Workout

Perform the following four exercises within 4 minutes. Continue to add additional rounds until you can no longer complete all the exercises as prescribed within the 4-minute time frame. If you finish before the 4-minute mark, use the additional time as rest.

Barbell front squat
- 6 reps × 50 percent body weight

Barbell bench press (#54)
- 10 reps × 50 percent body weight

Wide-grip pull-up (#117)
- 12 reps

Double-arm kettlebell swing (#13)
- 35 reps

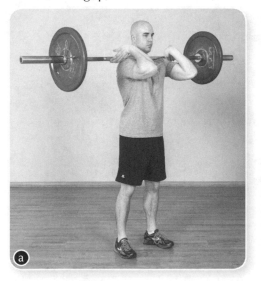

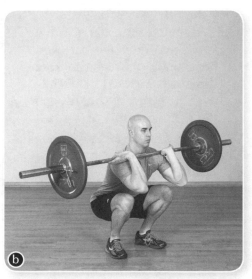

OPTIONS

Easy Option Reduce the number of pull-ups to 8 reps and the number of kettlebell swings to 25 reps.

Step It Up Perform the entire circuit in 3 minutes.

Cool-Down Standing quad stretch, 90-degree stretch, double lat stretch.

Inception

AMRAP stands for "as many reps as possible," and when you see that as the repetition prescription for a workout, you should certainly take a deep breath and say your prayers before the set begins. AMRAP workouts are brutal, but push yourself and you'll be rewarded by one of the best protocols to drive up work capacity and burn fat in a very time-efficient way. Just remember, it's as many reps as possible, not as many reps as you feel like doing. The goal is to push as hard as you can in the time allotted.

Warm-Up

4 reps per side of the world's greatest stretch, 5 reps of inchworm, 8 reps per side of shoulder sweeps

● Featured Exercise

Push Press

1. With your feet at hip width, grab a barbell at collarbone height with a double over-hand grip, just outside shoulder width.
2. Keeping your abs braced, bend slightly at the knees (a).
3. Simultaneously extend at the knees and drive the bar over-head until you reach lockout (b). The bar should be directly over the center of your head in the top position.
4. Return the bar to the starting position and repeat for reps.

Complete Workout

Perform 3 rounds of the following circuit.

Push press
- 1 minute × as many reps as possible
- 60 seconds of rest

Burpee (#7)
- 1 minute × as many reps as possible
- 60 seconds of rest

Push press
- 1 minute × as many reps as possible
- 3 minutes of rest

OPTIONS

Easy Option Perform each movement for 45 seconds.

Step It Up Add an additional round, completing a total of 4 circuits.

Cool-Down Pec stretch, double lat stretch, 90-degree stretch.

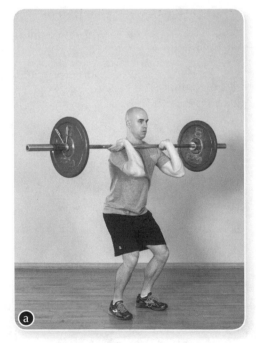
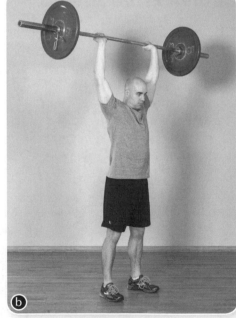

Fire in the Hole

Goal setting is as important a step in training as following a solid program, progressively getting stronger, and adhering to a good nutrition plan. Find a goal that is meaningful, measurable, and achievable; determine a timeline to reach that goal; and figure out what steps you have to put in place to make it a reality. Doing so will give your training much more focus and meaning.

Warm-Up

6 reps of squat to stand, 6 reps per side of quadruped T-spine rotation, 8 reps of glute bridge, 10 reps of cat–cow

● Featured Exercise

TRX Power Pull

1. With your TRX in single handle mode, grab the handle with your right hand with your feet in front of you, creating a straight line from head to heel.

2. Rotate your straight left arm away from the TRX anchor point and toward the floor (your body should look like a T that is perpendicular to the TRX) (*a*).

3. Rotate your body, bringing your left arm up toward the anchor point by rowing with your right arm, driving your right elbow behind you (*b*).

4. Reverse motion under control until you are back to the T position. Repeat until you complete all reps on one side before switching to the other.

Complete Workout

A. Barbell back squat (#63)
- 6 sets × 2 reps, 4 reps, 6 reps, 8 reps, 10 reps, 12 reps
- 60 seconds of rest between sets

B1. Incline dumbbell chest press (#210)
- 2 sets × 5 reps

B2. TRX power pull
- 2 sets × 8 reps/side

C. Rower (#212)
- 200 meters
- 2 sets
- 2 minutes of rest

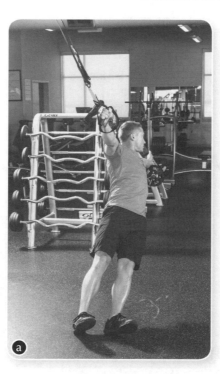
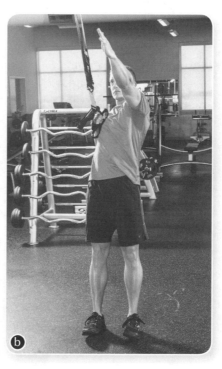

OPTIONS

Easy Option Eliminate the last 2 sets of the barbell back squat.

Step It Up Add an additional set to the B exercises.

Cool-Down Standing quad stretch, 90-degree stretch, double lat stretch.

Run and Gun

Want to excel at soccer, track, American football, and numerous other athletic endeavors? Then you are going to need the ability to sprint. And you certainly don't want to be just a "one and done" athlete. Being capable of explosive speed at the end of the game is what separates champions from everyone else. This workout will test both your sprinting abilities at various distances and your ability to recover. The running portion of this workout can be done on either a treadmill, a track, or a field.

Warm-Up

4 reps per side of the world's greatest stretch, 5 reps each of inchworm and inverted hamstring stretch, 10 reps of glute bridge

● Featured Exercise

Sprinting

1. Begin slowly running on a treadmill or a track.
2. Accumulate speed by striking your forefoot on the ground or treadmill and actively pulling your foot up toward your glutes (avoid striking your heel on the ground).
3. Prioritize longer strides and faster turnover to improve speed and performance during sprints.

Complete Workout

Perform one round of the following:

2-minute light jog

200-yard (200 m) sprint
- 3 minutes of rest

150-yard (150 m) sprint
- 2 minutes of rest

100-yard (100 m) sprint
- 1 minute of rest

75-yard (75 m) sprint
- 30 seconds of rest

50-yard (50 m) sprint

OPTIONS

Easy Option Add 1 minute to each of the rest periods. Eliminate the 200-yard (200 m) sprint.

Step It Up Repeat the workout by working back up the ladder, starting with the 50-yard (50 m) sprint and finishing with the 200-yard (200 m) sprint.

Cool-Down Double lat stretch, hamstring stretch, calf stretch.

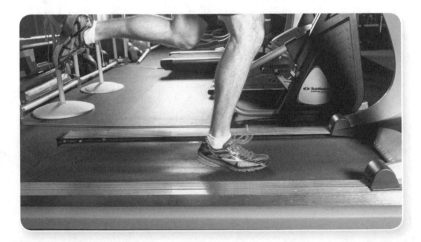

Super Circuit

When training for general fitness, strength, and mobility, always choose a high-bar barbell back squat as opposed to a low bar. The high bar, in which the barbell sits on your upper traps, allows for more range of motion as well as an upright torso position—both of which are advantageous in sport and everyday tasks. A low-bar squat should be chosen only as an occasional variation or if you are looking to compete in powerlifting. Otherwise keep the bar high and your chest tall.

Warm-Up

4 reps per side of the world's greatest stretch, 6 reps per side of hip rocker and inverted hamstring stretch, 8 reps per side of shoulder sweeps

● Featured Exercise

Super Squat Thrust

1. Place your hands straight up above your head, and squat as low as possible (*a*).
2. Place your hands on the ground in front of your feet (*b*) and bring your hips up in the air, straightening your legs as much as possible (*c*).

3. Bring your hips back down and kick both feet out directly behind you, as for the starting position of a push-up (*d*).
4. Bring your feet back in and lift your hands directly overhead.
5. Stand up and repeat for reps.

Complete Workout

Perform 5 rounds of the following circuit.

Barbell back squat (#63)
- 6 reps
- 10 seconds of rest

Neutral-grip pull-up (#237)
- 8 reps
- 10 seconds of rest

Super squat thrust
- 10 reps
- 10 seconds of rest

Push-up (#12)
- 12 reps
- 60 seconds of rest

OPTIONS

Easy Option   Perform 3 rounds of the circuit.

Step It Up   Add 2 reps per set to each of the exercises.

Cool-Down   Standing quad stretch, 90-degree stretch, double lat stretch.

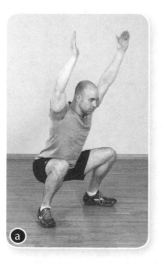
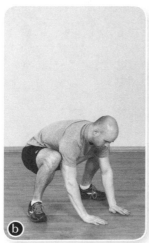
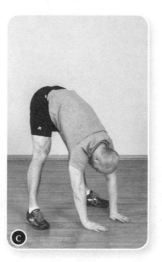
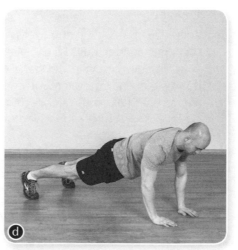

The Specialist

Certain medicine ball movements are designed to overcome the force of gravity (medicine ball sit-up throws, medicine ball squat throws), while others, such as the medicine ball slam featured in this workout, utilize gravity as part of the movement pattern. When throwing medicine balls toward the floor, it is much more appropriate to use a heavier ball because your muscles have to do much less work. However, when doing movements that overcome gravity, speed should be a priority and so lighter balls should be used.

Warm-Up

4 reps per side of the world's greatest stretch, 6 reps per side of hip rocker and inverted hamstring stretch, 8 reps per side of shoulder sweeps

Complete Workout

Complete 3 rounds of the following circuit, resting as little as possible between exercises and between circuits.

Pull-up (#231)
- 10 reps

Medicine ball slam
- 20 reps

Wall ball (#25)
- 30 reps

Double-arm kettlebell swing (#13)
- 40 reps

● Featured Exercise

Medicine Ball Slam

1. Grab a relatively heavy medicine ball and lift it directly over your head (*a*). (Relatively heavy could be a 6 lb ball for an untrained female or a 100 lb ball for an experienced heavyweight trainee. Choose a ball that is challenging but allows you to complete all reps without stopping.)

2. Keeping your head up and eyes forward, slam the ball into the floor (*b*). Make sure your spine stays in a neutral position during the entire movement and your feet remain flat on the floor (your body position should be similar to that of a squat at the bottom).

3. Catch the ball on a single bounce, and raise it above your head. Repeat for reps.

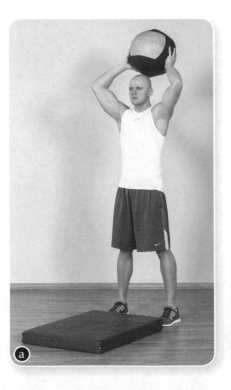
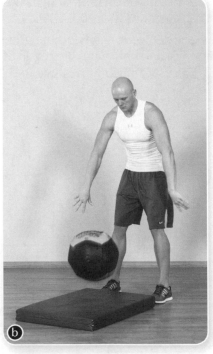

OPTIONS

Easy Option   Perform the circuit twice.

Step It Up   Perform the circuit four times.

Cool-Down   Standing quad stretch, 90-degree stretch, double lat stretch.

Over My Head

Holding a barbell overhead does several things. First, it guarantees core activation because you cannot hold any object overhead without core stabilization. Second, it encourages extension of the thoracic spine (middle back), which is something most people who sit slumped in chairs all day are certainly in need of to improve and optimize posture. Last, it trains stability in the shoulder, a notoriously unstable joint. Although these benefits will greatly aid your training, achieving them can be extremely demanding, so keep that in mind when choosing loads for any movements that include an overhead component.

Warm-Up

4 reps per side of the world's greatest stretch, 6 reps per side of hip rocker and inverted hamstring stretch, 8 reps per side of shoulder sweeps

● Featured Exercise

Snatch-Grip Overhead Reverse Lunge

1. Begin with the barbell across your upper traps as for the starting position of a barbell back squat. Slide your hands out so they are in a snatch-grip position, and press the bar overhead (a).

2. Keeping the bar slightly behind the back of your head, step back with the right leg, bending your knee until it reaches or is 1 inch (2.5 cm) above the floor. Your front leg should create a 90-degree angle at the bottom position (b).

3. Forcefully drive off of the front (left) foot to bring your feet back together.

4. Repeat the process, stepping back with the left leg (c). Continue to alternate in this manner until you have completed all reps.

Complete Workout

Perform 4 circuits of the following exercises, resting as little as possible.

Snatch-grip overhead reverse lunge
- 8 reps/leg

Neutral-grip pull-up (#237)
- 10 reps

200-yard (200 m) sprint (#41)

OPTIONS

Easy Option   Complete 2 circuits total.

Step It Up   Complete 6 circuits total.

Cool-Down   Standing quad stretch, 90-degree stretch, double lat stretch.

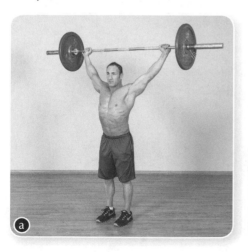
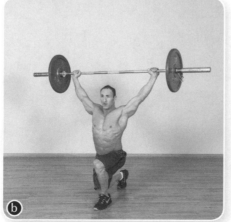
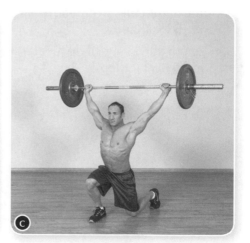

The Asylum

Complexes (stringing several exercises together using one implement such as a barbell, dumbbells, or kettlebells) are a great way to drive up the volume of a workout as well as increase metabolic demand. Essentially, they can deliver a lot of the fat-burning benefits associated with traditional cardio while being much more time efficient and encouraging muscle growth. Beware: Complexes are challenging and demanding. They might look simple on paper, but you need a lot of focus and desire to survive them.

Warm-Up

4 reps per side of the world's greatest stretch, 6 reps per side of hip rocker and inverted hamstring stretch, 8 reps per side of shoulder sweeps

● Featured Exercise

Dumbbell Push Press

1. Hold a pair of dumbbells with a neutral grip next to your shoulders. Your elbows should be bent and close to your sides.
2. Keeping your chest tall and back flat, bend at the knees until you are in a quarter-squat position (*a*).
3. Explosively drive up with your legs and press the dumbbells overhead until your arms reach lockout (*b*).
4. Return the dumbbells to the starting position and repeat for reps.

OPTIONS

Easy Option   Perform 3 rounds of the complex.

Step It Up   Perform 5 rounds of the complex, and reduce rest to 45 seconds between rounds.

Cool-Down   Standing quad stretch, 90-degree stretch, double lat stretch.

Complete Workout

Perform 4 rounds of the following exercises as a complex, using one set of dumbbells for all movements and without resting between exercises.

Goblet squat (#2)
- 10 reps

Dumbbell push press
- 10 reps

Alternating dumbbell row (#246)
- 10 reps

Dumbbell Romanian deadlift (#267)
- 10 reps
- 60 seconds of rest

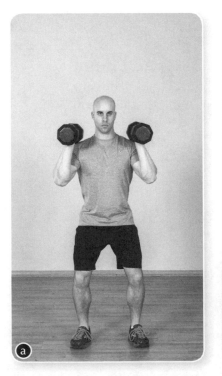
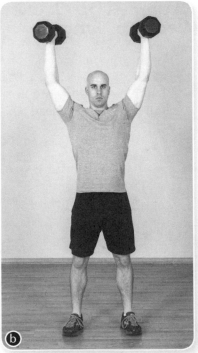

Come Clean

There is ever-increasing evidence that high-intensity interval training (HIIT) is superior to steady state training (SST) when it comes to fat loss. However, HIIT does not need to be performed solely on traditional cardio equipment. By utilizing a complex such as this one with a rest period between each set, you'll be getting the same effect as high-intensity cardio intervals (your heart rate will be sky high) with the added benefit of muscle gain by utilizing resistance (in this case, a barbell).

Warm-Up

4 reps per side of the world's greatest stretch, 6 reps per side of hip rocker and inverted hamstring stretch, 8 reps per side of shoulder sweeps

● Featured Exercise

Power Clean

1. Start by grabbing the barbell with an overhand grip, placing hands and feet slightly wider than shoulder-width apart (a).
2. Keeping the bar close to your shins, slowly pull your knees back while lifting the bar off the ground.

3. Once the bar gets to your midthighs, explosively jump upward, extending your body into triple extension—extending at the ankles, knees, and hips (b).
4. Aggressively pull your body under the bar, rotating your elbows around the bar. Catch the bar on your shoulders (c).
5. Catch the bar with flexed knees, but do not squat under the bar below parallel.
6. Stand up with the bar to complete the rep.

Complete Workout

Perform 5 rounds of the following complex, using one barbell.

Power clean
  • 6 reps
Push press (#16)
  • 8 reps
Barbell front squat (#44)
  • 10 reps
Barbell rollout (#228)
  • 12 reps
  • 90 seconds of rest

OPTIONS

Easy Option   Perform 6 rounds of the complex.

Step It Up   Perform 4 rounds of the complex.

Cool-Down   Hamstring stretch, calf stretch, pec stretch.

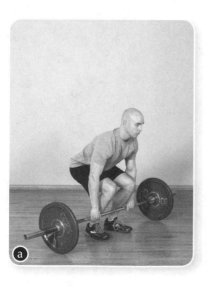

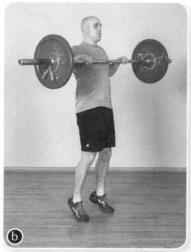

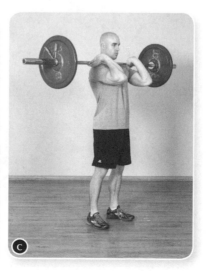

Beast Mode

Once you've got your mobility, proficiency with the movements, and base strength levels in check, the biggest thing you can bring to your workouts is a killer attitude—sometimes referred to as "beast mode." So rather than approaching your workout as if you are just trying to survive it, attack each set with intention and focus, and let out your inner beast.

Warm-Up

4 reps per side of the world's greatest stretch, 6 reps per side of hip rocker and inverted hamstring stretch, 8 reps per side of shoulder sweeps

Featured Exercise

Dumbbell Hang Clean and Press

1. Grab a dumbbell with your right hand, and assume a shoulder-width stance with your feet. Keeping your chest tall, bend at the knees and bring your hips back until the dumbbell is right above knee level (a).

2. Explosively drive your hips forward, shrug your right shoulder, and extend at the ankles, driving the dumb-

bell up to shoulder height (b). Be sure to keep the dumbbell close to your body for the entire movement.

3. Catch the dumbbell by bringing your elbow in tight to your rib cage (c). Rebend your knees and drive the dumbbell overhead (d).

4. Reverse the process to return the dumbbell to its original starting point. Complete all reps for one side before switching.

Complete Workout

Complete the following circuit four times, resting as little as possible between exercises and 2 minutes between circuits.

Prisoner jump squat (#4)
- 8 reps

Dumbbell hang clean and press
- 4 reps/side

Frog sit-up (#27)
- 15 reps

200-yard (200 m) sprint (#41)
- 2 minutes of rest

OPTIONS

Easy Option Perform the entire circuit 2 times.

Step It Up Add 2 reps to the prisoner jump squats and 1 rep per side on the dumbbell hang clean and press.

Cool-Down Hamstring stretch, calf stretch, pec stretch.

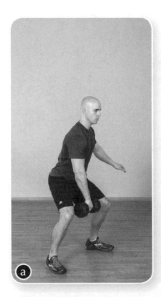
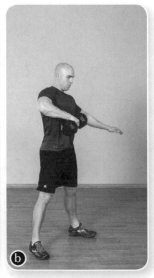
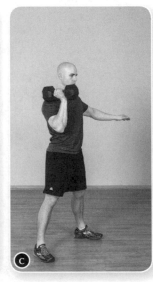
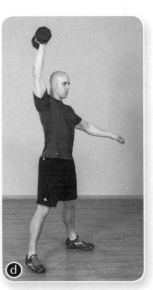

CHAPTER 5

Getting Stronger

Increasing strength is truly the foundation of all other fitness qualities. Getting stronger will help you develop more muscle mass, perform better on the athletic field, and drive up your daily metabolic rate, which, in turn, will allow you to burn more fat. Strength and power are also the two attributes we lose most quickly as we age, so you would be well served to develop them as much as you can now. In this chapter you will notice a smaller variety of movements per workout, allowing you to focus on adding weight to the bar. Do not let the increased rest periods or decreased volume (total number of sets and reps) fool you. A few reps of lifting heavy weights can be just as taxing on your body and lungs as any metabolic or cardiorespiratory training.

Minute on the Minute: Bench Press

Without a doubt, the bench press is the most popular exercise in the gym. But when done with bad form, it also poses the greatest risk of injury. To ensure safety, keep your feet on the floor and your head, upper back, and glutes on the bench. When lowering the bar, tuck your elbows in toward your rib cage as opposed to letting them flare out (flaring increases stress on the shoulder joint). If you haven't been using these techniques, you may need to back off the weight at first. This sacrifice is well worth it because you'll ultimately blast through plateaus and keep your joints happy and healthy.

Warm-Up

4 reps per side of the world's greatest stretch, 5 reps of inchworm, 8 reps per side of shoulder sweeps

● Featured Exercise

Barbell Bench Press

1. Lie back so your head, upper back, and glutes are in contact with the bench and your feet are flat on the floor. Begin with your eyes directly under the bar.

2. Grab the barbell with a double overhand grip just outside shoulder width (a).

3. Keeping your elbows tucked toward your rib cage, lower the bar until it makes contact with your mid-chest (b).

4. Drive the bar off your chest until you reach lockout.

Repeat for the prescribed number of reps then rerack the bar with your arms fully extended.

Complete Workout

Perform 3 reps of the bench press at the top of every minute for 20 minutes. If you can no longer complete 3 reps within that minute, end the workout. Use 75 to 80 percent of your 1RM.

Barbell bench press
  • As many sets as possible, as described

Warning: Even with lighter weights, it is suggested that you use a spotter while performing a bench press. You do not want to get stuck at the bottom of a rep with the bar on your chest and no means of escape.

OPTIONS

Easy Option Perform 2 reps of the bench press each minute.

Step It Up Perform 5 reps of the bench press each minute.

Cool-Down Pec stretch, double lat stretch, 90-degree stretch.

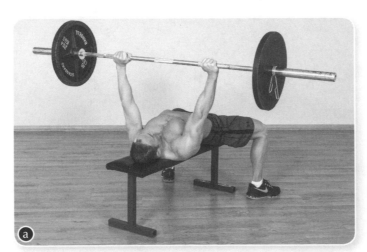
(a)

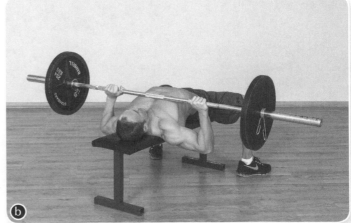
(b)

The Depths of Hell

There may be no exercise better suited for improving vertical leap than the depth jump. There also may be no exercise more demanding on your ankle and knee joints. Be sure to have mastered box jumps and bounding drills before taking on the depth jump. And when you do tackle this movement, start off on a low box (12 inches [30 cm] or lower), and limit the number of contacts until you gain experience with the exercise.

Warm-Up

5 reps of inchworm, 6 reps per side of quadruped T-spine rotation, 10 reps of cat–cow

Featured Exercise

Depth Jump

1. Stand with both feet at the edge of a 12-inch (30 cm) box (or lower).
2. Step off the box with one foot to start your descent (*a*), and land on both feet simultaneously (balls of your forefoot followed by your heels) (*b*). Keep your knees flexed in order to absorb impact and generate force.

3. As soon as you make contact with the ground, jump vertically as high as you can (as you would in a vertical jump) (*c*).
4. Land with both feet making contact with the ground at once, knees flexed to absorb impact.

Complete Workout

A. Depth jump
- 4 sets × 3 reps
- 90 seconds of rest

B. Snatch (#84)
- 3 sets × 3 reps
- 90 seconds of rest

C1. Plyo push-up (#165)
- 2 sets × 12 reps
- 60 seconds of rest

C2. Double-arm kettlebell swing (#13)
- 2 sets × 20 reps
- 60 seconds of rest

OPTIONS

Easy Option Substitute the push-up (#12) for the plyo push-up.

Step It Up Perform an additional set of the snatch, plyo push-up, and double-arm kettlebell swing.

Cool-Down Double lat stretch, cross-body stretch, hamstring stretch.

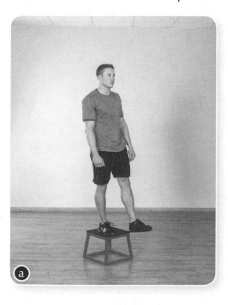
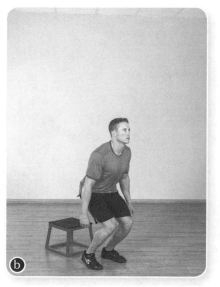
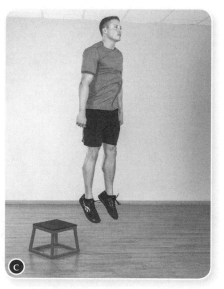

Dead on Arrival

If you've ever moved a television, installed an air conditioner, or picked up a toddler, you've performed some variation of a deadlift, one of the most functional exercises that can be performed in a gym. The deadlift trains your entire posterior chain (the muscles in the back of your body) to coordinate and work as a complete unit.

Warm-Up

4 reps per side of the world's greatest stretch, 5 reps each of inchworm and inverted hamstring stretch, 10 reps of glute bridge

● Featured Exercise

Conventional Deadlift

1. Utilize a hip-width stance, hinge at your hips (see chapter 1, Ramping Up, for a full description of the hip hinge), bend your knees slightly, and grab the bar with either a double overhand or mixed grip (a).

2. Keeping the bar close to your shins, pull it off the ground by extending at the knees and driving your hips forward.

3. Lock out fully at the hips, and maintain a neutral spine at the top of the movement (b).

4. Return the bar to the ground by first hinging at your hips and then slightly bending your knees as the bar gets closer to the ground. Repeat for reps.

Complete Workout

Complete each set at the repetition maximum for the reps prescribed. For example, the set of 5 should be performed with a weight you can lift with perfect form for no more than 5 reps. Increase the weight each set as the reps decrease.

Conventional deadlift
- 5 sets × 5, 4, 3, 2, 1 reps
- 2 minutes of rest between sets

OPTIONS

Easy Option   Eliminate the single rep.

Step It Up   Perform two additional singles with your heaviest weight.

Cool-Down   Double lat stretch, hamstring stretch, calf stretch.

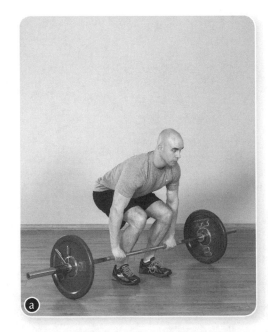
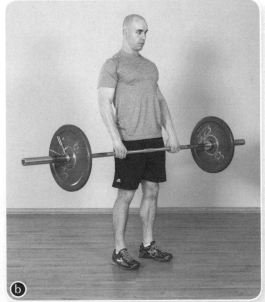

In Over Your Head

Although one of your goals should be to get strong in all the major movement patterns—presses, pulls, squats, and deadlifts—not all movement patterns are for everyone. If you cannot lift your arms directly overhead without over-extending your lower back, have poor hip control, cannot produce stiffness in your core, or don't have great rotation in your shoulder joints, overhead pressing is probably not a great movement pattern for you. Work on those mobility and stability issues first. Once you've got them squared away, you're free to safely develop your overhead pressing strength.

Warm-Up

4 reps per side of the world's greatest stretch, 5 reps of inchworm, 8 reps per side of shoulder sweeps

● Featured Exercise

Barbell Push Jerk

1. Begin in a standing position, feet at hip width, with a barbell directly in front of your collarbones. Hands should be just outside shoulders.
2. Bend your knees slightly (a), and utilize your legs to explosively drive the bar overhead.
3. Catch the bar in the top position with slightly bent knees before standing up to complete lockout (b).
4. Lower the barbell back to its original position and repeat for reps.

Complete Workout

For the barbell overhead press, begin with a weight you can comfortably complete for 3 or 4 reps. Perform 1 rep. Rest 60 seconds and add weight for set number 2; continue in this manner (adding weight each set) until you have completed 5 singles. Using the same weights you used for the 5 sets of the barbell overhead press, perform 3 reps per set of the barbell push press. When you have completed those 5 sets, use the same weights to complete all 5 sets of the barbell push jerk. For example, if you used 135 lb, 155 lb, 165 lb, 175 lb, and 180 lb for the overhead press singles, use those same weights for the sets of push press and push jerk (but with the increased number of reps).

A. Barbell overhead press (#36)
   - 5 sets × 1, 1, 1, 1, 1 reps
   - 60 seconds of rest
B. Barbell push press (#280)
   - 5 sets × 3, 3, 3, 3, 3 reps
   - 60 seconds of rest
C. Barbell push jerk
   - 5 sets × 5, 5, 5, 5, 5 reps
   - 60 seconds of rest

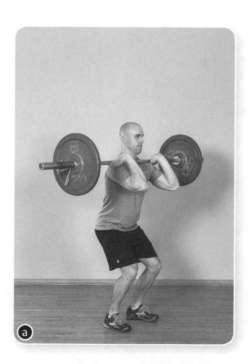
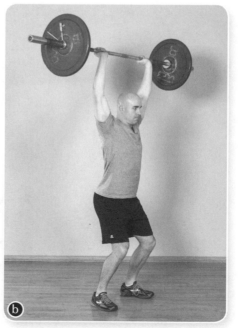

OPTIONS

Easy Option Begin by using your 6-7RM on your first set of the barbell overhead press.

Step It Up Add another set to each exercise.

Cool-Down Pec stretch, double lat stretch, 90-degree stretch.

The Thrust of It

Barbell thrusters are most often utilized as a metabolic exercise because they recruit many different muscle groups and get the heart rate elevated very quickly. However, the ability to develop strength and power with combo exercise should not be overlooked. This workout has you performing several low-rep sets with a decent amount of rest between efforts. Attempt to add weight to the bar each set, and really test your strength on this one.

Warm-Up

5 reps of squat to stand; 6 reps per side of kneeling adductor stretch, hip rocker, and quadruped T-spine rotation

Featured Exercise

Barbell Thruster

1. Rack a barbell on your shoulders with a double overhand grip. Your elbows should be forward of the bar.

2. Unlock your hips and squat down toward the floor, keeping your chest tall and eyes forward throughout the entire movement (a).

3. Once you've reached the bottom of your range of motion (your upper legs should be at or below parallel to the floor), reverse your motion, driving your hips forward (b).

4. As you return to the standing position, drive the barbell overhead until reaching full lockout (c).

5. Rerack the barbell at your shoulders and repeat for reps.

Complete Workout

Barbell thruster
- 9 sets × 3, 3, 3, 2, 2, 2, 1, 1, 1 reps
- 90 seconds of rest between each set

OPTIONS

Easy Option Perform 6 sets total by eliminating the single-rep sets.

Step It Up Add an additional set of a single rep at the end.

Cool-Down Standing quad stretch, 90-degree stretch, cross-body stretch.

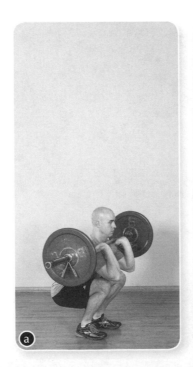
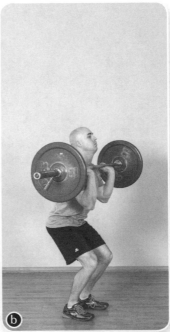
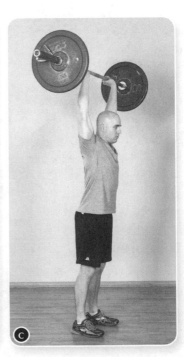

Snatched

One of the most underrated aspects of training recovery is a proper night's sleep. In fact, research shows that if you are working on training a specific skill (such as the paused snatch featured in this workout) and do not get a minimum amount of sleep (about 6 hours), you may not gain any benefit from the training session. In other words, without this critical aspect of recovery, you will not solidify any of the movement skills you just busted your butt to learn. So, if you are working on perfecting a new, technically demanding lift, make sure you shut off all your electronic devices and get a good night's sleep.

Warm-Up

5 reps of inchworm, 6 reps per side of quadruped T-spine rotation, 10 reps of cat–cow

● Featured Exercise

Paused Snatch

1. With a loaded barbell on the floor, grab the barbell with a snatch grip, bend your knees, and pull your hips down toward the ground. Keep your chest up and eyes forward. Your shoulders should be even with or slightly behind the bar.

2. Keeping your chest tall, lift the bar toward your knees (your back angle should not change). Once the bar reaches just below your knees, pause for 2 seconds (a).

3. Drive your knees back and your hips forward to continue bringing the bar up toward your hips.

4. As the bar nears the top of your thighs, explosively drive your hips forward in an effort to drive the bar vertically (b).

5. Simultaneously shuffle your feet outward and allow the bar to travel overhead.

6. Pull yourself under the bar and catch it in the bottom of the overhead squat position, or complete a full overhead squat if you catch the bar higher (c).

7. Return the bar to the starting position, reset, and complete for reps.

Complete Workout

Paused snatch
- 8 sets × 2 reps
- 2 minutes of rest

OPTIONS

Easy Option   Reduce to 6 sets total.

Step It Up   Increase the length of the pause to 3 seconds.

Cool-Down   Double lat stretch, cross-body stretch, hamstring stretch.

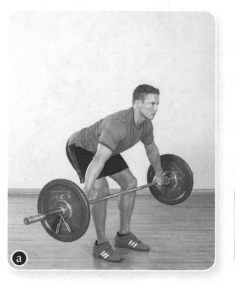

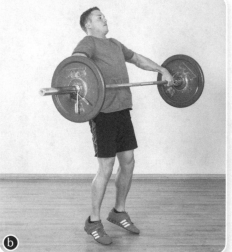

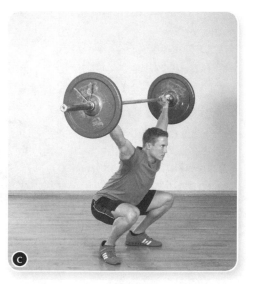

Right Said Dead

The phrase *don't judge a book by its cover* is clearly a cliché, but when it comes to a workout, it's good advice to take. Just because a workout may look easy on paper, don't be fooled until you get under the bar and give it a try. In fact, almost any workout can be easy or challenging. It just depends on how much weight you are willing to use and how much effort you are willing to put in.

Warm-Up

5 reps of inchworm, 6 reps per side of quadruped T-spine rotation, 10 reps of cat–cow

⦿ Featured Exercise

Snatch-Grip Deadlift

1. Begin with your feet under a loaded barbell at hip width. Reach down and grab the barbell with a snatch grip (the same wide grip you would use to perform a barbell snatch).

2. Bring your shins to the bar and your hips down, keeping your chest tall (a).

3. Keeping a neutral spine, lift the bar along your body, bringing your hips forward.

4. Once you reach the top position with the barbell directly in front of your hip bones (b), reverse the motion and bring the barbell back to the floor. Note that you need increased mobility over the conventional deadlift to perform this exercise correctly.

Complete Workout

Add weight each set, and try to use the same weight for each set of each exercise (e.g., if you used 220 lb, 235 lb, 245 lb, 250 lb, and 255 lb for the snatch-grip deadlift singles, use those same weights for the sets of 3-rep conventional deadlifts and sets of 5-rep sumo deadlifts).

A. Snatch-grip deadlift
- 5 sets × 1 rep
- 60 seconds of rest

B. Conventional deadlift (#5)
- 5 sets × 3 reps
- 60 seconds of rest

C. Sumo deadlift (#82)
- 5 sets × 5 reps
- 60 seconds of rest

OPTIONS

Easy Option   Reduce each exercise to 3 sets.

Step It Up   Increase the weights used for the conventional deadlift and sumo deadlift.

Cool-Down   Double lat stretch, cross-body stretch, hamstring stretch.

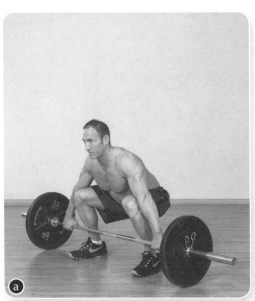
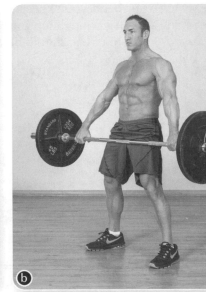

Snatch Complex

Olympic lifting pulls can be done from various positions (from the floor, from the midshin, from the hang) and employ the same techniques as the full Olympic lifts minus the catching phase. There are several benefits to performing pulls. They can help you master different phases of the lift that you may be struggling with as well as allow you to load the bar with more weight than you would be able to use in the full lift. This can ultimately lead to breakthroughs in plateaus and new personal records, so don't shortchange using pulls in your program.

Warm-Up

6 reps of squat to stand, 6 reps per side of quadruped T-spine rotation, 8 reps of glute bridge, 10 reps of cat–cow

● Featured Exercise

Hang Snatch Pull

1. Grab a barbell at approximately double shoulder width (when your arms are straight and you are standing tall, the barbell should rest about 2 inches [5 cm] below your navel).

2. Bend your knees and bring your hips back so the bar rests just below your knees. This will be the starting position (a).

3. Drive your hips forward, shrug your shoulders, and extend at the ankles simultaneously, driving the bar upward (b).

4. Once you have completed this triple extension, pull your elbows up and back, bringing the bar to your midchest (note: the bar should stay close to your body throughout the entire movement, which should be performed explosively).

Complete Workout

Complete 8 rounds of the following complex, moving from one exercise to the next without rest. Rest 90 seconds between rounds. Increase the weight (when possible) from one round to the next.

Hang snatch pull
- 1 rep

Snatch (#84)
- 1 rep

Overhead squat (#167)
- 1 rep
- 90 seconds of rest

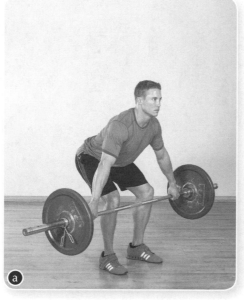
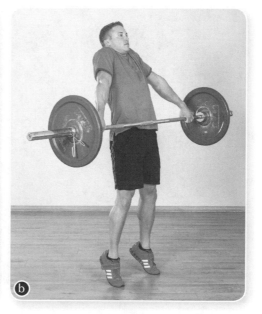

OPTIONS

Easy Option   Perform 6 rounds of the complex.

Step It Up   Perform 2 rounds of the complex before resting.

Cool-Down   Standing quad stretch, 90-degree stretch, double lat stretch.

Absolute Bench Press

Developing a strong bench press is a gym rite of passage. This workout utilizes lower reps for several sets in an effort to drive up your bench numbers. As a general rule, the lower the reps per set, the more total sets you should perform—particularly in a workout focusing on strength.

Warm-Up

4 reps per side of the world's greatest stretch, 5 reps of inchworm, 8 reps per side of shoulder sweeps

● Featured Exercise

High-to-Low Cable Fly

1. Attach two D handles to the ends of a cable station set in the high position.
2. Grab one handle with each hand, and step forward so you are positioned directly between both handles and in front of the weight stacks.

3. With only a slight bend in your elbows, begin with your hands at shoulder height (*a*) and pull both cables until your hands end up in front of your lower abdomen (*b*).
4. Return to the starting position and repeat for reps.

Complete Workout

Barbell bench press (#54)
- 6 sets × 3 reps
- 2 minutes of rest

Incline dumbbell chest press (#210)
- 3 sets × 6 reps
- 90 seconds of rest

High-to-low cable fly
- 3 sets × 6 reps
- 90 seconds of rest

OPTIONS

Easy Option   Reduce to 4 sets of the barbell bench press.

Step It Up   Increase to 8 sets of the barbell bench press.

Cool-Down   Pec stretch, double lat stretch, 90-degree stretch.

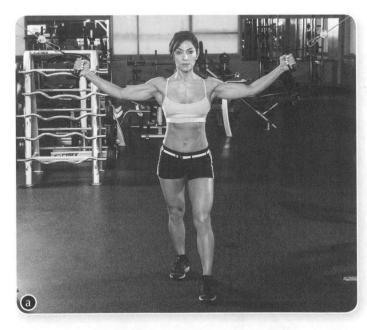

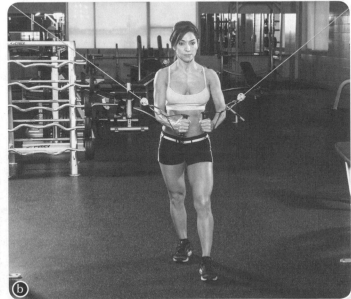

Total War

Determining your benchmarks in certain lifts or workouts is a great way to realize where you currently stand in your training, and it also lets you set performance goals that you can shoot for over a specific period. When it comes to strength gains, there may be no better benchmark than a "total," which is the combined weight of two or three lifts—usually ones you use very often in training. Rather than getting hung up on one lift, your total can still improve whether or not you hit a plateau in a certain exercise.

Warm-Up

4 reps per side of the world's greatest stretch, 6 reps per side of hip rocker and inverted hamstring stretch, 8 reps per side of shoulder sweeps

● **Featured Exercise**

Barbell Back Squat

1. Utilizing a shoulder-width stance, step under a bar in a squat rack, with the barbell resting on your upper traps. Take one step back with each foot (*a*).

2. Maintaining a neutral or slightly arched lower back, unlock your hips and begin bringing them back. Almost instantaneously, bend at your knees.

3. Keeping your entire foot on the ground, continue to lower yourself to as deep a level as possible (you want your hip crease to be at least below your knee) (*b*).

4. When you reach your full range of motion, forcefully drive your feet into the ground and stand up, returning to the starting position.

Complete Workout

Take 8 minutes in each lift to warm up and find your 1RM (you can find more information on finding your 1RM in chapter 1, Ramping Up). Once you do, add up all the lifts to determine your total.

A. Barbell back squat
   • 1 rep
B. Barbell overhead press (#36)
   • 1 rep
C. Conventional deadlift (#5)
   • 1 rep

⚠️ **Warning:** Finding multiple 1RMs in the same workout can be extremely demanding. Make sure you are very familiar with all of the movement patterns and ensure that you are using good technique on each rep.

OPTIONS

Easy Option   None.

Step It Up   None.

Cool-Down   Double lat stretch, cross-body stretch, hamstring stretch.

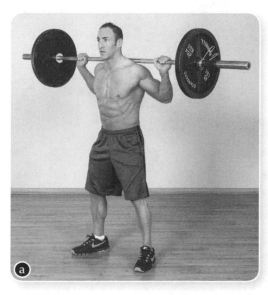

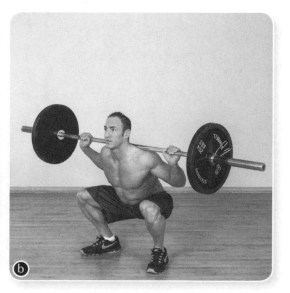

Bench Max

Correctly warming up for a maximal lift can mean the difference between just another heavy single and a personal record. Start with 50 percent of your projected 1RM, and perform 5 reps. Add weight to the bar, and perform a number of sets between 60 percent and 80 percent, getting 2 or 3 reps per set. Once you get to the 85 percent mark, start going for singles and keep working your way. Although this progression won't guarantee a new best lift, it will put you in a position to hit the biggest number possible for that day.

Warm-Up

5 reps of inchworm, 6 reps per side of quadruped T-spine rotation, 10 reps of cat–cow

Complete Workout

Take 12 minutes to find your 1RM in the barbell bench press, using as many sets and as much rest as you deem necessary. The goal is to hit the heaviest single possible for that day.

A. Barbell bench press (#54)
   - 12 minutes × as many sets as needed to find your 1RM

B. Triceps rope press down
   - 3 sets × 12 reps
   - 60 seconds of rest

● Featured Exercise

Triceps Rope Press Down

1. Attach a rope to a high pulley at a cable station. Grab the rope with a neutral grip (palms facing each other), lean forward slightly and unlock your knees.

2. Keeping your elbows locked in toward your rib cage, start with your arms approximately parallel to the floor (a).

3. Pull the rope down toward your lap and slightly out to the sides (b).

4. Return the rope to the start position. Be sure to not allow your upper arms to move forward.

5. Repeat for reps.

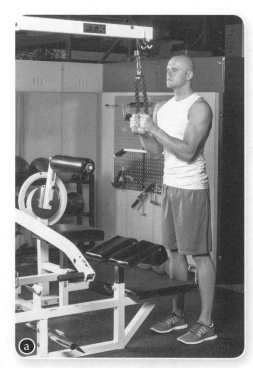
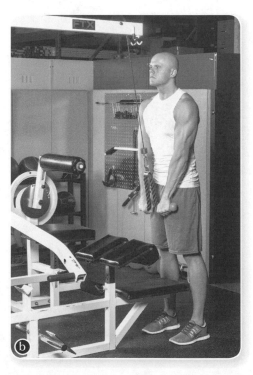

OPTIONS

Easy Option   Instead of working up to a heavy single, try to find your heaviest triple.

Step It Up   Once you establish your heaviest single, reduce the weight by 15 percent and perform a set of as many reps as possible.

Cool-Down   Double lat stretch, cross-body stretch, hamstring stretch.

Body-Weight Front Squat

There are several standards of fitness that everyone should strive to accomplish. One of the most valuable may be performing a front squat that is equal to your own body weight. In this workout, you'll have 5 sets in which your goal is to front squat your body weight as many times as possible. Remember that front squats are truly a total-body exercise, demanding a lot of stabilization of the abs, upper back, and lower back as well as strength from your quad, glutes, and calves. So even if your legs feel as if they have more in the tank, pay attention to the posture of your upper body during each set. If you find you can't maintain good form, end the set.

Warm-Up

6 reps of squat to stand, 6 reps per side of quadruped T-spine rotation, 8 reps of glute bridge, 10 reps of cat–cow

Complete Workout

Load a bar with your body weight for the front squat. Be sure to include several ramp-up sets before attempting the prescribed work sets.

A. Barbell front squat (#44)
- 5 sets × as many reps as possible
- 2 minutes of rest

B. TRX hamstring curl
- 3 sets × 12 reps
- 60 seconds of rest

Featured Exercise

TRX Hamstring Curl

1. Place your heels inside the stirrups of a TRX or other suspension trainer that is set to approximately 12 inches (30 cm) off the floor.
2. Lie on your back with your hands out to the sides, palms facing up (*a*).
3. Simultaneously lift your hips while pulling your heels toward your butt.
4. Once you have reached your full range of motion (*b*), return to the starting position and repeat for reps.

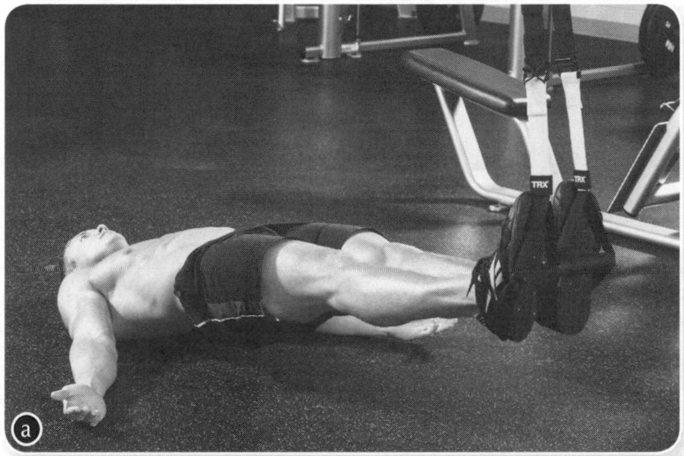

a

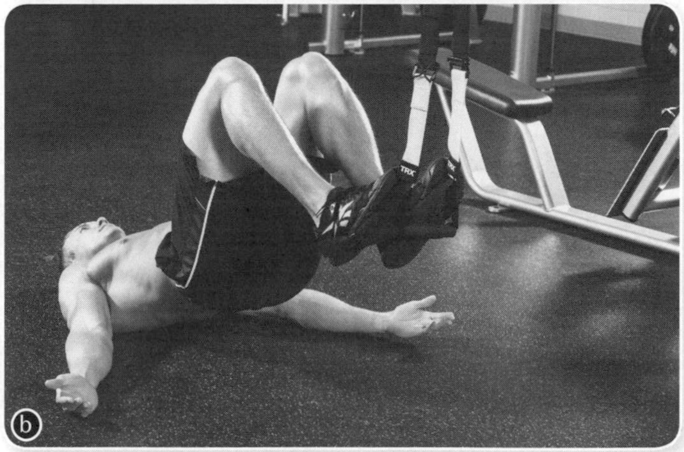

b

OPTIONS

Easy Option Use 50 percent of your body weight for the front squat.

Step It Up Use 125 percent of your body weight for the front squat.

Cool-Down Standing quad stretch, 90-degree stretch, double lat stretch.

Muscle Beach

The hang muscle snatch (featured in this workout) is great for developing the power, pulling ability, and shoulder stability critical for performing the full version of the snatch without as much need for mobility. Breaking down complex lifts such as the snatch into their components (snatch-grip deadlift, snatch pull, hang muscle snatch, overhead squat) is really an excellent way to develop the foundational components of the lift.

Warm-Up

5 reps of inchworm, 6 reps per side of quadruped T-spine rotation, 10 reps of cat–cow

● Featured Exercise

Hang Muscle Snatch

1. Place a barbell at the creases of your hips (about 2 to 3 inches [5 to 8 cm] below your navel), and grab it with a straight-arm snatch grip.
2. Keeping your torso tall and your weight on your heels, bend your knees 3 to 4 inches (8 to 10 cm) (do not bend at the hips).

3. From this point, bring your hips back until the bar is directly below your knees (a).
4. Keep the bar close to your legs as you return to the tall posture described at the beginning of step. Without pausing, explosively extend your knees and hips, shrug your traps, and allow the bar to travel overhead (b).
5. Catch the bar in a high position overhead, with your knees locked out (c).
6. Return the bar to the starting position and repeat for reps.

Complete Workout

A. Hang muscle snatch
- 5 sets × 3 reps
- 90 seconds of rest

B. Overhead squat (#167)
- 5 sets × 3 reps
- 75 seconds of rest

C. Face pull (#127)
- 5 sets × 8 reps
- 75 seconds of rest

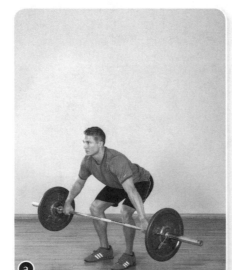

(a)

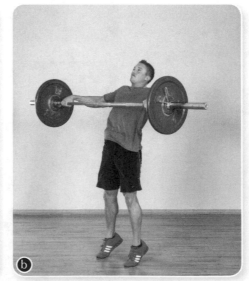

(b)

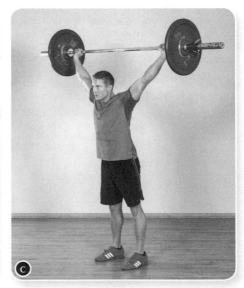

(c)

Perfect Pause

Pausing in the middle of any rep can be disadvantageous to building momentum and expressing strength. However, in the case of the Olympic lifts that rely on precise bar positioning, pauses can help you establish a good bar path, which will result in huge benefits when returning to the full (nonpaused) version of the lift. So be sure to add some paused lifts to your training, and watch your overall technique improve.

Warm-Up

5 reps of squat to stand; 6 reps per side of kneeling adductor stretch, hip rocker, and quadruped T-spine rotation

● Featured Exercise

Paused Clean

1. With a loaded barbell on the floor, grab the barbell with a clean grip, bend your knees, and pull your hips down toward the ground. Keep your chest up and eyes forward. Your shoulders should be even with or slightly behind the bar (a).

2. Keeping your chest tall, lift the bar toward your knees (your back angle should not change). Once the bar reaches just below your knees, pause for 2 seconds (b).

3. Drive your knees back and your hips forward to continue bringing the bar up toward your hips.

4. As the bar nears the top of your thighs, explosively drive your hips forward in an effort to drive the bar vertically (c).

5. Simultaneously shuffle your feet outward and whip your elbows around in order to catch the bar in the front rack position.

6. Pull yourself under the bar and catch it in the bottom of the front squat position, or complete a full front squat if you catch the bar higher (d).

7. Return the bar to the starting position, reset, and complete for reps.

Complete Workout

Paused clean
- 8 sets × 2 reps
- 2 minutes of rest

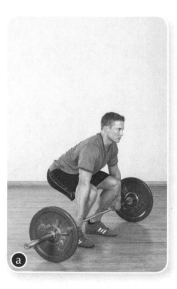
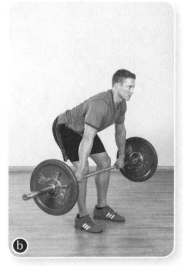
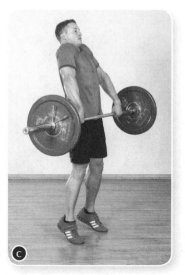
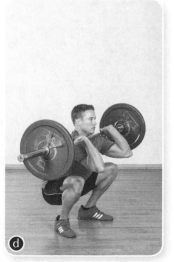

OPTIONS

Easy Option   Reduce to 6 sets total.

Step It Up   Increase the length of the pause to 3 seconds.

Cool-Down   Standing quad stretch, 90-degree stretch, cross-body stretch.

Crazy 8s: Push Press

Your shoulder joint is one of the most mobile in your body. And although this is very useful for accomplishing many tasks, it also makes it one of the body's most vulnerable joints. For the vast majority of movements that you perform in the gym, externally rotating at the shoulder joint will keep it in a safer position. You can do this in many ways, including rotating your armpits out during any variation of overhead pressing. This can be accomplished by thinking about bending the bar in the bench press and screwing your hands into the floor on the push-up.

Warm-Up

4 reps per side of the world's greatest stretch, 5 reps of inchworm, 8 reps per side of shoulder sweeps

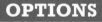 **Featured Exercise**

Shoulder Sweep

1. Lie on your back on the floor, bend your left knee to 90 degrees, and cross it over your right leg, keeping your entire upper body in contact with the floor (if you cannot reach the floor with your left knee, place a medicine ball or yoga block underneath it to limit the range of motion).

2. Place your left hand on your right knee to keep it in contact with the floor. Extend your right arm directly overhead (a).

3. Sweep your right arm along the floor, attempting to internally rotate at the shoulder to bring your hand toward your middle back (b).

4. When you've reached the end of the range of motion (c), sweep your arm (trying to keep as much of it in contact with the floor as possible) toward your right ear.

5. Continue to sweep back and forth to these end positions until you complete all reps for one side before repeating the process for the other side.

Complete Workout

A1. Push press (#16)
- 8 sets × 2 reps
- 60 seconds of rest

A2. Shoulder sweep
- 8 sets × 4 reps/side
- 60 seconds of rest

OPTIONS

Easy Option Perform 6 sets of the exercises.

Step It Up Perform 10 sets of the exercises.

Cool-Down Pec stretch, double lat stretch, 90-degree stretch.

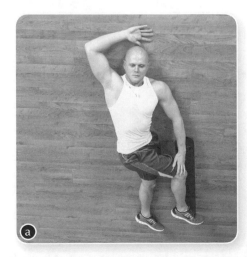
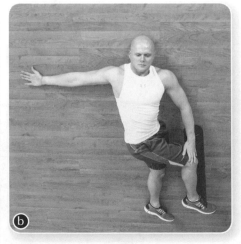
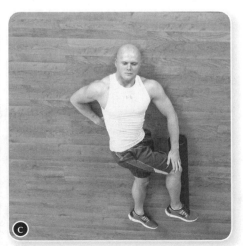

Row and Go

To get the most out of your rowing movements, do your best to keep your shoulders away from your ears. Given that so many people spend their days with their upper backs rounded and shoulders hunched, this may be easier said than done. By keeping your shoulder blades depressed and retracted, you'll be utilizing the often underdeveloped muscles of the upper and midback as opposed to the over-used upper traps and subscapularis. It may be hard to get the hang of it at first, and you may need to use a bit less weight, but in the long run this postural correction will be worth your while.

Warm-Up

4 reps per side of the world's greatest stretch, 5 reps of inchworm, 8 reps per side of shoulder sweeps

● Featured Exercise

Underhand-Grip Seated Cable Row

1. Attach a straight bar or handles to the cable at a seated row machine. Grab the handles with a double underhand grip. Brace your feet against the support, with your knees slightly bent, shoulder blades down, and chest tall (a).
2. Pull the bar to your sternum, making sure not to extend at the hips.
3. Pause at the end position (b), and contract your lats before returning the bar to the starting position (do not flex at the hips when returning the bar). Repeat for reps.

Complete Workout

A. Conventional deadlift (#5)
- 4 sets × 4 reps
- 90 seconds of rest

B1. Wide-grip pull-up (#117)
- 3 sets × 10 reps
- 45 seconds of rest

B2. Underhand-grip seated cable row
- 3 sets × 10 reps
- 45 seconds of rest

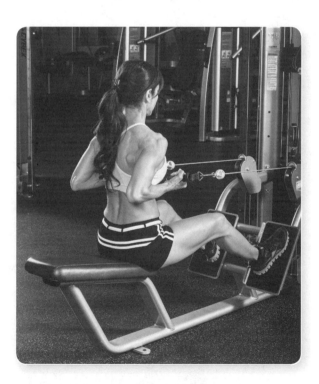

OPTIONS

Easy Option   Perform 2 sets of the wide-grip pull-up and under-hand-grip seated cable row.

Step It Up   Add 2 reps to each set of the wide-grip pull-up.

Cool-Down   Pec stretch, double lat stretch, 90-degree stretch.

Fade to Black

In our desire to make training sessions more difficult or challenging, we often rely on the tried and true methods of either adding weight to the bar or reps to the set. But there are other methods of increasing the difficulty of any given exercise, including taking advantage of mechanical disadvantages such as bar placement or grip and inserting pauses at different phases of the lift. The snatch-grip deadlift uses a wide hand placement, making the lift much more challenging.

Warm-Up

4 reps per side of the world's greatest stretch, 5 reps each of inchworm and inverted hamstring stretch, 10 reps of glute bridge

Featured Exercise

Glute–Ham Raise

1. Set up a glute–ham machine so your thighs are against the front pads, your feet are flat against the back platform, and your shins are parallel to the floor.

2. Begin with your legs straight and your upper body bent forward at the hip (a).

3. Forcefully drive your thighs into the pad and use your glutes and hamstrings to lift your torso beyond parallel.

4. You should end with your shoulders directly over your hips (b).

5. Lower yourself to the start position and repeat for reps.

Complete Workout

A. Snatch-grip deadlift (#60)
- 6 sets × 3 reps
- 2 minutes of rest

B1. Seated cable face pull (#251)
- 3 sets × 8 reps
- 90 seconds of rest

B2. Glute–ham raise
- 3 sets × 8 reps
- 90 seconds of rest

 Warning: Performing any movement with a snatch grip from the floor requires an increased need for mobility. If you perform these movements without proper spinal alignment, you put yourself at risk for injury. Be sure you can maintain a neutral spine position before attempting this or any other snatch-grip movement from the floor.

OPTIONS

Easy Option   Reduce to 4 sets of the snatch-grip deadlift.

Step It Up   Add an additional set to the seated cable face pull.

Cool-Down   Double lat stretch, hamstring stretch, calf stretch.

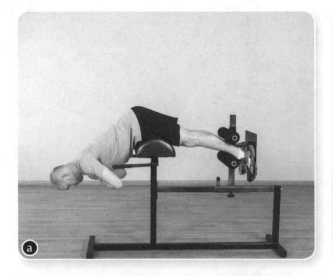
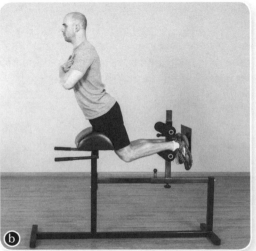

Pressed for Time

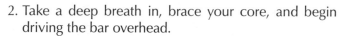

Your lungs can't tell if you are running on a treadmill or lifting a barbell. All they know is that when you exercise with intensity, they need to work harder to supply more oxygen to your system. Don't be fooled into thinking that cardio has to be performed on a treadmill, rowing machine, or stair climber. Working with weights at an intensity that drives up your heart rate is just as beneficial to your cardiorespiratory system as any running program.

Warm-Up

5 reps of inchworm, 6 reps per side of quadruped T-spine rotation, 10 reps of cat–cow

● Featured Exercise

Barbell Overhead Press

1. Grab a loaded bar just outside shoulder width at collarbone height. The bar should be resting on top of your anterior deltoids (front of your shoulders) (*a*).

2. Take a deep breath in, brace your core, and begin driving the bar overhead.

3. As the bar passes over the top of your head, drive your body slightly forward so the bar is over the center of your foot (do not, however, jut your chin out or extend your neck).

4. Continue to press the bar overhead until you have achieved full lockout (*b*). Return the bar to the starting position and repeat for reps.

Complete Workout

Take 12 minutes to find your 1RM in the barbell overhead press, using as many sets and as much rest as you deem necessary. The goal is to hit the heaviest single possible for that day.

Barbell overhead press

- 12 minutes × as many sets as needed to find your 1RM

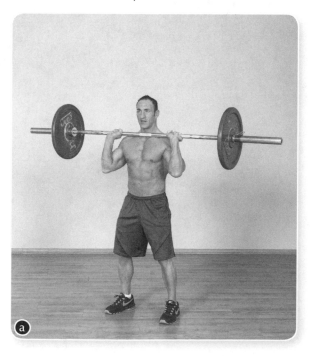

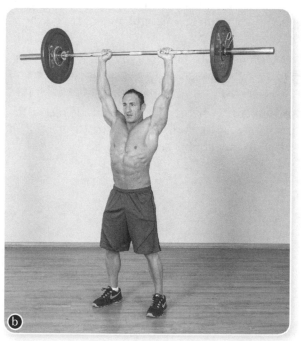

OPTIONS

Easy Option   Instead of working up to a heavy single, try to find your heaviest triple.

Step It Up   Once you establish your heaviest single, reduce the weight by 15 percent and perform a set of as many reps as possible.

Cool-Down   Double lat stretch, cross-body stretch, hamstring stretch.

Crazy 8s: Front Squat

Doubles (sets of 2 reps) may be one of the most overlooked yet beneficial protocols when it comes to developing strength. You can utilize nearly your 1RM (or approximately 95 percent) without the risk factors of lifting your true max. Plus you'll often achieve better range of motion on the second repetition because your nervous and muscular systems tend to be more accepting of the weight after you perform the first rep. This workout uses 8 sets of 2 with an active recovery movement between sets to facilitate mobility.

Warm-Up

5 reps of squat to stand; 6 reps per side of kneeling adductor stretch, hip rocker, and quadruped T-spine rotation

Featured Exercise

Pillar Bridge March

1. Assume a plank position, with your elbows directly under your shoulders, your forearms flat on the floor, and your body forming a straight line from your head to your heels (a).

2. Without rotating your hips, lift your right arm off the floor and press it straight out so your biceps is next to your ear and your arm is parallel to the floor (b).

3. Return your arm to the starting position, and repeat the process with your left arm (c). Continue to alternate in this manner until all reps are complete.

OPTIONS

Easy Option   Perform 6 sets of the exercises.

Step It Up   Perform 10 sets of the exercises.

Cool-Down   Standing quad stretch, 90-degree stretch, cross-body stretch.

Complete Workout

Barbell front squat (#44)
- 8 sets × 2 reps

Pillar bridge march
- 8 sets × 8 reps per side

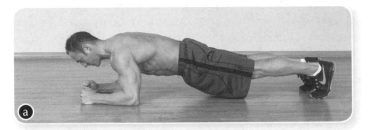

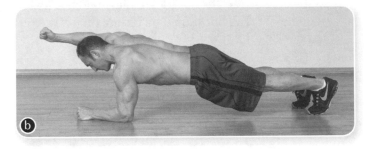

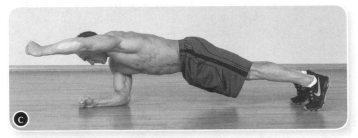

Minute on the Minute: Chin-Up

One of the key mistakes in chin-up technique is arming-up the rep, meaning you leave your back disengaged and loose, forcing your arms to do all the work of getting your chin above the bar. There are two reasons to avoid this misstep: (1) Performing the reps in this way completely removes one of the key benefits of chin-ups—building a bigger, stronger back. (2) Using your smaller arm muscles as opposed to your bigger back muscles almost guarantees you'll fatigue much faster. Be sure to depress your shoulder blades and focus on pulling with your mid- and upper back during your chin-ups. You may have a few more reps in the tank than you'd expect.

Warm-Up

5 reps of inchworm, 6 reps per side of quadruped T-spine rotation, 10 reps of cat–cow

● Featured Exercise

Chin-Up

1. Grab a pull-up bar with a supinated grip (palms facing you) at shoulder width.
2. Start in a dead hang (your arms should be straight) (*a*), and begin the movement by depressing your shoulder blades.
3. Drive your elbows down and behind you, bending at the elbows in order to pull your chest up toward the bar.
4. Once your chin clears the bar (*b*), return to the starting position under control. Repeat for reps.

Complete Workout

Perform 3 reps of a chin-up at the top of every minute for 20 minutes. If you can no longer complete 3 reps within that minute, end the workout. Use additional load if needed.

Chin-up
- As many sets as possible, as described

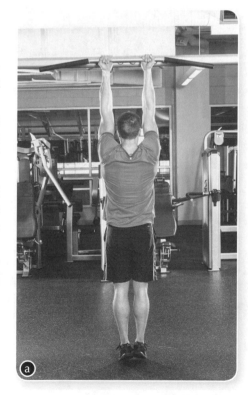
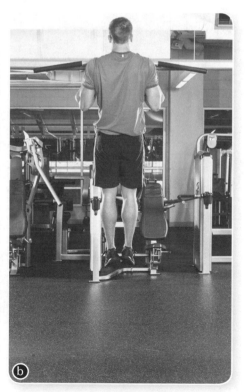

(a)   (b)

OPTIONS

Easy Option   Perform 2 reps of the chin-up each minute.

Step It Up   Perform 5 reps of the chin-up each minute.

Cool-Down   Double lat stretch, cross-body stretch, hamstring stretch.

12 Minutes to Dead

Taking a specific amount of time to work up to your heaviest single rep does several things. First, it forces you to be strategic because you have only a limited number of sets you'll be able to perform in this time frame. Second, it demands that you stay focused because there is no time for daydreaming or people watching around the gym. Last, it adds a conditioning component to a strength workout because you will likely not be fully recovered before stepping up to the bar for the next set.

Warm-Up

4 reps per side of the world's greatest stretch, 5 reps each of inchworm and inverted hamstring stretch, 10 reps of glute bridge

● Featured Exercise

Conventional Deadlift

1. Approach a barbell set up on the floor by placing your feet under the bar until it is 2 to 3 inches (5 to 8 cm) in front of your shins. Your stance should be approximately hip width.

2. Bend down and grab the bar just outside your legs with either a double overhand or mixed grip.

3. Pull your hips down and bring your shins in contact with the bar. Keep your chest tall and maintain a neutral spine (a).

4. Stand up by raising simultaneously at your hips and shoulders, driving your hips forward until you reach lockout (b).

Complete Workout

Take 12 minutes to find your 1RM in the conventional deadlift, using as many sets and as much rest as you deem necessary. The goal is to hit the heaviest single possible for that day.

Conventional deadlift
- 12 minutes × as many sets as needed to find your 1RM

OPTIONS

Easy Option   Instead of working up to a heavy single, try to find your heaviest triple.

Step It Up   Once you establish your heaviest single, reduce the weight by 15 percent and perform a set of as many reps as possible.

Cool-Down   Double lat stretch, hamstring stretch, calf stretch.

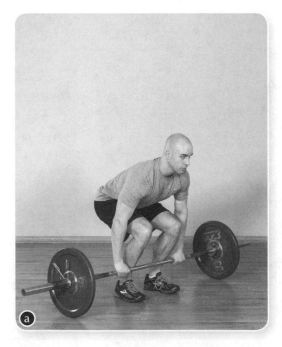
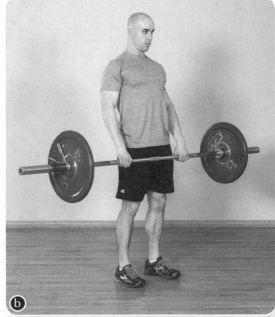

Body-Weight Bench

There are several standards of fitness that everyone should strive to accomplish. One such standard is being able to bench press your own body weight. This workout gives you five opportunities to bench press your body weight as many times as possible. As with any workout that either has you lifting close to your 1RM or has you performing as many reps as possible, it is highly recommended that you use a spotter.

Warm-Up

4 reps per side of the world's greatest stretch, 5 reps of inchworm, 8 reps per side of shoulder sweeps

Complete Workout

Load a bar with your body weight for the bench press. Be sure to include several ramp-up sets before attempting the prescribed work sets.

A1. Barbell bench press (#54)
- 5 sets × as many reps as possible
- 2 minutes of rest

A2. TRX Y
- 3 sets × 12 reps
- 60 seconds of rest

● Featured Exercise

TRX Y

1. Grab the handles of a TRX or other suspension trainer, and step away from the anchor point until you remove the slack from the straps.

2. Begin with your arms straight in front of you at shoulder height. Your front foot should be closer to the anchor point than to your head (*a*).

3. Keeping a straight line from shoulder to heel and your arms straight, pull your arms back and overhead. Your body should form a Y shape at the top of the movement (*b*).

4. Lower yourself back to the starting position under control. Repeat for reps.

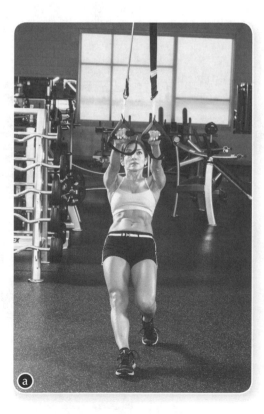
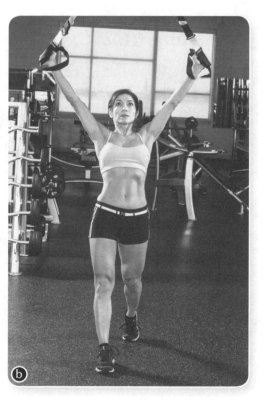

OPTIONS

Easy Option Use 75 percent of your body weight for the barbell bench press.

Step It Up Use 125 percent of your body weight for the barbell bench press.

Cool-Down Pec stretch, double lat stretch, 90-degree stretch.

Two Times Dead

There are several standards of fitness that everyone should strive to accomplish. One such standard is being able to deadlift two times your own body weight. This workout gives you five opportunities to deadlift twice your body weight as many times as possible. Although this workout certainly demands that you push your limits of strength, keep in mind that deadlifts are very demanding and can have negative physical consequences once form breaks down. Therefore, go for another rep only if you believe you can keep integrity on the technique.

Warm-Up

4 reps per side of the world's greatest stretch, 5 reps each of inchworm and inverted hamstring stretch, 10 reps of glute bridge

Featured Exercise

TRX Hamstring Curl

1. Set up a TRX or other suspension trainer so that the handles are 12 to 16 inches (30 to 40 cm) above the ground.

2. Place the heels of your feet in the stirrups, and lift your hips until you are forming a straight line from your heels to your shoulders (a).

3. Pull your heels toward your glutes while simultaneously driving your hips up.

4. Once you have reached your end range of motion (b), reverse back to the starting position. Keep in mind that the farther you set up from the anchor point, the more challenging the exercise.

Complete Workout

Load a bar with twice your body weight for the conventional deadlift.

A. Conventional deadlift (#5)
- 5 sets × as many reps as possible
- 2 minutes of rest

B. TRX hamstring curl
- 3 sets × 12 reps
- 60 seconds of rest

 Warning: The deadlift is a very demanding exercise that can put you at risk for injury if done with bad form. End each set when you can no longer perform the reps with correct technique.

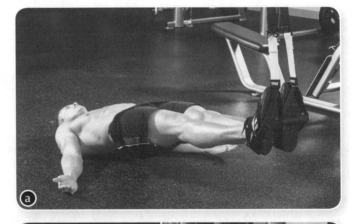

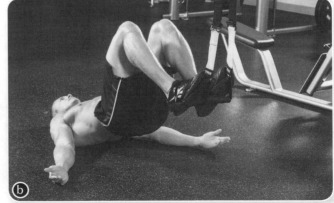

OPTIONS

Easy Option Use 100 percent of your body weight for the conventional deadlift.

Step It Up Use 225 percent of your body weight for the conventional deadlift.

Cool-Down Double lat stretch, hamstring stretch, calf stretch.

Front Squat Max

Sometimes you just want to know how much weight you can manage in any given exercise. The set and rep protocol in front squat max will get you to that maximal load safely but before you burn out from doing a bunch of warm-up sets. The goal is to increase weight used on all the singles of the front squat, hitting your max by the last set.

Warm-Up

5 reps of squat to stand; 6 reps per side of kneeling adductor stretch, hip rocker, and quadruped T-spine rotation

● **Featured Exercise**

Single-Leg Press

1. Begin with your butt firmly in the seat of a leg press machine. Maintain a slight arch (as you would during a squat) in your low back throughout the set.
2. Place your right foot flat near or at the center of the platform. Given that this is a single-leg variation, you should keep your foot closer to the center than you would in the standard bilateral leg press.
3. Unlock the leg press, and bring your knee toward your shoulder, trying to achieve a full range of motion (a).

4. Drive through your entire foot to press the platform back to its original starting position (b). Try to keep your knee just short of lockout in order to maintain tension in your quads. Repeat all reps for one leg before switching to the other.

Complete Workout

Increase the weight used on each set of the front squat until you reach your maximum weight.

A. Barbell front squat (#44)
- 5 sets × 5, 3, 1, 1, 1 reps
- 90 seconds of rest

B1. Dumbbell Romanian deadlift (#267)
- 2 sets × 10 reps
- 60 seconds of rest

B2. Single-leg press
- 2 sets × 10 reps (5 per leg)
- 60 seconds of rest

B3. Leg press calf raise (#136)
- 2 sets × 10 reps
- 60 seconds of rest

OPTIONS

Easy Option Eliminate one of the singles on the front squat.

Step It Up Perform two additional singles with your heaviest weight on the front squat.

Cool-Down Standing quad stretch, 90-degree stretch, cross-body stretch.

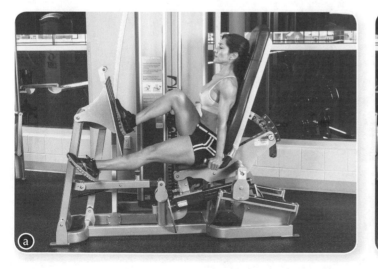

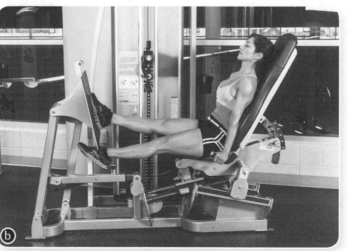

Recondo

Training multiple strength qualities at once (strength, endurance, power) is a great way to gain an overall competency and a solid fitness base. However, if your goal is more specific (get stronger, get bigger, become a great Olympic lifter), your time is much better spent practicing and perfecting those movement patterns and developing those qualities. Putting significant time and effort into one specific goal will certainly make sure you are optimally progressing toward that goal.

Warm-Up

6 reps of squat to stand, 6 reps per side of quadruped T-spine rotation, 8 reps of glute bridge, 10 reps of cat–cow

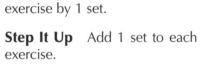 **Featured Exercise**

Snatch Balance

1. Place a barbell across your upper traps (as in the beginning of a back squat), and grab the bar with the same grip you would use for a snatch (a).

2. Keep your chest tall, quickly flex your knees, and drop under the bar as you explosively extend your arms (the goal is to hit the bottom position of the overhead squat as you simultaneously lock the bar out overhead) (b-c).

3. Stand up and carefully lower the bar back to the starting position (when you catch the bar on your traps, flex your knees to help you safely receive the bar). Repeat for reps.

Complete Workout

A. Snatch balance
- 4 sets × 2 reps
- 90 seconds of rest

B1. Neutral-grip pull-up* (#237)
- 3 sets × 4 reps
- 60 seconds of rest

B2. Trap bar deadlift (#8)
- 3 sets × 6 reps
- 60 seconds of rest

C. Rower (#212)
- 1 set × 200 meters

*Add weight if needed

OPTIONS

Easy Option Reduce each exercise by 1 set.

Step It Up Add 1 set to each exercise.

Cool-Down Standing quad stretch, 90-degree stretch, double lat stretch.

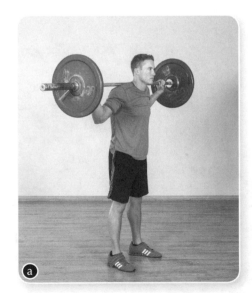
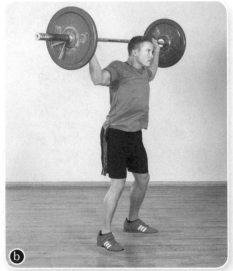
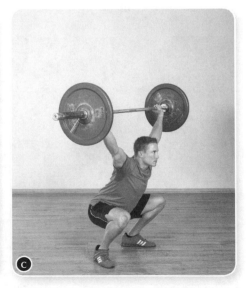

Minute on the Minute: Clean and Push Press

Combination lifts (such as the barbell clean and push press featured in this workout), which combine two separate lifts into one movement, can be a very challenging yet efficient technique to add to your training. Most combo lifts use a large amount of muscle mass, making them metabolically demanding while allowing you to strength-train multiple muscle groups at the same time.

Warm-Up

4 reps per side of the world's greatest stretch, 5 reps of inchworm, 8 reps per side of shoulder sweeps

● Featured Exercise

Barbell Clean and Push Press

1. Start by holding the barbell with an overhand grip, placing your hands and feet slightly wider than shoulder-width apart. The bar should be on the floor directly over your midfoot (a).

2. With a flat back and your chest tall, lift the bar until it reaches your midthighs. Transition by explosively jumping upward, extending your body into triple extension—extending at the ankles, knees, and hips (b).

3. Aggressively pull your body under the bar, rotating your elbows around the bar. Catch the bar on your shoulders (c) while moving into a squat position.

4. Upon hitting the bottom of your squat, stand up immediately. Flex at the knees and, using leg drive, press the bar directly overhead (d).

5. Bring the bar back to your shoulders then return to the floor (or, if you are in a gym that's friendly to Olympic lifting, drop the weight from overhead to the floor).

Complete Workout

Perform 3 reps of the barbell clean to push press at the top of every minute for 20 minutes. If you can no longer complete 3 reps within that minute, end the workout.

Barbell clean and push press
- As many sets as possible, as described

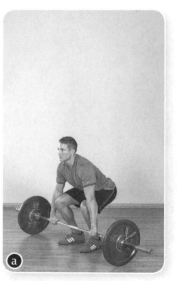 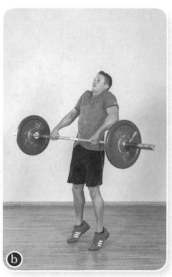 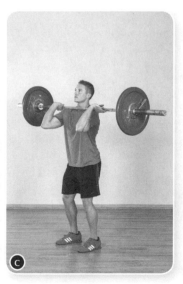 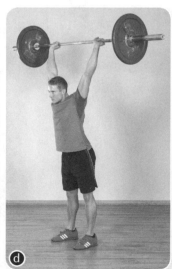

OPTIONS

Easy Option Perform 2 reps of the barbell clean to push press each minute.

Step It Up Perform 5 reps of the barbell clean to push press each minute.

Cool-Down Pec stretch, double lat stretch, 90-degree stretch.

Rack 'Em

A great way to get stronger is to perform lifts in a partial range of motion (ROM). This allows you to use more weight than you would in a full ROM lift and should carry over to more strength when you return to the full ROM movement.

Warm-Up

4 reps per side of the world's greatest stretch, 5 reps each of inchworm and inverted hamstring stretch, 10 reps of glute bridge

● Featured Exercise

Rack Pull

1. Set the safety bars in a squat rack to just above knee height, and place a barbell across the bars.

2. Bending your knees slightly, bring your hips back and grab the barbell with either a mixed (over and under) or overhand grip. Your thighs (just above your knees) should be against the bar (a).

3. Tighten your abs and legs, retract your shoulder blades, keep your arms straight, and lift the bar directly up so it stays in contact with your legs until you are completely upright (b).

4. Return to the starting position and repeat for reps.

Complete Workout

Perform all sets of the rack pull using 90 to 110 percent of your usual deadlift weight.

A. Rack pull
- 5 sets × 3 reps
- 2 minutes of rest

B1. Lying hamstring curl (#168)
- 4 sets × 6 reps

B2. Barbell walking lunge (#112)
- 4 sets × 6 reps/side
- 75 seconds of rest

OPTIONS

Easy Option   Perform 3 sets of the lying hamstring curl and barbell walking lunge.

Step It Up   Work up to 130 percent+ of your deadlift max for the rack pulls.

Cool-Down   Double lat stretch, hamstring stretch, calf stretch.

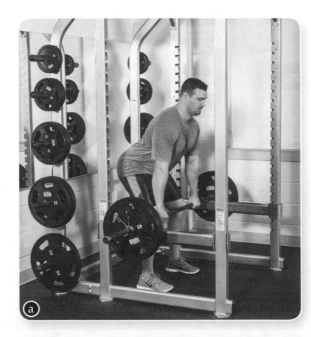
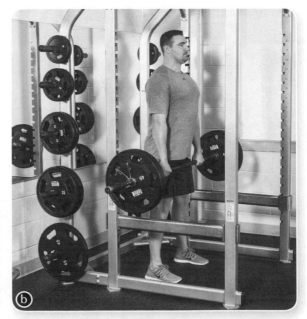

The Military

Performing an explosive or speed exercise directly before performing a strength exercise that uses a similar movement pattern may allow you to actually lift more weight than usual in the second movement. This is referred to as neural potentiation, which, in a nutshell, is a way to fire up your central nervous system (via the explosive lift) so it is more optimally prepared for the heavier load to come.

Warm-Up

4 reps per side of the world's greatest stretch, 5 reps of inchworm, 8 reps per side of shoulder sweeps

● Featured Exercise

Push Jerk

1. Begin in a standing position, feet at hip width, with a barbell directly in front of your collarbones. Hands should be just outside shoulders.

2. Bend your knees slightly (*a*), and utilize your legs to explosively drive the bar overhead.

3. Catch the bar in the top position with slightly bent knees (*b*) before standing up to complete lockout.

4. Lower the barbell back to its original position and repeat for reps.

Complete Workout

Perform 6 rounds of the following exercise pairing. Be sure to perform the push jerk explosively with 60 to 70 percent of the weight you will be using for the barbell overhead press.

Push jerk
- 3 reps
- 30 seconds of rest

Barbell overhead press (#36)
- 8 reps
- 2 minutes of rest

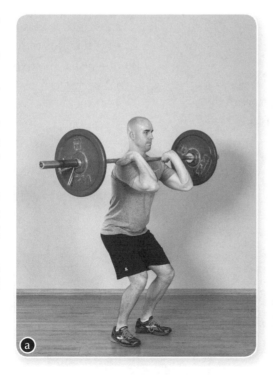

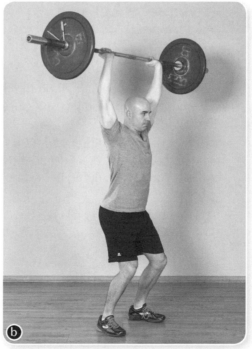

OPTIONS

Easy Option   Reduce the push jerk to 50 percent of your barbell overhead press weight.

Step It Up   Perform 8 rounds of the pairing.

Cool-Down   Pec stretch, double lat stretch, 90-degree stretch.

The Sumo

Sumo deadlifts (featured in this workout) differ from conventional deadlifts in several key areas. First, the sumo uses a much wider stance, with toes pointed outward. Sumos also utilize an arms-inside-of-knees position. Both these differences in setup allow the sumo deadlifter a much taller posture at the start of the lift. The sumo also utilizes the quads and adductors to a greater degree than the conventional, which focuses more on glutes, hamstrings, and upper back. The verdict: It's beneficial to use both types of deadlifts in your training program for overall leg development and strength.

Warm-Up

4 reps per side of the world's greatest stretch, 5 reps each of inchworm and inverted hamstring stretch, 10 reps of glute bridge

● Featured Exercise

Sumo Deadlift

1. Step up to a loaded barbell on the floor with an outside-shoulder-width stance and toes pointing out at 45 degrees.
2. Reach down with either a double overhand or mixed grip and grab the barbell. Your arms should be inside your knees.
3. Bend at the knees and pull your hips down toward the floor (a).

4. Drive your feet into the ground, keep your arms locked, and drive your hips forward until you've reached a standing position (b).
5. Reverse the motion, bringing your hips back and bending at the knees. Bring the bar to a complete stop on the floor before attempting additional reps.

Complete Workout

A. Sumo deadlift
- 5 sets × 4 reps
- 2 minutes of rest

B1. Lying hamstring curl (#168)
- 2 sets × 8 reps
- 60 seconds of rest

B2. Alternating step-back lunge (#24)
- 2 sets × 8 reps/side
- 60 seconds of rest

B3. Reverse hyperextension (#263)
- 2 sets × 8 reps
- 60 seconds of rest

OPTIONS

Easy Option   Perform 4 sets of the sumo deadlift.

Step It Up   Perform 3 sets of the B exercises.

Cool-Down   Double lat stretch, hamstring stretch, calf stretch.

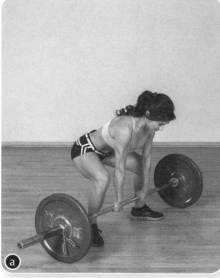
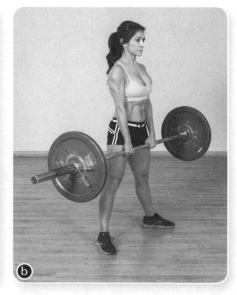

Clean Complex

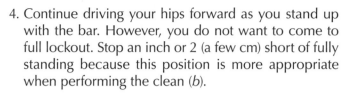

Performing several partial phases of an Olympic lift will certainly lead to greater fatigue than simply performing the full lift for a single rep. However, using this technique can force you to be more technically efficient in your cleans and snatches because you can't get away with muscling-up the bar and other flaws when you are already a bit fatigued. Feel free to use submaximal weights in these types of workouts to really focus on improving technical efficiency. This will lead to bigger numbers the next time you perform the full lift.

Warm-Up

5 reps of squat to stand; 6 reps per side of kneeling adductor stretch, hip rocker, and quadruped T-spine rotation

Featured Exercise

Clean Deadlift

1. With your feet at hip width, grab a barbell with a double overhand grip just outside shoulder width.

2. Pull your hips down toward the floor, keeping your chest tall, shoulders just in front of the bar, and eyes forward (*a*).

3. Keep your entire foot on the ground and lift the bar, keeping it close to your body. Your hips and shoulders should rise at the same time.

4. Continue driving your hips forward as you stand up with the bar. However, you do not want to come to full lockout. Stop an inch or 2 (a few cm) short of fully standing because this position is more appropriate when performing the clean (*b*).

Complete Workout

The following four movements are meant to be done as a complex—back to back with no rest in between. Once you have completed one round of the complex, rest 90 seconds and repeat for 8 total rounds. Increase the load each set until you've achieved the maximum you can use.

Clean deadlift
- 1 rep

Power clean (#52)
- 1 rep

Hang clean (#15)
- 1 rep

Split jerk (#17)
- 1 rep
- 90 seconds of rest

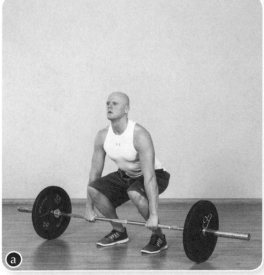

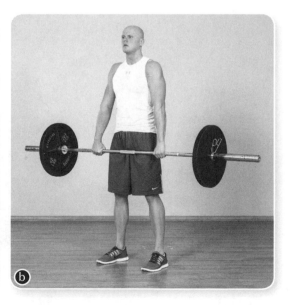

OPTIONS

Easy Option   Perform 6 sets of the complex.

Step It Up   Perform 2 rounds of the complex before resting.

Cool-Down   Standing quad stretch, 90-degree stretch, cross-body stretch.

The Third World

When it comes to Olympic weightlifting, one of the most challenging aspects can be the third pull—the ability to finish with your hips and, seemingly instantaneously, pull yourself under to receive the barbell in a low position. The complex featured in this workout is designed to help you drill this bottom position. As noted several times in this book, weightlifting is a complex sport unto itself. If you are just starting out, seek a qualified coach to help you with technique.

Warm-Up

5 reps of inchworm, 6 reps per side of quadruped T-spine rotation, 10 reps of cat–cow

Featured Exercise

Snatch

1. Begin with the barbell on the floor. Grab the barbell with a double overhand snatch grip. Bring your hips down, keeping your chest tall and your shoulders in line with the bar (a).

2. Keeping your chest tall, push your knees back and lift your hips, bringing the bar up toward the knees (b).
3. Once the bar has passed your knees and reached midthigh, begin dropping your hips.
4. As the bar continues to travel upward, explosively extend at your hips and knees (c), sending the bar directly overhead.
5. As the bar travels overhead, aggressively pull your body under the bar, catching it in a full overhead squat (d).
6. Stand with the bar overhead to complete the rep.

Complete Workout

Perform this series of exercises as a complex, transitioning from one movement to the next. Complete 6 total complexes.

Snatch
- 1 rep

Overhead squat (#167)
- 2 reps

Snatch balance (#78)
- 1 rep

OPTIONS

Easy Option Perform 1 rep per set of the overhead squat.

Step It Up Perform 2 reps of the snatch.

Cool-Down Double lat stretch, cross-body stretch, hamstring stretch.

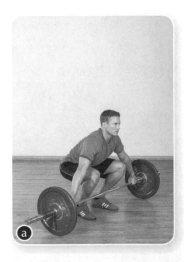 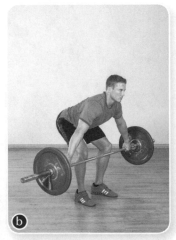 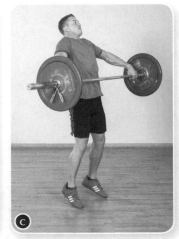 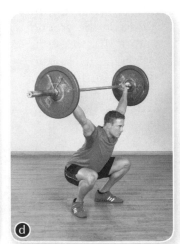

The Reaper

The Grim Reaper is often referred to simply as Death. He sneaks up on you, taps you on the shoulder, and lets you know your time is up. And although you may not see a shadowy figure in a cloak holding a staff while performing this workout, you might feel his presence as you push the limits of your strength. This one may look easy on paper, but you've been warned. Perform all sets of the barbell overhead press, increasing the load used while decreasing the reps per sets as described.

Warm-Up

4 reps per side of the world's greatest stretch, 5 reps each of inchworm and inverted hamstring stretch, 10 reps of glute bridge

Featured Exercise

Barbell Overhead Press

1. Grab a loaded bar just outside shoulder width at collarbone height. The bar should be resting on top of your anterior deltoids (front of your shoulders) (*a*).

2. Take a deep breath in, brace your core, and begin driving the bar overhead.

3. As the bar passes over the top of your head, drive your body slightly forward so the bar is over the center of your foot (do not, however, jut your chin out or extend your neck).

4. Continue to press the bar overhead until you have achieved full lockout (*b*). Return the bar to the starting position and repeat for reps.

Complete Workout

Perform all sets, increasing the load used while decreasing the reps/distance per set as described.

Barbell overhead press
- 5 sets × 10, 8, 6, 4, 2 reps
- 60 seconds of rest

Farmer's walk (#187)
- 5 sets × 60 yards (60 m), 50 yards (50 m), 40 yards (40 m), 30 yards (30 m), 20 yards (20 m)
- 60 seconds of rest

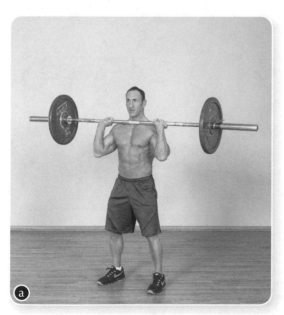

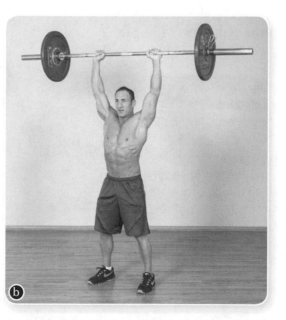

OPTIONS

Easy Option Reduce the number of farmer's walks to 3 sets (40 yards [40 m], 30 yards [30 m], and 20 yards [20 m]).

Step It Up Increase the length of the farmer's walks to 80 yards (80 m), 70 yards (70 m), 60 yards (60 m), 50 yards (50 m), and 40 yards (40 m).

Cool-Down Double lat stretch, hamstring stretch, calf stretch.

Absolute Deadlift

Training the strength quality known as *absolute strength* requires low reps and high loads and has the greatest carry over to improving your one repetition maximum (1RM). If getting stronger is a priority to you, much of your training should involve absolute strength rather than getting dominated by the more typical high-rep training schemes.

Warm-Up

Perform 4 reps per side of world's greatest stretch, 5 reps each of inchworm and inverted hamstring stretch, 10 reps of glute bridge

● Featured Exercise

Conventional Deadlift

1. Approach a barbell set up on the floor by placing your feet under the bar until it is 2 to 3 inches in front of your shins. Your stance should be approximately hip width.

2. Bend down and grab the bar just outside your legs with either a double overhand or mixed grip.

3. Pull your hips down and bring your shins in contact with the bar (*a*). Keep your chest tall and maintain a neutral spine.

4. Stand up by raising simultaneously at your hips and shoulder, driving your hips forward until your reach lock out (*b*).

Complete Workout

Perform all sets and reps for exercise A before moving on to the superset of B1 and B2, resting between sets as prescribed below

A. Conventional deadlift
  - 6 sets × 3 reps
  - 2 minutes of rest

B1. Lying hamstring curl (#168)
  - 3 sets × 6 reps
  - 90 seconds of rest

B2. Glute–ham raise (#70)
  - 3 sets × 6 reps
  - 90 seconds of rest

OPTIONS

Easy Option   Reduce to 4 sets of the deadlift.

Step It Up   Increase to 8 sets of the deadlift.

Cool-Down   Double lat stretch, hamstring stretch, calf stretch.

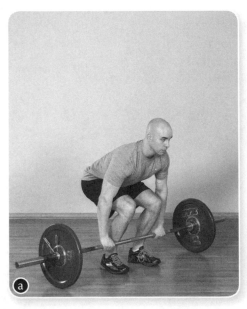

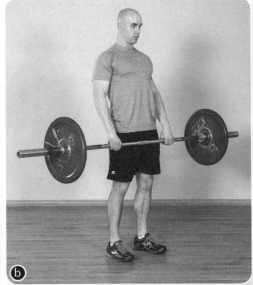

Insurance

Supplementation is a fantastic way to provide your body with nutrition insurance. Taking certain supplements will ensure you are getting vitamins, minerals, and other micronutrients of which you may have a deficiency. However, supplementation is not a replacement for a solid nutrition plan, so make sure you have that in place first. Also, it's better to focus on the supplements that benefit health such as vitamin D, omega 3s, zinc, and magnesium over supposed performance enhancers or hormone boosters. Prioritizing the health of your system is a great way to ensure your ability to perform and maintain good body composition.

Warm-Up

6 reps of squat to stand, 6 reps per side of quadruped T-spine rotation, 8 reps of glute bridge, 10 reps of cat–cow

● Featured Exercise

Snatch-Grip Barbell Back Extension

1. Load a barbell and place it in front of the back extension station. Step into the back extension machine, and grab the bar with a snatch grip (outside shoulder width) (a).

2. Keeping your back flat, extend at your hips until you are creating a straight line from head to heels (b). Be sure to contract your glutes and hamstrings in the top position (this will take stress off your lower back).

3. Slowly lower by flexing at the hips until the bar is just above the floor. Repeat for reps.

Complete Workout

A. Hang clean (#15)
- 4 sets × 4 reps
- 90 seconds of rest

B1. Goblet squat (#2)
- 2 sets × 12 reps
- 60 seconds of rest

B2. Snatch-grip barbell back extension
- 2 sets × 12 reps
- 60 seconds of rest

B3. Push-up (#12)
- 2 sets × 12 reps
- 60 seconds of rest

OPTIONS

Easy Option Perform 10 reps per set of each of the B exercises.

Step It Up Add an extra set to each of the B exercises.

Cool-Down Standing quad stretch, 90-degree stretch, double lat stretch.

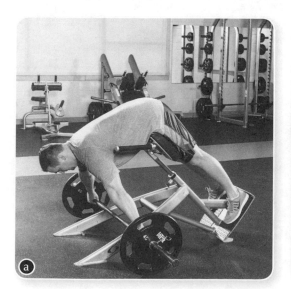

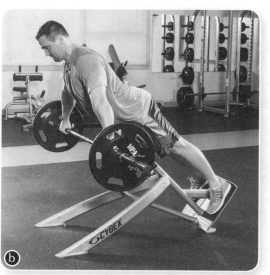

Crazy 8s: Deadlift

Adding mobility work between sets of heavier compound movements is an excellent way to ensure you are gaining proper range of motion and muscle activation during these primary lifts. Consider what muscle groups are being used in your big movements, and choose mobility work or activation drills that target these same muscles.

Warm-Up

4 reps per side of the world's greatest stretch, 5 reps each of inchworm and inverted hamstring stretch, 10 reps of glute bridge

● Featured Exercise

Yoga-Plex

1. Place a 12-inch (30 cm) box approximately 3 feet (1 m) in front of you (if you do not have a box, a bench will do).

2. From a tall standing position, step forward with your right foot, bending your knee into a lunge. Keep your back leg as straight as possible, and place both hands on the box (a).

3. Keep your right hand on the box while you reach your left arm up and over your head (b), rotating your torso and reaching toward your rear hip (c).

4. Bring your left hand back to the box, and push off your right foot to return to the standing position.

5. Lunge forward with your left leg, and repeat the sequence on the opposite side. Continue to alternate until you have completed all reps.

Complete Workout

A1. Conventional deadlift (#5)
- 8 sets × 2 reps
- 60 seconds of rest

A2. Yoga-plex
- 8 sets × 4 reps/side
- 60 seconds of rest

OPTIONS

Easy Option   Perform 6 sets of the exercises.

Step It Up   Perform 10 sets of the exercises.

Cool-Down   Double lat stretch, hamstring stretch, calf stretch.

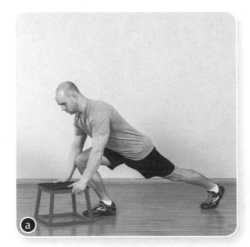
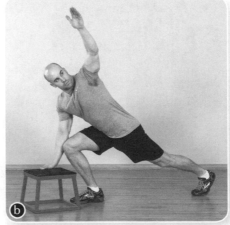
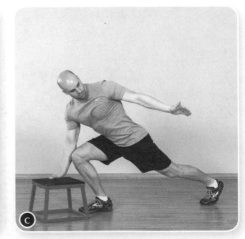

Olympic Complex

Olympic weightlifters are some of the strongest, most powerful, and most dynamic athletes you will find anywhere. Yet, their training utilizes very little exercise variety and focuses on low-rep sets. The Olympic complex combines several key weightlifting movements into one continuous circuit to drive up not only explosive power but mobility and conditioning as well.

Warm-Up

5 reps of squat to stand; 6 reps per side of kneeling adductor stretch, hip rocker, and quadruped T-spine rotation

● Featured Exercise

Push Jerk

1. Begin with the barbell resting across the front of your shoulders. Hands should be grasping the bar just outside shoulder width. Your elbows should be in front of you, with your upper arm parallel to the floor.

2. Dip down into a quarter-squat position by driving your knees forward (do not bring your hips back as you would at the beginning of a traditional squat) (a).

3. Forcefully reverse the motion, generating power from your legs as you explosively lift the bar overhead to lockout (b).

4. Lower the barbell back to its original position and repeat for reps.

Complete Workout

Perform 8 rounds of this complex, completing 1 rep of each movement directly after the other before resting as prescribed.

Power snatch (#35)
- 1 rep

Overhead squat (#167)
- 1 rep

Barbell front squat (#44)
- 1 rep

Push jerk
- 1 rep
- 90 seconds of rest

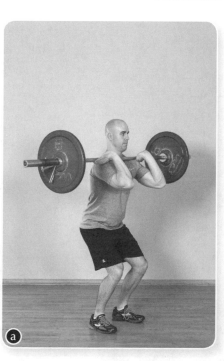

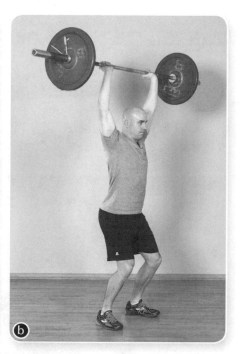

OPTIONS

Easy Option Perform 6 rounds of this complex.

Step It Up Add an additional rep of the overhead squat and front squat.

Cool-Down Standing quad stretch, 90-degree stretch, cross-body stretch.

Push Press Max

The push press is a great exercise to do when transitioning from the more stable lifts such as bench presses and squats to the more dynamic lifts such as snatches, cleans, jerks, and jumps. The push press uses aspects of the dynamic lifts by utilizing leg drive to gain momentum while requiring you to finish with the more familiar upper body strength used in other overhead pressing movements. Focus on this transition from dynamic to stable in your warm-up sets because getting this balance correct will allow you to drive up strength on this great exercise much more quickly.

Warm-Up

6 reps of squat to stand, 6 reps per side of quadruped T-spine rotation, 8 reps of glute bridge, 10 reps of cat–cow

● Featured Exercise

Tall Kneeling Face Pull

1. Kneel with both knees on the ground, facing a cable station with the rope attachment set at nose height.
2. Grab the rope with a double handshake grip (a).
3. Keeping your upper arms parallel to the floor, your shoulder blades down, and your back and traps depressed, simultaneously pull the rope toward your ears and rotate your thumbs downward.
4. Full range of motion is achieved when your hands are equal to or just past your ears (b). Squeeze your shoulder blades together, and return the rope to the starting position.

Complete Workout

Increase the weight used on each set of the push press until you reach your maximum weight on the final set.

A. Push press (#16)
- 5 sets × 5, 3, 1, 1, 1 reps
- 90 seconds of rest

B1. Alternating dumbbell row (#246)
- 2 sets × 10 reps per side
- 60 seconds of rest

B2. Tall kneeling face pull
- 2 sets × 10 reps
- 60 seconds of rest

B3. Alternating dumbbell hammer curl (#230)
- 2 sets × 10 reps
- 60 seconds of rest

OPTIONS

Easy Option   Remove the final single in the push press.

Step It Up   Add two more singles with your max weight for the push press.

Cool-Down   Standing quad stretch, 90-degree stretch, double lat stretch.

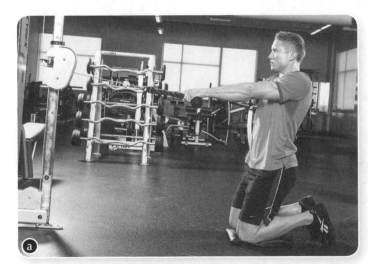

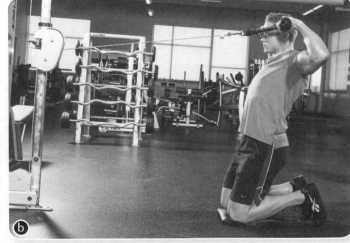

Popeye's Revenge

Grip musculature can be trained in an incredibly wide variety of ways. And although there will be some carryover between gripping heavy barbells, gripping a chin-up bar, using fat grips in your training, and grabbing the side of a cliff during a weekend mountain climbing trip, you should be training grip for both variety and specificity of needs. This will not only improve performance in nearly any movement in which grip is a factor but also contribute to strong and well-developed forearms.

Warm-Up

4 reps per side of the world's greatest stretch, 5 reps each of inchworm and inverted hamstring stretch, 10 reps of glute bridge

● Featured Exercise

Pinch-Grip Farmer's Walk

1. Grab two 10 lb (4.5 kg) metal weight plates, and put them together so the smooth sides are facing out. Repeat this process with two additional weight plates (you will be using two plates per hand).

2. Grip the plates together at the very top with the tips of your fingers and the tip of your thumb (*a*). Repeat with the other hand.

3. Standing tall, walk forward with your arms at your sides, actively pinching the plates together for the entire distance (*b*).

Complete Workout

A. Conventional deadlift (#5)
- 4 sets × 3 reps
- 90 seconds of rest

B1. Neutral-grip pull-up (#237)
- 3 sets × 8 reps
- 60 seconds of rest

B2. Alternating dumbbell row (#246)
- 3 sets × 8 reps/side

B3. Pinch-grip farmer's walk
- 3 sets × 50 yards (50 m)

⚠️ **Warning:** If you feel your grip being compromised, bend at the knees and lower the weight to the floor. Avoid dropping plates on your feet.

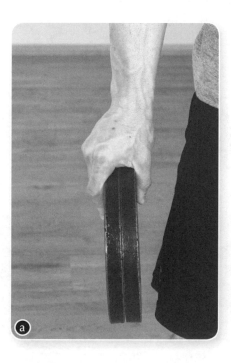

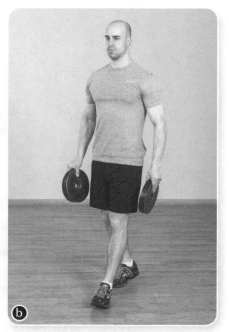

OPTIONS

Easy Option Reduce the B exercises to 3 sets, and perform the pinch-grip farmer's walk for 40 yards (40 m).

Step It Up Increase the distance of the pinch-grip farmer's walk to 100 yards (100 m).

Cool-Down Double lat stretch, hamstring stretch, calf stretch.

The Jumper

When performing a barbell back squat (or any squat with a barbell, for that matter), make sure the barbell's path is aligned with the middle of your feet during the entire range of motion. This will reduce the risk of injury while also keeping you in the strongest position possible to drive up the weight.

Warm-Up

6 reps of squat to stand, 6 reps per side of quadruped T-spine rotation, 8 reps of glute bridge, 10 reps of cat–cow

⦿ Featured Exercise

Jump Squat

1. Begin in a standing position, feet at hip width and turned out slightly.
2. Unlock your hips and bend your knees in order to lower yourself into the bottom of a squat position (*a*).
3. Explode out of the bottom position, and jump as high as possible (*b*).
4. Land with your knees slightly bent (*c*). Return to the starting position and repeat for reps.

Complete Workout

Perform 6 rounds of the following circuit.

Jump squat
- 3 reps
- 30 seconds of rest

Barbell back squat (#63)
- 8 reps
- 2 minutes of rest

OPTIONS

Easy Option Reduce the number of reps of the barbell back squat to 6 per set.

Step It Up Use a light barbell in the back squat position for the jump squat.

Cool-Down Standing quad stretch, 90-degree stretch, double lat stretch.

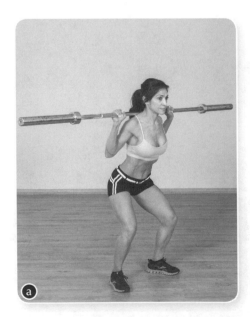

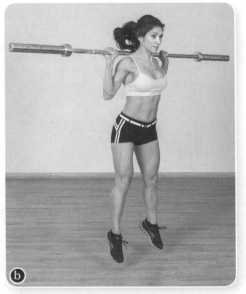

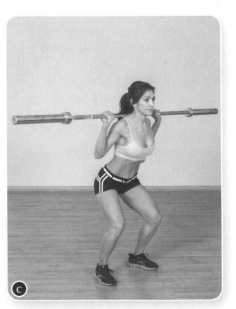

To the Death

Although some workouts should focus on higher reps (and there are plenty of workouts in this book that do), don't shortchange the benefits of timed circuits with lower reps and heavier loads. Doing so will increase your ability to repeatedly express strength as well as deliver massive cardiovascular benefits. If you think a set of 5, 3, or even 1 rep can't drive your heart rate through the roof, think again. You do, however, need to be more conscious of form in these types of workouts because using heavier weights when fatigued poses a risk. So be safe, train hard, and don't underestimate how much work capacity you can develop from a 45-rep workout.

Warm-Up

5 reps of inchworm, 6 reps per side of quadruped T-spine rotation, 10 reps of cat–cow

● Featured Exercise

Hang Power Clean

1. Start by holding the barbell with an overhand grip, placing your hands and feet slightly wider than shoulder-width apart. The bar should rest just below your knees (*a*).
2. Explosively drive the bar upward by extending at the knees and hips (*b*).

3. Aggressively shuffle your feet out and pull your body under the bar, rotating your elbows around the bar. Catch the bar on your shoulders while moving into a half-squat position (you should catch the bar with your upper legs parallel to the floor or above).
4. Stand up, locking out your legs (*c*).
5. Flex your knees slightly, and return the barbell to the starting position in front of your thighs. Repeat for reps.

Complete Workout

Perform 5 rounds of the following circuit, starting with 5 reps of each in the first round and reducing by 1 rep each set. Use 75 percent of body weight for the hang power clean, 1.5 × body weight for the trap bar deadlift, and 1 × body weight for the barbell bench press. Complete the circuit in as little time as possible, being sure to use good form on each rep.

Hang power clean
- 5 sets × 5, 4, 3, 2, 1 reps

Trap bar deadlift (#8)
- 5 sets × 5, 4, 3, 2, 1 reps

Barbell bench press (#54)
- 5 sets × 5, 4, 3, 2, 1 reps

OPTIONS

Easy Option Use 50 percent of your body weight (or less) for the hang power clean, 1 × body weight for the trap bar deadlift, and 75 percent body weight for the barbell bench press.

Step It Up Use 1 × body weight for the hang power clean, 2 × body weight for the trap bar deadlift, and 1.25 × body weight for the barbell bench press.

Cool-Down Double lat stretch, cross-body stretch, hamstring stretch.

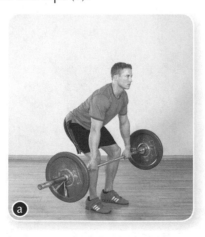
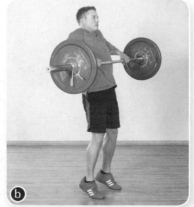
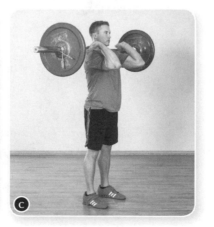

Tonnage

Although most timed workouts call for a certain number of reps to be performed as quickly as possible, this is not the only way to design a program that measures performance over time. In this workout, you'll be using tonnage—the total amount of load lifted in a workout. The goal of tonnage workouts is to lift a certain amount of weight in an exercise in as little time as possible. You can use heavier weight for fewer reps, lighter weight for more reps, or any combination of the two. The goal is to then lift the total amount of weight in less time the next time you do the workout.

Warm-Up

5 reps of squat to stand; 6 reps per side of kneeling adductor stretch, hip rocker, and quadruped T-spine rotation

● Featured Exercise

Barbell Back Squat

1. Utilizing a shoulder-width stance, step under a bar in a squat rack, with the barbell resting on your upper traps (a). Take one step back with each foot.

2. Maintaining a neutral or slightly arched lower back, unlock your hips and begin bringing them back. Almost instantaneously, bend at your knees.

3. Keeping your entire foot on the ground, continue to lower yourself to as deep a level as possible (you want your hip crease to be at least below your knee) (b).

4. When you reach your full range of motion, forcefully drive your feet into the ground and stand up, returning to the starting position.

Complete Workout

This is a tonnage workout featuring the barbell back squat; you are trying to lift a total of 10,000 lb (4,500 kg) throughout the entire workout. You can use whatever weight you wish throughout the workout and perform as many reps per set as you'd like. For example, if you performed 10 sets of 10 reps with 100 lb (45 kg) on the barbell, you would reach the 10,000 lb ($10 \times 10 \times 100 = 10,000$). The goal is to lift a total of 10,000 lb in as little time as possible (note your time to see if you can beat it in future workouts).

Barbell back squat
- 10,000 lb (4,500 kg) total in as little time as possible

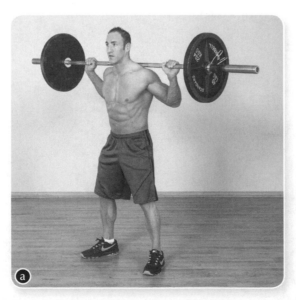
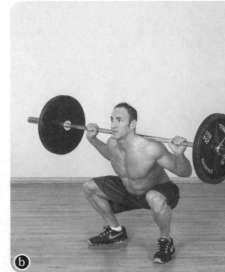

Leatherneck

Jerking or pressing a barbell overhead from the behind-the-neck position has several advantages. First, the bar remains in the same plane of motion throughout the entire movement (as opposed to an overhead press, which starts under your chin and has to loop around your head). Second, the bar starts and ends directly above your center of mass, placing you in a very strong position. This end position best mimics the desired end position of the clean and jerk. However, to be able to press from behind the neck, you need proper shoulder stability, good range of motion in the shoulder joint, and a properly functioning rotator cuff and other structures of the shoulder girdle. In simple terms, this lift is not for everyone, so proceed with caution.

Warm-Up

4 reps per side of the world's greatest stretch, 5 reps each of inchworm and inverted hamstring stretch, 10 reps of glute bridge

Complete Workout

A. Behind-the-neck jerk
- 6 sets × 2 reps
- 90 seconds of rest

B1. Trap bar deadlift (#8)
- 4 sets × 6 reps
- 90 seconds of rest

B2. Weighted chin-up (#160)
- 4 sets × 6 reps
- 90 seconds of rest

● Featured Exercise

Behind-the-Neck Jerk

1. Begin with a loaded barbell resting across your upper traps. Your hands should be just outside shoulder width (a).

2. Simultaneously press the bar upward while dropping your body underneath the bar by splitting your legs into a lunge stance.

3. Once you catch the bar overhead (b), straighten your legs and bring your feet back to their starting position.

4. Lower the bar back to your upper traps with flexed knees to absorb the weight. Repeat for reps.

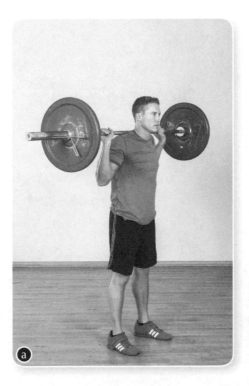

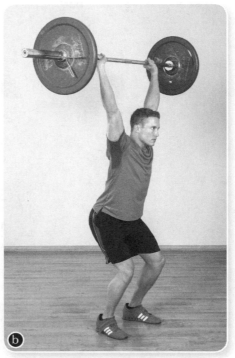

OPTIONS

Easy Option Substitute a kneeling lat pull-down (#120) for the weighted chin-up.

Step It Up Add another set to the trap bar deadlift and weighted chin-up.

Cool-Down Double lat stretch, hamstring stretch, calf stretch.

High Heels

For many people, achieving full range of motion in the back squat is difficult because of lack of ankle mobility. The heel-elevated back squat helps overcome this problem by allowing for a greater range of motion. Place small (think 5 or 10 lb [2.5 or 4.5 kg]) weight plates under your heels, and you should notice an ability to get deeper into your squat. Keep working on your ankle and hip mobility through activation and mobilization drills in order to keep this depth even without the weight plates.

Warm-Up

5 reps of squat to stand; 6 reps per side of kneeling adductor stretch, hip rocker, and quadruped T-spine rotation

● Featured Exercise

Heel-Elevated Back Squat

1. Place a small pad or two small weight plates under your heels and have a barbell resting on your upper traps (*a*).

2. Unlock your hips, and slowly descend into a squat by bringing your hips back and bending your knees.

3. Once you reach full range of motion (you are attempting to get the crease of your hips below the height of your knee) (*b*), reverse the motion to return to standing. Repeat for reps.

Complete Workout

After you have completed the six sets of the three reps (A), reduce the weight and perform as many heel-elevated back squats as possible for 20 seconds. Rest for 10 seconds and repeat. Continue to work for 20 seconds and rest for 10 seconds for a total of 8 rounds (4 minutes). Choose a load that is 50 percent of the maximum load you used for the first round of heel-elevated back squats.

A. Heel-elevated back squat
  • 6 sets × 3 reps

B. Heel-elevated back squat Tabata

OPTIONS

Easy Option   Cut the Tabata in half, completing 4 rounds.

Step It Up   Strive to get a minimum of 8 reps in every set during the Tabata portion of the workout.

Cool-Down   Standing quad stretch, 90-degree stretch, cross-body stretch.

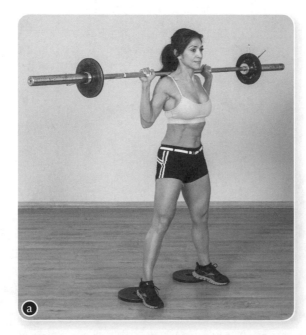

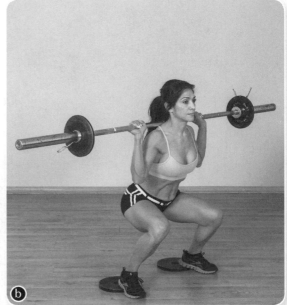

Olympic Total

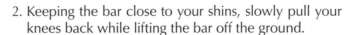

Olympic weightlifting (technically referred to simply as *weightlifting*) is a sport in which the goal is to perform a maximal effort in two lifts—the snatch and the clean and jerk. In this workout, you get to play the role of a competing weightlifter, attempting to determine your 1RM in both lifts. Once you do, add these numbers up to determine your total. This is a great benchmark to try improving through your training. And although you may not be ready for a trip to the Olympics, working toward new personal bests will give you the determination and motivation of an athlete.

Warm-Up

4 reps per side of the world's greatest stretch, 6 reps per side of hip rocker and inverted hamstring stretch, 8 reps per side of shoulder sweeps

● Featured Exercise

Clean and Jerk

1. Start by grabbing the barbell with an overhand grip, placing your hands and feet slightly wider than shoulder-width apart (*a*).

2. Keeping the bar close to your shins, slowly pull your knees back while lifting the bar off the ground.

3. Once the bar gets to your midthighs (*b*), explosively extend at your knees and hips to drive the bar upward.

4. Aggressively pull your body under the bar into a full squat, rotating your elbows around the bar. Catch the bar on your shoulders (*c*).

5. Stand up with the bar, bend at the knees (keeping your chest tall), and explosively drive the bar overhead. You can catch the bar with your legs split (as in the split jerk) (*d*) or your feet parallel (power jerk).

6. Traditionally, the bar is dropped from overhead, but follow the rules of the facility where you are training and control the weight when necessary by bringing it back to your shoulders and then to the floor.

Complete Workout

Take 12 minutes in each lift to warm up and find your 1RM. Once you do, add the two lifts to determine your total.

Snatch (#84)
- 1 rep

Clean and jerk
- 1 rep

OPTIONS

Easy Option   None.

Step It Up   None.

Cool-Down   Standing quad stretch, 90-degree stretch, double lat stretch.

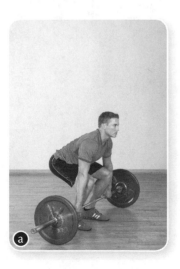
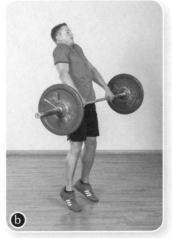
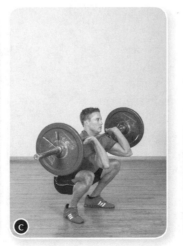
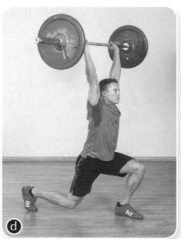

Crazy 8s: Bench Press

Specific warm-up sets are an important part of any training program but are particularly important when lifting loads close to your repetition maximum. A good rule of thumb is that the closer to your 1RM your work sets will be, the more warm-up sets you will need. Therefore, a workout that features doubles (such as the bench press in this workout) can require as many as 5 warm-up sets, while a workout that has you working in the 10- to 12-rep range may require only one or two warm-ups. Bottom line: The fewer reps per set (and, therefore, the heavier load being used), the more warm-up sets are needed.

Warm-Up

4 reps per side of the world's greatest stretch, 5 reps of inchworm, 8 reps per side of shoulder sweeps

● Featured Exercise

Scapulae Wall Slide

1. Place your butt, back, and head against an empty wall. Lift your arms overhead in a V shape (*a*).
2. Pull your elbows down toward your rib cage, attempting to keep as much of your lower back, upper arms, forearms, wrists, and hands against the wall at all times.
3. Pull your elbows down as low as you can while maintaining contact with the wall. Your arms should resemble a W in the bottom position (*b*).
4. Keep contact with the wall, and press your arms back up to the original position. Repeat for reps.

Complete Workout

A1. Barbell bench press (#54)
  • 8 sets × 2 reps
A2. Scapulae wall slide
  • 8 sets × 8 reps

OPTIONS

Easy Option   Perform 6 sets of the exercises.

Step It Up   Perform 10 sets of the exercises.

Cool-Down   Pec stretch, double lat stretch, 90-degree stretch.

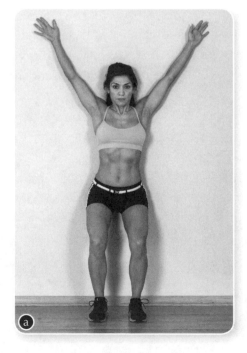
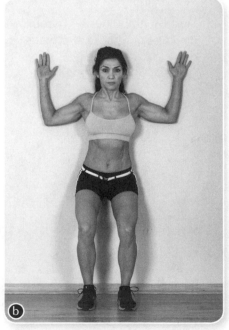

National Pride

As a general rule of thumb, if a movement is named after a country, it's going to be tough because national pride is on the line. This workout combines three of the greatest of these exercises: the Romanian deadlift, which may be the purest example of the hip hinge; Bulgarian split squats, which challenge the entire musculature of the legs and hips; and the Turkish get-up, one of the great total-body integrated moves.

Warm-Up

4 reps per side of the world's greatest stretch, 5 reps each of inchworm and inverted hamstring stretch, 10 reps of glute bridge

Complete Workout

A. Trap bar Romanian deadlift (#248)
- 6 sets × 3 reps
- 2 minutes of rest

B1. Bulgarian split squat (#200)
- 3 sets × 6 reps per leg
- 90 seconds of rest

B2. Turkish get-up
- 3 sets × 4 reps per side
- 90 seconds of rest

● Featured Exercise

Turkish Get-Up

1. Lie on your back with your right knee bent 90 degrees (so your foot is flat on the floor) and your right arm, holding a kettlebell, extended straight up toward the ceiling.

2. Rotate to the left, posting up on your left elbow (*a*).

3. Continue rotating to the left, extending your left arm so your hand is on the ground. Extend at your hips so you are creating a straight line from your left ankle to your right shoulder (*b*).

4. Slide your left leg behind you (*c*), and extend your torso as if you were in the bottom position of a lunge (*d*). Be sure to keep the kettlebell above you at all times.

5. Stand up and bring your feet together. Reverse the process until you are back in the starting position. Repeat all reps on one side before switching.

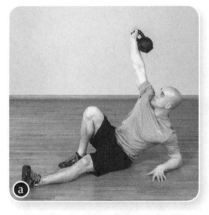
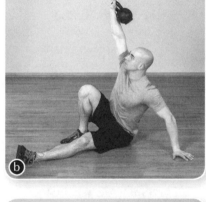
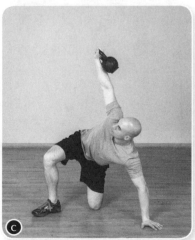
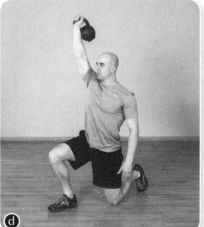

OPTIONS

Easy Option Complete 4 sets of the Romanian deadlift.

Step It Up Increase to 4 sets of the Bulgarian split squat and Turkish get-up.

Cool-Down Double lat stretch, hamstring stretch, calf stretch.

Russian Complex

For many years, Russia dominated Olympic weightlifting by virtue of their groundbreaking methodologies and thorough analysis of training methods. This complex is very similar to ones being used by today's top Russian athletes, who still display a passion for, and excellence in, the sport.

Warm-Up

4 reps per side of the world's greatest stretch, 6 reps per side of hip rocker and inverted hamstring stretch, 8 reps per side of shoulder sweep

● Featured Exercise

Split Jerk

1. Begin with the barbell resting across the front of your shoulders. Hands should be grasping the bar just outside shoulder width. Your elbows should be in front of you, with your upper arm parallel to the floor (*a*).

2. Dip down into a quarter-squat position by driving your knees forward (do not bring your hips back as you would at the beginning of a traditional squat).

3. Forcefully reverse the motion, splitting your legs so one foot lands in front of you and the other behind (as if in the middle of a lunge) as the bar locks out overhead (*b*).

4. Recover by bringing your front foot back to a neutral position, followed by your back foot. Lower the bar back to your shoulders.

OPTIONS

Easy Option   Perform 6 rounds of the complex.

Step It Up   Perform 2 reps of each movement per round.

Cool-Down   Standing quad stretch, 90-degree stretch, double lat stretch.

Complete Workout

Perform 8 rounds of the following complex, performing 1 rep of each exercise in succession and resting 90 seconds between rounds.

Conventional deadlift (#5)
- 1 rep

Power clean (#52)
- 1 rep

Barbell front squat (#44)
- 1 rep

Push press (#16)
- 1 rep

Split jerk
- 1 rep
- 90 seconds of rest

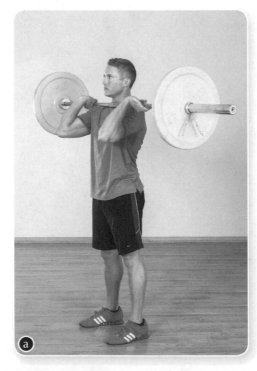
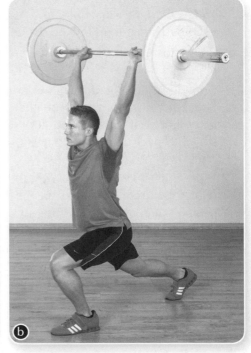

Max and Drop

Drop sets, as featured in this workout, are a great way to add additional volume and intensity of effort without increasing the length of a workout. A drop set is achieved by lifting a weight a certain number of times, reducing the load by a certain percentage, and lifting the weight again, with minimal rest between sets. The weight can be dropped as little as once or several times, resulting in multiple sets. Since drop sets do not allow for a long recovery between sets, be prepared for a big performance drop-off from one set to the next.

Warm-Up

4 reps per side of the world's greatest stretch, 5 reps of inchworm, 8 reps per side of shoulder sweeps

● Featured Exercise

Narrow-Grip Bench Press

1. Set up in a bench press station with your eyes directly under the bar; feet on the floor; and butt, upper back, and head on the bench.
2. Grab the bar exactly at shoulder width (*a*).
3. Lower the bar under control until it touches the middle of your chest. Keep your elbows tucked toward your rib cage (not flaring out) (*b*).
4. Forcefully drive the bar back up to the starting position and repeat for reps.

Complete Workout

Take 10 minutes to work up to your heaviest bench press.

Narrow-grip bench press
- 80 percent of your 1RM (as many reps as possible)
- 30 seconds of rest
- Reduce by 20 percent and perform as many reps as possible
- 30 seconds of rest
- Reduce by 20 percent and perform as many reps as possible

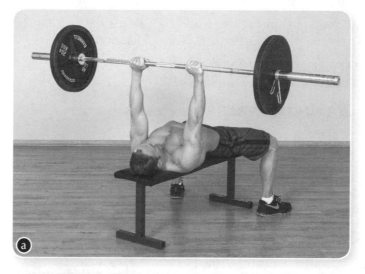

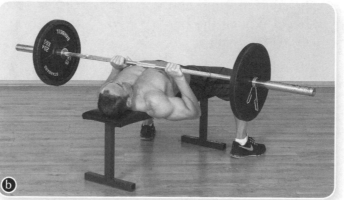

OPTIONS

Easy Option Begin the drop sets at 70 percent of your 1RM.

Step It Up Include one more drop set, reducing the weight by an additional 20 percent and performing as many reps as possible.

Cool-Down Pec stretch, double lat stretch, 90-degree stretch.

Strict Press Plus

Overtraining can lead to depression, loss of desire to train, weight fluctuations, increased risk of injury, restless sleep, altered appetite, and mood swings. However, overtraining is actually a fairly rare phenomenon usually reserved for those who are training at a high level for multiple hours or sessions in a day. In fact, the majority of the population probably has to worry more about undertraining than overtraining. However, if you're experiencing any of the symptoms just identified and have been hitting it particularly hard lately, try reducing training and life stress for several days until things return to normal.

Warm-Up

4 reps per side of the world's greatest stretch, 5 reps of inchworm, 8 reps per side of shoulder sweeps

Featured Exercise

Barbell Overhead Press

1. Grab a loaded bar just outside shoulder width at collarbone height. The bar should be resting on top of your anterior deltoids (front of your shoulders) (a).
2. Take a deep breath in, brace your core, and begin driving the bar overhead.

3. As the bar passes over the top of your head, drive your body slightly forward so the bar is over the center of your foot (do not, however, jut your chin out or extend your neck).
4. Continue to press the bar overhead until you have achieved full lockout (b). Return the bar to the starting position and repeat for reps.

Complete Workout

Load 30 percent of your 1RM for the barbell overhead press onto a barbell. Perform 2 reps every minute on the minute (start at the top of each minute, and rest whatever remains of that minute after your set is complete). Increase the weight on the bar by 10 lb (4.5 kg) every minute. Continue until you hit a weight where you can no longer complete 2 reps.

Barbell overhead press
- As many sets as possible, as described

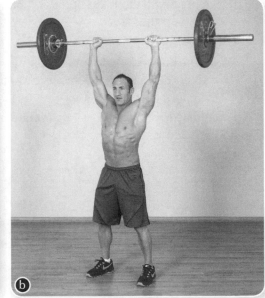

Walk the Plank

As exhilarating and empowering as deadlifting or bench pressing huge weights can be, there are other movements that are so seemingly simple yet so humbling when you actually try to perform them. The side plank with leg raise (featured in this workout) is one of those movements. It challenges coordination between your inner and outer obliques and the lateral muscles in your hip—muscles that are often undertrained. It's also common to perform much better on one side than the other. Keep working on this movement because integrating these muscle groups and having them coordinate will carry over to improved strength in other exercises

Warm-Up

6 reps of squat to stand, 6 reps per side of quadruped T-spine rotation, 8 reps of glute bridge, 10 reps of cat–cow

● Featured Exercise

Side Plank With Leg Raise

1. Lying on your side, put your elbow directly under your shoulder, and press your body up into a side plank. Your heels should be stacked (a).

2. Keeping your hips high and a straight line from your shoulder to your heels, raise your top leg as high as possible (b).

3. Lower your leg back to the starting position and repeat for reps. Complete all reps for one side before switching to the other.

Complete Workout

A. Conventional deadlift (#5)
- 4 sets × 5 reps
- 90 seconds of rest

B1. Alternating step-back lunge (#24)
- 3 sets × 8 reps/side
- 30 seconds of rest

B2. Side plank with leg raise
- 3 sets × 10 reps/side
- 30 seconds of rest

B3. Alternating-arm seated cable row (#142)
- 3 sets × 10 reps/side
- 30 seconds of rest

OPTIONS

Easy Option Complete 2 sets of each of the B exercises.

Step It Up Add 2 reps to each set of the B exercises.

Cool-Down Standing quad stretch, 90-degree stretch, double lat stretch.

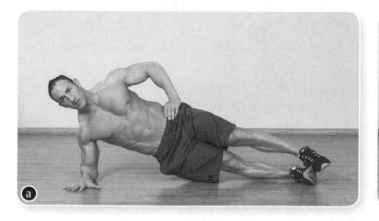

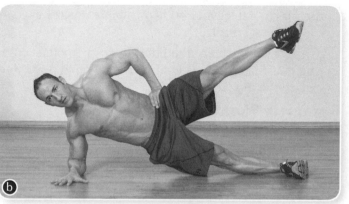

Reach Out

Ever notice how a push-up looks a lot like a plank? Truth is, push-ups are a great way to train your abs, lats, and glutes. Wanna make them an even better core exercise? Add a reach (as described here in the push-up with reach). By creating a longer lever, the reach will require your abdominals to stabilize to an even greater extent so you don't end up falling on your face. Guaranteed, you'll never look at push-ups as strictly a chest exercise ever again.

Warm-Up

4 reps per side of the world's greatest stretch, 6 reps per side of hip rocker and inverted hamstring stretch, 8 reps per side of shoulder sweeps

● Featured Exercise

Push-Up With Reach

1. Begin in a push-up position with your hands slightly wider than your shoulders, your arms straight, and your body forming a straight line from your head to your heels (*a*).

2. Bend at the elbows to lower yourself toward the floor (keep your elbows tucked back toward your rib cage) (*b*). Press yourself back up to the starting position. Extend your left hand out and hold for one second (*c*). Try to not let your body rotate (particularly at your hips) as you reach.

3. Return your hand to the floor; perform another push up, this time reaching with your right hand once you reach the top. That is one rep.

Complete Workout

A. Barbell front squat (#44)
- • 6 sets × 4 reps
- • 90 seconds of rest

B1. Chin-up (#73)
- • 2 sets × 10 reps
- • 30 seconds of rest

B2. Push-up with reach
- • 2 sets × 8 reps/side
- • 30 seconds of rest

B3. Side plank (#175)
- • 2 sets × 20 seconds per side
- • 30 seconds of rest

OPTIONS

Easy Option   Perform 4 sets of the front squat.

Step It Up   Add 2 reps to the chin-up and push-up with reach and 10 to the side plank.

Cool-Down   Standing quad stretch, 90-degree stretch, double lat stretch.

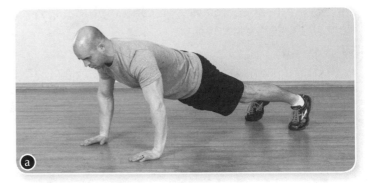

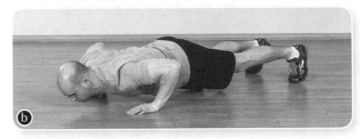

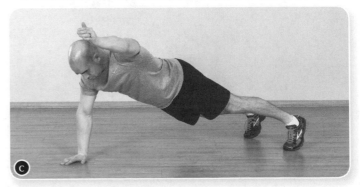

Untouchable

The hip snatch (featured in this workout) trains one of the most critical components of the Olympic lifts—the ability to fully extend at the hips and knees in order to generate the power that drives the bar overhead. It is also a great exercise for practicing getting under the bar quickly as it travels upward. Use this exercise to work on your timing, and you will see a huge carryover to the full versions of both the snatch and the clean.

Warm-Up

4 reps per side of the world's greatest stretch, 6 reps per side of hip rocker and inverted hamstring stretch, 8 reps per side of shoulder sweeps

● Featured Exercise

Hip Snatch

1. Place a barbell at the creases of your hips (about 2 to 3 inches [5 to 8 cm] below your navel), and grab it with a straight-arm snatch grip (a).

2. Keeping your torso tall and the weight on your heels, bend your knees 3 to 4 inches (8 to 10 cm) (do not bend at the hips).

3. Explosively extend your knees and hips, shrug your traps, and allow the bar to travel upward (b).

4. As the bar travels upward, pull yourself under the bar and catch it with arms fully extended at the bottom or in an overhead squat position (c).

5. Stand up with the bar overhead. Return the bar to the starting position and repeat for reps.

Complete Workout

Hip snatch
- 5 sets × 5 reps
- 90 seconds of rest

Hang snatch pull (#61)
- 5 sets × 5 reps
- 90 seconds of rest

OPTIONS

Easy Option Perform 3 reps per set of the hip snatch.

Step It Up Add an additional set of the hip snatch and hang snatch pull.

Cool-Down Hamstring stretch, calf stretch, pec stretch.

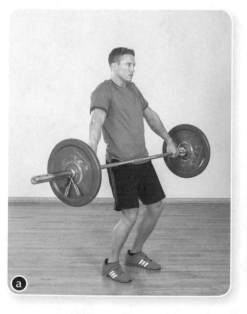

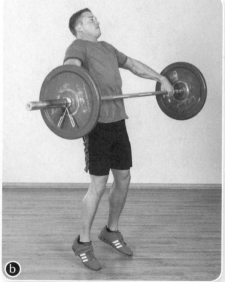

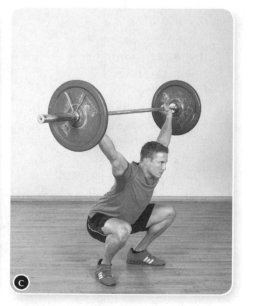

The Sniper

A sniper never announces his arrival. He just sneaks in, attacks, leaves his deadly mark, and retreats. A workout can be much like a sniper. It can sneak up on you, and before you know it, your muscles are burning, your lungs are on fire, and you think you are left for dead. Don't let sniper workouts get the best of you. Fight to the finish, and escape with the victory of knowing you put everything you had in it.

Warm-Up

5 reps of inchworm, 6 reps per side of quadruped T-spine rotation, 10 reps of cat–cow

● **Featured Exercise**

Barbell Overhead Press

1. Grab a loaded bar just outside shoulder width at collarbone height. The bar should be resting on top of your anterior deltoids (front of your shoulders) (*a*).

2. Take a deep breath in, brace your core, and begin driving the bar overhead.

3. As the bar passes over the top of your head, drive your body slightly forward so the bar is over the center of your foot (do not, however, jut your chin out or extend your neck).

4. Continue to press the bar overhead until you have achieved full lockout (*b*). Return the bar to the starting position and repeat for reps.

Complete Workout

This is a tonnage workout featuring the barbell overhead press; you are trying to lift a total of 8,000 lb (3,600 kg) throughout the entire workout. You can use whatever weight you wish throughout the workout and perform as many reps per set as you'd like. For example, if you performed 10 sets of 8 reps with 100 lb (45 kg) on the barbell, you would reach the 8,000 lb ($10 \times 8 \times 100 = 8,000$). The goal is to lift a total of 8,000 lb in as little time as possible (note your time to see if you can beat it in future workouts).

Barbell overhead press
- 8,000 lb (3,600 kg) total in as little time as possible

OPTIONS

Easy Option Lift a total of 6,000 lb (2,700 kg) for the entire workout.

Step It Up Get to 8,000 lb in fewer than 50 reps.

Cool-Down Double lat stretch, cross-body stretch, hamstring stretch.

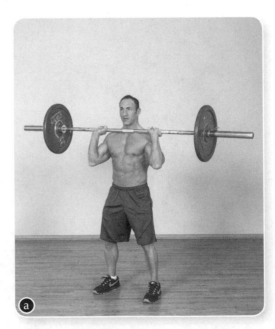
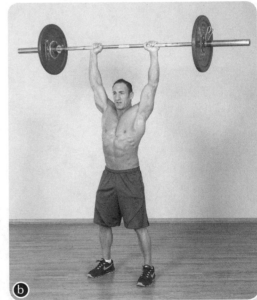

Minute on the Minute: Trap Bar Deadlift

Work capacity? Check. Strength? Check. Wondering how so much sweat is pouring into your eyes given that you are doing only three reps at a time? Check. Minute-on-the-minute protocols such as the one featured in this workout deliver a lot of bang for your buck. You can use relatively heavy weights while still getting your workout in a short period of time. The only catch? It's hard as hell.

Warm-Up

6 reps of squat to stand, 6 reps per side of quadruped T-spine rotation, 8 reps of glute bridge, 10 reps of cat–cow

Complete Workout

Perform 3 reps of the trap bar deadlift at the top of every minute for 20 minutes. If you can no longer complete 3 reps within that minute, end the workout. Use 75 to 80 percent of your 1RM.

Trap bar deadlift
- As many sets as possible, as described

● Featured Exercise

Trap Bar Deadlift

1. Step into a loaded trap bar with your feet at shoulder width.
2. Grab the handles at their center, bend your knees, pull your hips down, and retract your shoulder blades (*a*).
3. Lift the bar by simultaneously extending your knees and driving your hips forward.
4. Complete the movement by fully locking out your hips at the top (*b*).
5. Reverse the motion by first bringing your hips back and then flexing the knees. Maintain a tall chest and neutral spine in all phases of the movement.

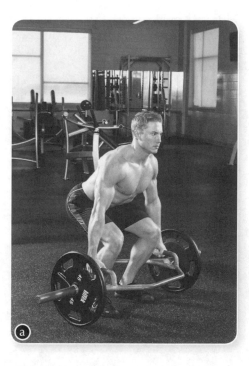

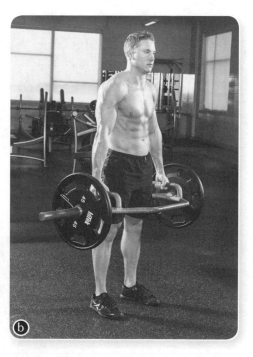

OPTIONS

Easy Option   Perform 2 reps of the trap bar deadlift each minute.

Step It Up   Perform 5 reps of the trap bar deadlift each minute.

Cool-Down   Standing quad stretch, 90-degree stretch, double lat stretch.

Absolute Front Squat

The very definition of strength is the ability to lift heavy loads. In order to train for strength, you need to systematically add weight to the bar. This can most efficiently and effectively be done by using lower-rep sets of compound lifts. With low-rep sets, you can not only lift more weight but also focus more on technique as well as mental and physical intensity.

Warm-Up

5 reps of squat to stand; 6 reps per side of kneeling adductor stretch, hip rocker, and quadruped T-spine rotation

● Featured Exercise

Barbell Front Squat

1. Set up a barbell just below collarbone height in a squat rack.
2. Step under the bar so it sits on your front deltoids (shoulders), and grab the bar with a clean grip, with your elbows high and your upper arms parallel to the ground. Unrack the bar, and take one step back with each foot (a).

3. Tighten up your upper body, unlock your hips, bend your knees, and lower your body toward the ground, trying to sit as low as possible while keeping the bar over the center of your foot (for more on proper squat technique, see chapter 1, Ramping Up) (b).
4. Once you reach the bottom of your range, reverse the motion and stand up. Repeat for reps.

Complete Workout

A. Barbell front squat
   - 6 sets × 3 reps
   - 2 minutes of rest

B1. Heel-elevated back squat (#96)
   - 3 sets × 6 reps

B2. Leg press (#114)
   - 3 sets × 6 reps
   - 90 seconds of rest

OPTIONS

Easy Option   Reduce to 4 sets of the front squat.

Step It Up   Increase to 8 sets of the front squat.

Cool-Down   Standing quad stretch, 90-degree stretch, cross-body stretch.

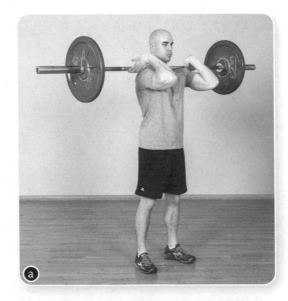

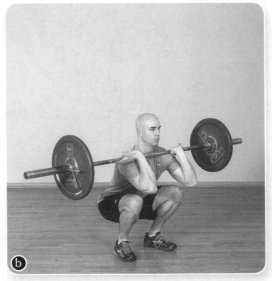

CHAPTER 10

Targeted Muscle Builders

For years body-part splits, in which you trained one or two body parts per workout, were the standard training protocol in gyms across the world. Then in the late 1990s, when functional fitness became the craze, people started focusing more on total-body or movement pattern–based training and left the body-part splits to aspiring bodybuilders. Truth is there is no need to throw out the baby with the bathwater. Both functional and body-part training are effective, and I encourage you to use both methodologies in your training. Targeting specific muscle groups is a great way to bring up lagging body parts—for instance, developing bigger calves or shapelier triceps—and increase hypertrophy (muscle size). The bottom line is that all these training modalities lead to what you want: a stronger, leaner, and more capable body.

Five-Star General

Although many people place too much of an emphasis on pressing movements in their programs (not a good thing), they are usually choosing pressing movements that take place in the horizontal plane (think barbell bench press or incline dumbbell bench press). This workout combines several overhead pressing movements in the vertical plane across a variety of strength qualities (power, strength, hypertrophy), allowing you to tap into some new muscle motor units.

Warm-Up

4 reps per side of the world's greatest stretch, 5 reps of inchworm, 8 reps per side of shoulder sweeps

● Featured Exercise

Flat Dumbbell Bench Press

1. Grab a set of dumbbells and lay back on a flat bench. Be sure your head, upper back and glutes are on the bench and your feet are on the floor.

2. With your palms facing each other, start with your arms fully extended and the dumbbells directly over your shoulders (a).

3. Lower the dumbbells keeping your elbows tucked in towards your ribcage.

4. Once the dumbbells reach chest level (b), drive them back up to the start position (c).

5. Repeat for reps.

Complete Workout

Push press (#16)
- 5 sets × 3 reps
- 60 seconds of rest

Barbell overhead press (#36)
- 5 sets × 6 reps
- 60 seconds of rest

Flat dumbbell bench press
- 5 sets × 8 reps
- 60 seconds of rest

Lateral raise (#147)
- 5 sets × 10 reps
- 2 minutes of rest

OPTIONS

Easy Option   Perform 3 sets of each exercise.

Step It Up   Add an additional set, bringing the total to 6 sets per movement.

Cool-Down   Pec stretch, double lat stretch, 90-degree stretch.

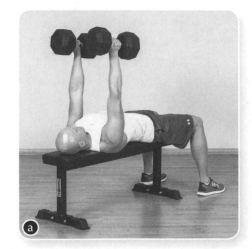
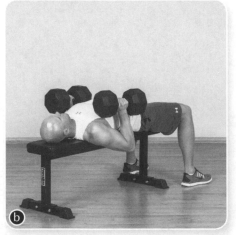
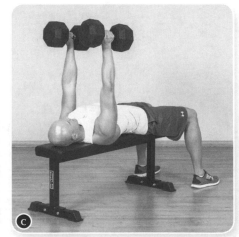

What happens when a workout combines a rep range associated with strength (6), one that prioritizes size (12), and one that focuses on endurance (25)? You get a great workout that will leave you walking (or in this case, crawling) away with a serious pump.

Warm-Up

4 reps per side of the world's greatest stretch, 5 reps each of inchworm and inverted hamstring stretch, 10 reps of glute bridge

● Featured Exercise

Stability Ball Hamstring Curl

1. Lie on your back with the heels of your feet on top of a stability ball. You should form a straight line from your ankles to your shoulders (a).

2. Drive your heels into the ball, and curl toward your glutes. Your hips should rise as the ball gets closer to your torso, maintaining a straight line from your knee to shoulder (b).

3. Squeeze your hamstrings at the end of the range of motion, and return the ball to its starting position. Repeat for reps.

Complete Workout

Perform the following three exercises as a circuit, resting 10 seconds between exercises and 100 seconds between rounds. Repeat the circuit a total of 4 times.

Conventional deadlift (#5)
- 6 reps
- 10 seconds of rest

Dumbbell Romanian deadlift (#267)
- 12 reps
- 10 seconds of rest

Stability ball hamstring curl
- 25 reps
- 100 seconds of rest

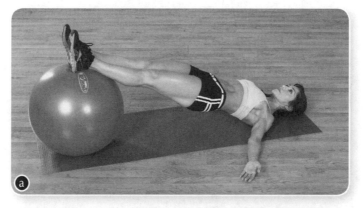

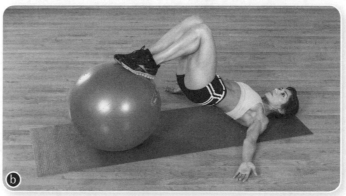

OPTIONS

Easy Option   Perform 15 reps of the stability ball hamstring curl.

Step It Up   Add an additional round, bringing the total number of circuits up to five.

Cool-Down   Double lat stretch, hamstring stretch, calf stretch.

Back Attack

It is very easy to turn movements that are designed to target your back into movements that overutilize your arms. Conquer this technique flaw in your rowing variations and pulling movements by keeping your shoulders down and chest out by and initiating the movement from your lats and the muscles that surround your scapulae. This will ensure you are getting the desired effect from your back training.

Warm-Up

5 reps of inchworm, 6 reps per side of quadruped T-spine rotation, 10 reps of cat–cow

● Featured Exercise

Chest-Supported Dumbbell Row

1. Grab a set of dumbbells, and lie chest down on a bench set to a 45-degree incline.
2. With your arms hanging straight down (*a*), retract your shoulder blades and simultaneously row both dumbbells up toward your rib cage (*b*).
3. Squeeze your lats at the top of the movement before returning to the starting position. Repeat for reps.

OPTIONS

Easy Option   Complete 3 sets of each exercise.

Step It Up   Complete 5 sets of each exercise.

Cool-Down   Double lat stretch, cross-body stretch, hamstring stretch.

Complete Workout

Perform these three exercises as a superset, resting 60 seconds between movements and 2 minutes between rounds.

Weighted chin-up (#160)
- 4 sets × 4 reps
- 60 seconds of rest

Seated cable row with hip flexion (#174)
- 4 sets × 4 reps
- 60 seconds of rest

Chest-supported dumbbell row
- 4 sets × 12 reps
- 2 minutes of rest

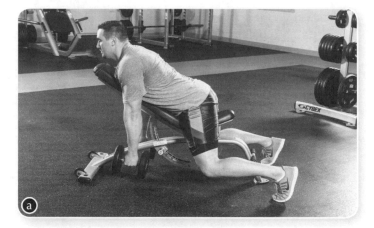

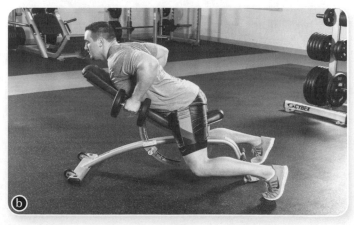

Boxed In

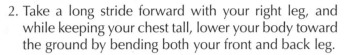

Box jumps are a great exercise to build explosive power and improve vertical jump. However, many people choose a box that is too high and end up developing their hip mobility (by bringing their knees up to their chest in order to land on the box) rather than their jumping ability. Choose a box height that allows you to express your full jumping ability without overemphasizing hip mobility. You'll end up a better athlete in the long run.

Warm-Up

5 reps of squat to stand; 6 reps per side of kneeling adductor stretch, hip rocker, and quadruped T-spine rotation

● Featured Exercise

Barbell Walking Lunge

1. Place a loaded bar on your upper back, across your traps as you would in the barbell back squat (*a*).

2. Take a long stride forward with your right leg, and while keeping your chest tall, lower your body toward the ground by bending both your front and back leg.

3. When your back knee either touches or is an inch (2.5 cm) above the floor (*b*), drive off the front foot to return to the standing position.

4. Repeat the movement, this time starting with the left leg forward. Continue to alternate in this fashion until all reps are complete for both legs.

Complete Workout

Box jump (#198)
- 8 sets × 6 reps
- 60 seconds of rest

Barbell walking lunge
- 8 sets × 5 reps/side
- 60 seconds of rest

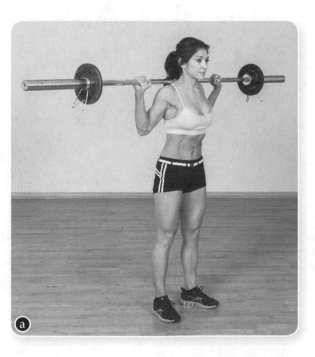

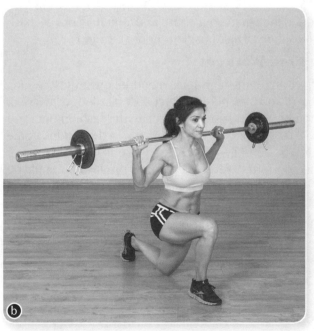

OPTIONS

Easy Option   Reduce the number of sets to 5 for each exercise.

Step It Up   Increase the number of reps for the barbell walking lunge to 8 per side.

Cool-Down   Standing quad stretch, 90-degree stretch, cross-body stretch.

Chest Blaster

Setting a bench press at a high incline allows you to focus more on the musculature of the anterior and medial deltoids (front and top of the shoulders) as well as the top of the chest and triceps, as compared with a traditional flat bench press. Be warned, however, that this position is not as advantageous to moving big weight as the flat barbell bench press, so adjust your load accordingly.

Warm-Up

4 reps per side of the world's greatest stretch, 5 reps of inchworm, 8 reps per side of shoulder sweeps

Featured Exercise

High-Incline Barbell Press

1. At an adjustable bench press station, set the bench at a 60-degree angle.
2. Start with your eyes directly under the bar (a). Lower the bar to your chest just above your nipple level (b). Keep your elbows tucked in toward your rib cage.
3. Touch the bar to your chest, and forcefully drive it back up to the starting position. Repeat for reps.

Complete Workout

Perform 1 rep of the high-incline barbell press. Rest as long as needed, and then perform 2 reps. Rest as long as needed, and then perform 3 reps. Continue in this fashion until you reach 10 reps. Once you reach the top of this ladder, come back down, starting with 10 reps. Rest as long as needed, and then perform 9 reps. Continue in this fashion until you reach 1 rep. Use approximately 60 percent of your 1RM for all sets.

High-incline barbell press
- 1 to 10 reps and back down, as described
- Rest as needed

OPTIONS

Easy Option Perform the ladder up to 6 reps and then back down.

Step It Up Take 3 seconds to lower the bar with each rep.

Cool-Down Pec stretch, double lat stretch, 90-degree stretch.

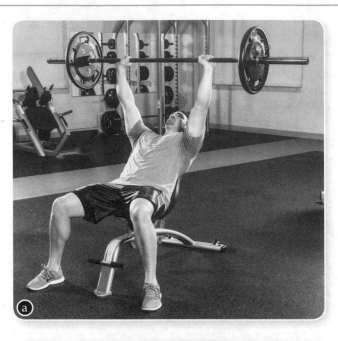

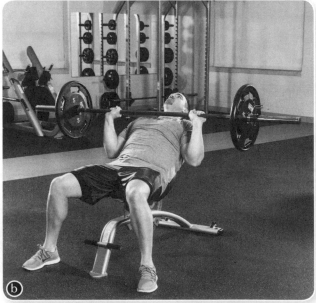

Quadzilla

Since 1954 the movie monster Godzilla has battled such villains as Mothra and Megaguirus in an effort to save Tokyo from destruction. In this workout you will tackle the front squat, back squat, and leg press in an effort to turn your quads into absolute monsters. Get ready to roar.

Warm-Up

5 reps of squat to stand; 6 reps per side of kneeling adductor stretch, hip rocker, and quadruped T-spine rotation

● Featured Exercise

Leg Press

1. Place your feet flat on a leg press platform, assuming the same stance you would use in a squat.

2. Keeping a slight arch in your lower back, unrack the weight and lower the platform under control (a).

3. Utilize a full range of motion by allowing your upper legs to break parallel, keeping your butt on the seat for the entire movement.

4. Once you reach the bottom of the range of motion, drive the platform away by straightening your legs (b). Repeat for reps.

Complete Workout

Complete 4 rounds of the following circuit.

Barbell front squat (#44)
- 4 reps
- 10 seconds of rest

Barbell back squat (#63)
- 4 reps
- 10 seconds of rest

Leg press
- 12 reps
- 2 minutes of rest

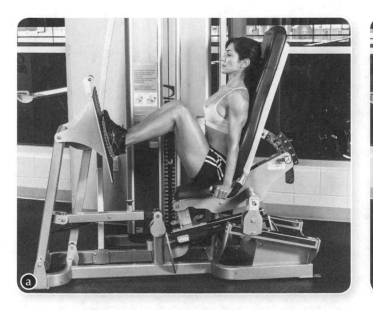

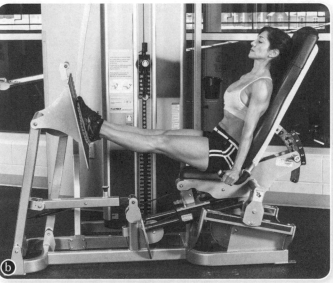

OPTIONS

Easy Option Perform 3 rounds of the circuit.

Step It Up Perform 4 rounds of the circuit.

Cool-Down Standing quad stretch, 90-degree stretch, cross-body stretch.

Push Push Push

Whether it's because of travel, a holiday, or a family event, some days you just can't make it to the gym. That doesn't mean you can't still train. This routine using only body weight works your shoulders and chest efficiently, with no equipment needed (besides a band and a dining room chair, your living room couch, or a bench).

Warm-Up

5 reps of squat to stand; 6 reps per side of kneeling adductor stretch, hip rocker, and quadruped T-spine rotation

● Featured Exercise

Incline Push-Up

1. Facing a bench, chair, or sofa, place your hands firmly on the edge, with your toes on the floor. Maintain a straight line from your head all the way down to your heels (a).
2. Lower your body until your chest touches the edge of the bench, sofa, or chair (b).
3. Return to the starting position and repeat for reps.

Complete Workout

Perform 4 rounds of the following circuit, resting as little as possible between exercises and rounds.

Banded push-up (#3)
- As many reps as possible to failure

Push-up (#12)
- As many reps as possible to failure

Incline push-up
- As many reps as possible to failure
- 2 minutes of rest

OPTIONS

Easy Option Perform sets of 10 reps for each exercise.

Step It Up Add an additional round of the circuit.

Cool-Down Pec stretch, double lat stretch, 90-degree stretch.

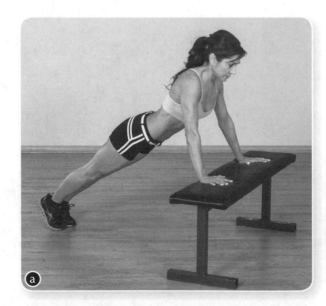
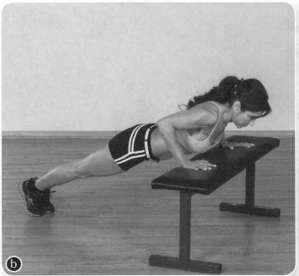

Ham and Aches

Why is this workout called Ham and Aches? Because your hamstrings will be aching by the time you are done. Be sure to utilize the hip hinge (described in chapter 1, Ramping Up) for the Romanian deadlift. This will ensure the emphasis is on the hamstrings (where it belongs) and not on your lower back. If there is no back extension machine in your gym, you can perform the back extensions on a stability ball.

Warm-Up

4 reps per side of the world's greatest stretch, 5 reps each of inchworm and inverted hamstring stretch, 10 reps of glute bridge

● **Featured Exercise**

Back Extension

1. Place your feet securely into a back extension machine.
2. Place your hands across your chest with elbows bent, and lower yourself by folding at the waist (a).
3. Once you reach the bottom of your range, reverse the motion, bringing your body back into a straight line from your head to your heels (b). Fire your glutes and hamstrings at the top (you should not feel stress in your lower back). Repeat for reps.

Complete Workout

Perform 4 rounds of this circuit, resting 30 seconds between exercises and 90 seconds between rounds.

Dumbbell Romanian deadlift (#267)
- 10 reps

Lying hamstring curl (#168)
- 10 reps

Glute–ham raise (#70)
- 10 reps

Back extension
- 10 reps

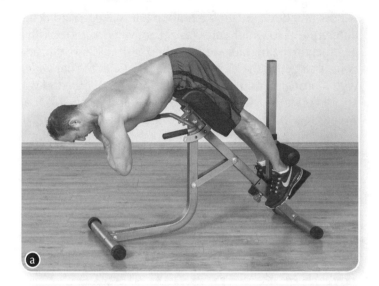

(a)

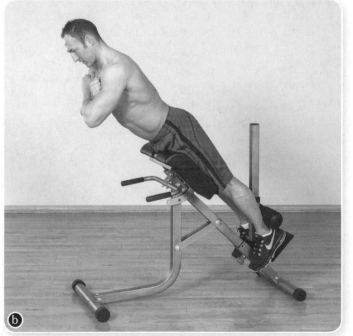

(b)

OPTIONS

Easy Option Replace the lying hamstring curl with a stability ball hamstring curl (#110).

Step It Up Extend a weighted medicine ball overhead during the back extensions.

Cool-Down Double lat stretch, hamstring stretch, calf stretch.

Back Blaster

Where and how you grab a pull-up bar makes a significant difference as to which muscles get activated. Grab it with a neutral grip (palms facing each other) at shoulder width, and you are targeting the biceps and the lats. Grab the bar wider, with a pronated grip (arms facing away from you), and you are targeting much more of the mid- and upper back as well as the forearms. Since the muscles used for pulling in a wide grip are smaller and, usually, less developed, this is often the most challenging position to pull from.

Warm-Up

5 reps of inchworm, 6 reps per side of quadruped T-spine rotation, 10 reps of cat–cow

● Featured Exercise

Wide-Grip Pull-Up

1. Grab a pull-up bar well outside shoulder width.
2. Start every rep in a dead hang (arms totally straight) (*a*).
3. Begin pulling yourself up to the bar by retracting your scapulae and using the muscles in your mid- and upper back as well as your lats and biceps.
4. Bring your chest up to the bar (*b*), and lower yourself with control back to the starting position. Repeat for reps.

Complete Workout

Perform 1 rep of the wide-grip pull-up. Rest as long as needed, and then perform 2 reps. Rest as long as needed, and then perform 3 reps. Continue in this fashion until you reach 10 reps. Once you reach the top of this ladder, come back down, starting with 10 reps. Rest as long as needed, and then perform 9 reps. Continue in this fashion until you reach 1 rep.

Wide-grip pull-up
- 1 to 10 reps and back down, as described

OPTIONS

Easy Option   Perform the ladder up to 6 reps and then back down.

Step It Up   Take 3 seconds to lower yourself with each rep.

Cool-Down   Double lat stretch, cross-body stretch, hamstring stretch.

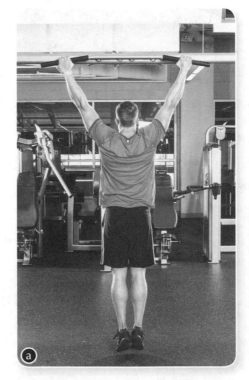
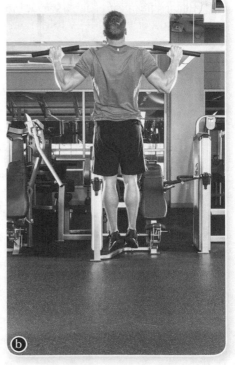

Squat-a-Lot

Possibly more than any other exercise, squat stance and squat depth are very individualized. Because of your specific anatomy, strength, and comfort, you will need to experiment with foot position and angle until you find the optimal setup. And although you should try to squat as deeply as possible (you will get the most athletic benefit and leg development from deep squats), not everyone has the mobility to get down in the hole. Work on increasing your ankle and hip mobility, and if you find you aren't making progress, definitely seek the advice of an experienced lifter or trainer who can troubleshoot your form. The squat is too essential, beneficial, and potentially risky a movement not to be done correctly.

Warm-Up

5 reps of inchworm, 6 reps per side of quadruped T-spine rotation, 10 reps of cat–cow

Complete Workout

Complete 4 rounds of the following circuit.

Goblet squat
- 10 reps
- 30 seconds of rest

Barbell back squat (#63)
- 8 reps
- 30 seconds of rest

Barbell front squat (#44)
- 6 reps
- 30 seconds of rest

Overhead squat (#167)
- 4 reps
- 30 seconds of rest

● Featured Exercise

Goblet Squat

1. Grab a dumbbell at one end by placing your hands in a V and wrapping your hands around the edges (*a*).
2. Keeping your feet slightly turned out at shoulder width, your chest tall and the weight directly in front of your collarbones, unlock your hips and knees and lower your body toward the floor.
3. In a controlled manner, sit as low as possible while maintaining an upright torso (*b*). Once depth is achieved, reverse the movement back to the starting position. Repeat for reps.

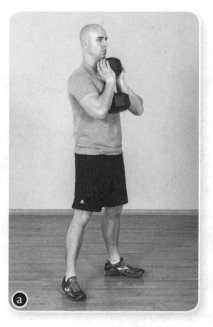
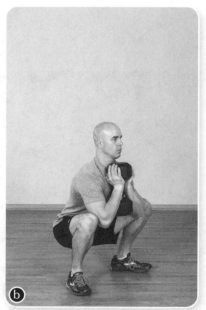

OPTIONS

Easy Option   Perform 3 rounds of the circuit.

Step It Up   Add 2 reps per set to each of the exercises.

Cool-Down   Double lat stretch, cross-body stretch, hamstring stretch.

Mechanical Bench Drop

This workout is for those of you who love the bench press (which, last I checked, is pretty much everyone). You will utilize a mechanical drop set featuring three different angles of the barbell bench press, beginning with the most challenging (incline), progressing to flat, and finishing up with decline.

Warm-Up

4 reps per side of the world's greatest stretch, 5 reps of inchworm, 8 reps per side of shoulder sweeps

● Featured Exercise

Decline Bench Press

1. At a decline bench press station, grab the bar just outside shoulder width, and unrack it from the barbell catches (a).

2. Keeping a slight natural arch in your lower back, lower the bar until it touches your torso at midchest level. Keep your elbows tucked toward your side as you lower the bar (b).

3. Forcefully drive the weight back up until you achieve lockout of your elbows. Repeat for reps.

Complete Workout

Perform 5 rounds of the following circuit, keeping the same weight on the bar for each movement.

Incline barbell bench press (#179)
- 6 reps
- 15 seconds of rest

Barbell bench press (#54)
- 6 reps
- 15 seconds of rest

Decline bench press
- 12 reps
- 2 minutes of rest

OPTIONS

Easy Option   Reduce to 4 rounds of the circuit.

Step It Up   Increase reps to 8 for both the incline barbell bench press and barbell bench press.

Cool-Down   Pec stretch, double lat stretch, 90-degree stretch.

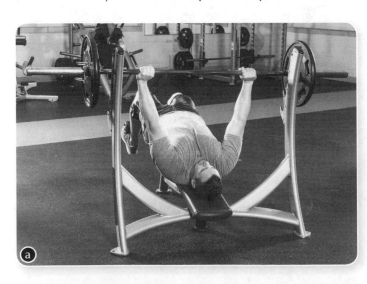

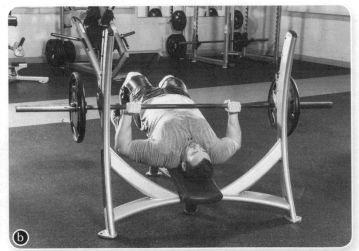

Lots of Lats

Although there is no substituting for the pull-up, there are many people who simply cannot perform this tough movement for higher-rep sets. Enter the lat pull-down, which can be a great substitution until you have built up strength in the pull-up. Even better is the kneeling lat pull-down (featured in this workout) because it more closely mimics the positioning of your body in the pull-up, allowing your glutes to fire in conjunction with your lats—an important muscular relationship.

Warm-Up

5 reps of inchworm, 6 reps per side of quadruped T-spine rotation, 10 reps of cat–cow

● Featured Exercise

Kneeling Lat Pull-Down

1. Grab a lat pull-down bar with a wider than shoulder-width overhand grip.
2. Kneel with your knees on the floor directly behind the seat (a).
3. Keep your chest tall, squeeze your glutes, and pull the bar down to your collarbones (b).
4. Return the bar to the starting position and repeat for reps.

Complete Workout

A. Chin-up (#73)
- 4 sets × 4 reps
- 60 seconds of rest

B1. Kneeling lat pull-down
- 2 sets × 8 to 10 reps
- 60 seconds of rest

B2. Alternating dumbbell row (#246)
- 2 sets × 6 to 8 reps/side
- 60 seconds of rest

B3. Straight-arm cable pull-down (#139)
- 2 sets × 8 to 10 reps
- 60 seconds of rest

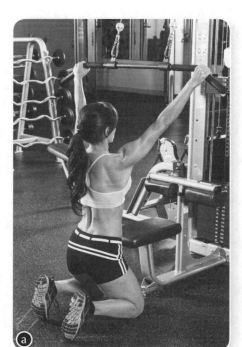

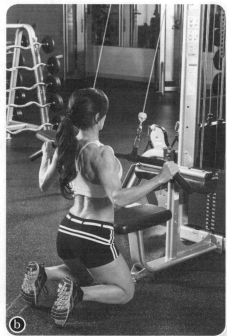

OPTIONS

Easy Option   Complete 3 reps per set of the chin-up.

Step It Up   Perform 3 sets of the kneeling lat pull-down, alternating dumbbell row, and straight-arm cable pull-down.

Cool-Down   Double lat stretch, cross-body stretch, hamstring stretch.

Get a Leg Up

If walking is important to you over the next day or two, you may want to reconsider giving this workout a try. By combining a series of movements that all focus on knee flexion (bending at the knee), your quads will certainly feel as if they've been crushed long after the workout has finished.

Warm-Up

5 reps of squat to stand; 6 reps per side of kneeling adductor stretch, hip rocker, and quadruped T-spine rotation

● Featured Exercise

Dumbbell Step-Up

1. Choose a set of dumbbells and stand in front of a step or plyo box (a). Place your left foot on the plyo box. Your knee should be at a 90-degree angle (b).
2. Drive the heel of your left foot down into the box to straighten your left leg. Lift your right foot and bring it alongside your left on top of the box (c).

3. Lower your right foot down to the floor, followed by your left foot. Step your right foot back up to the box and then repeat all the steps, this time focusing on driving the heel of your right foot to straighten your right leg, bringing your left foot alongside it.
4. Bring your left foot down, followed by your right. That is one complete repetition.

Complete Workout

Barbell front squat (#44)
- 4 sets × 6 reps
- 90 seconds of rest

Dumbbell step-up
- 4 sets × 10 reps per leg
- 60 seconds of rest

Leg press (#114)
- 4 sets × 15 reps
- 60 seconds of rest

OPTIONS

Easy Option   Utilize a goblet squat (#2) instead of the front squat.

Step It Up   Complete an additional set of each of the exercises.

Cool-Down   Standing quad stretch, 90-degree stretch, cross-body stretch.

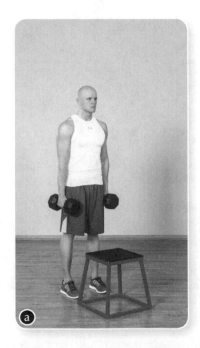
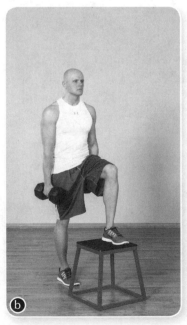
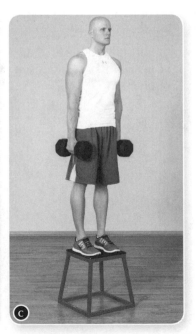

Shoulder Shredder

Whether you are looking for bowling ball delts to help you fill out a T-shirt or shapely shoulders to hold up the straps of your sundress, this shoulder shredder is the answer to your prayers. Just don't blame me if you have a hard time raising your hand in class or hailing a taxi for the rest of the day.

Warm-Up

4 reps per side of the world's greatest stretch, 5 reps of inchworm, 8 reps per side of shoulder sweeps

● Featured Exercise

Front Raise

1. Grab a pair of dumbbells and hold them in front of your thighs with your arms straight and palms facing you (*a*).
2. Lift both dumbbells simultaneously up to shoulder height being sure to keep your arms straight (*b*).
3. Return to start position and repeat for reps.

Complete Workout

Perform all three movements back to back using one set of dumbbells.

A. Push press (#16)
   - 4 sets × 3 reps
   - 60 seconds of rest

B1. Incline dumbbell chest press (#210)
   - 2 sets × 8 reps

B2. Cable diagonal raise (#137)
   - 2 sets × 8 reps
   - 45 seconds of rest

C. Front raise, lateral raise (#147), and seated dumbbell shoulder press (#209)
   - 2 sets of 15 reps per movement

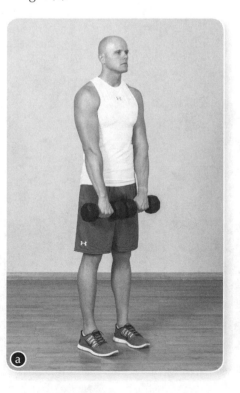

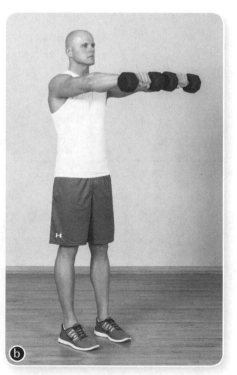

OPTIONS

Easy Option Perform 1 set of the final circuit.

Step It Up Add 1 set to the incline dumbbell chest press and the cable diagonal raise.

Cool-Down Pec stretch, double lat stretch, 90-degree stretch.

Medicine Man

Although many explosive movements, such as the snatch and the clean, require that you decelerate the barbell, medicine ball training allows for a more full expression of power by allowing you to release the ball at the end range of motion. This difference in technique also has greater carryover to pitching, throwing, leaping, and other athletic activities.

Warm-Up

4 reps per side of the world's greatest stretch, 5 reps of inchworm, 8 reps per side of shoulder sweeps

● Featured Exercise

Medicine Ball Chest Pass

1. Begin in a standing position, feet at hip width and facing forward.

2. Grab a medicine ball (4-8 lbs) and hold it to your chest with your elbows tucked toward your rib cage (a).

3. Explosively throw the ball forward by fully extending your arms to either a partner (b) or padded wall. Repeat for reps.

Complete Workout

Perform 6 sets of the following exercise combination.

Medicine ball chest pass
- 3 reps
- 30 seconds of rest

Barbell bench press (#54)
- 8 reps
- 2 minutes of rest

OPTIONS

Easy Option Reduce the number of reps of the barbell bench press to 6 per set.

Step It Up Increase the number of medicine ball chest passes to 5 per set.

Cool-Down Pec stretch, double lat stretch, 90-degree stretch.

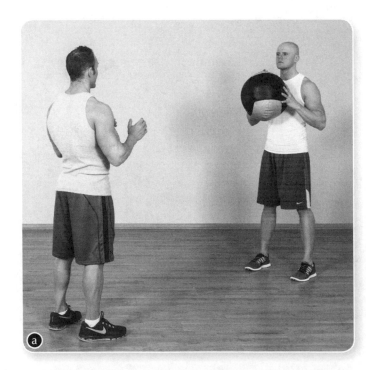

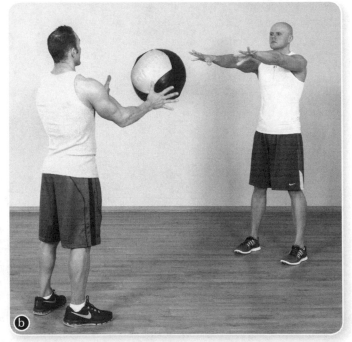

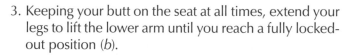

6-12-25 Quads

Whether your goal is a massive set of quads to pop out of your shorts or a pair of sexy gams to put on top of 4-inch stiletto heels, this workout will help you get the legs you are looking for. But be warned: No one said getting the legs you always dreamed of was going to be easy, so be prepared for a bit of postworkout soreness for a couple of days after you finish this one.

Warm-Up

5 reps of squat to stand; 6 reps per side of kneeling adductor stretch, hip rocker, and quadruped T-spine rotation

● Featured Exercise

Leg Extension

1. Adjust the back pad at a leg extension station so that, when you sit, your knee joint is aligned with the hinge joint of the machine (your knees should be just off the end of the seat).

2. Sit with your chest tall and your shins touching the ankle pad (a).

3. Keeping your butt on the seat at all times, extend your legs to lift the lower arm until you reach a fully locked-out position (b).

4. Control the lever arm back to the start position and repeat for reps.

Complete Workout

Perform the following three exercises as a circuit, resting 10 seconds between exercises and 100 seconds between rounds. Repeat the circuit a total of 4 times.

Barbell front squat (#44)
- 6 reps
- 10 seconds of rest

Barbell walking lunge (#112)
- 12 reps
- 10 seconds of rest

Leg extension
- 25 reps
- 100 seconds of rest

OPTIONS

Easy Option   Perform 15 reps of the leg extension.

Step It Up   Add an additional round, bringing the total number of circuits to 5.

Cool-Down   Standing quad stretch, 90-degree stretch, cross-body stretch.

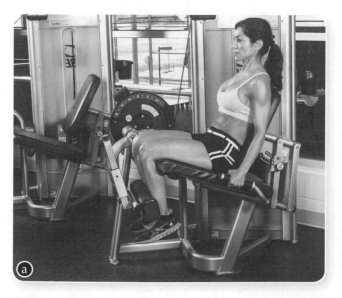

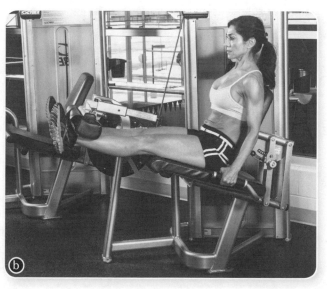

Back in Action

Is a rear lateral raise a shoulder exercise or a back exercise? The answer is both. A rear lateral raise certainly hits the posterior deltoid, which is often the least worked aspect of the shoulder. But it also works the rhomboids, middle traps, teres major, and other important muscles of the upper back. The underhand version of the movement (featured in this workout) also hits the rotator cuff, smaller muscles that are key to keeping your shoulders healthy.

Warm-Up

5 reps of inchworm, 6 reps per side of quadruped T-spine rotation, 10 reps of cat–cow

● Featured Exercise

Standing Underhand Rear Lateral Raise

1. Grab a pair of dumbbells, and bend forward at the hips until your torso is almost parallel to the floor. Maintain a slight bend in your knees.

2. Start with the dumbbells hanging down directly beneath your shoulders, with your palms facing forward (*a*).

3. Raise your arms straight out to the sides until they are in line with your body (*b*). Maintain the position of your torso, and do not bend your arms as you raise them.

4. Control the dumbbells back to the starting position. Repeat for reps.

Complete Workout

A. Neutral-grip pull-up (#237)
   - 3 sets × 8 reps
   - 60 seconds of rest

B1. Face pull (#127)
   - 3 sets × 8 reps
   - 60 seconds of rest

B2. Standing underhand rear lateral raise
   - 3 sets × 12 reps
   - 60 seconds of rest

OPTIONS

Easy Option   Perform 2 sets of each movement.

Step It Up   Perform 4 sets of each movement.

Cool-Down   Double lat stretch, cross-body stretch, hamstring stretch.

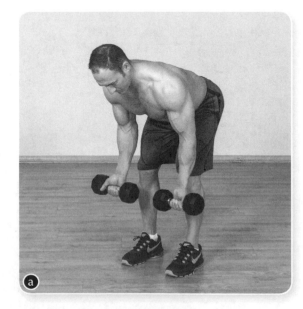

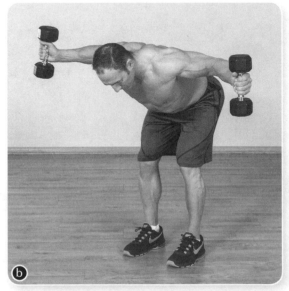

Spider-Man

Some exercises work well as strength exercises in their own right or can be incorporated into your dynamic warm-up. The Spider-Man push-up (featured in this workout) is one such exercise. To use it in the warm-up, perform the hands-walking-out portion of the inchworm (see chapter 1, Ramping Up), perform one Spider-Man push-up per leg, and then walk yourself up to standing. Complete all remaining reps in this manner.

Warm-Up

4 reps per side of the world's greatest stretch, 5 reps of inchworm, 8 reps per side of shoulder sweeps

Featured Exercise

Spider-Man Push-Up

1. Start in a push-up position with your hands slightly wider than your shoulders, your arms straight, and your body forming a straight line from your head to your heels.

2. Bend at the elbows to lower yourself toward the floor (keep your elbows tucked back toward your rib cage). As you are lowering, simultaneously lift your left foot off the floor, swing your left leg out to the side, and try to touch your knee to your elbow (a).

3. Reverse the movement of your leg. Once your foot reaches the floor, push yourself back up to the starting position (b). Repeat on the opposite side (c), and continue to alternate for reps.

Complete Workout

A. Barbell bench press (#54)
- 5 sets × 4 reps
- 90 seconds of rest

B1. Incline dumbbell chest press (#210)
- 3 sets × 10 reps
- 60 seconds of rest

B2. Spider-Man push-up
- 3 sets × 8 reps/side
- 60 seconds of rest

B3. Low-to-high cable chest fly (#157)
- 3 sets × 12 reps
- 60 seconds of rest

OPTIONS

Easy Option Perform 2 sets of the incline dumbbell bench press, Spider-Man push-up, and low-to-high cable chest fly.

Step It Up Add 2 reps to each set of the incline dumbbell bench press, Spider-Man push-up, and low-to-high cable chest fly.

Cool-Down Pec stretch, double lat stretch, 90-degree stretch.

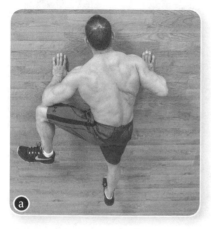
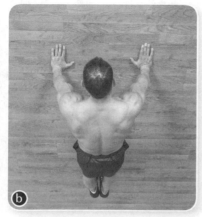
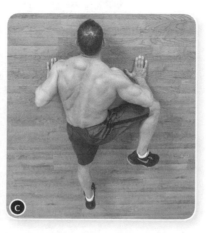

In Your Face

Shoulder health and improved posture are two of the most overlooked aspects of many training programs. Keeping your shoulder joints functioning and injury free are obviously critical for progressing your pressing movements such as the bench press. And improving posture will instantly give you the appearance of improved body composition. The face pull, which is a featured exercise in this workout, helps solve both these issues by strengthening the musculature of the rotator cuff and upper back while training a tall, shoulders-down posture.

Warm-Up

5 reps of inchworm, 6 reps per side of quadruped T-spine rotation, 10 reps of cat–cow

● Featured Exercise

Face Pull

1. Attach a rope handle at slightly below forehead height at a cable station.
2. Utilizing a parallel stance, grab each end of the rope with an overhand grip (*a*).

3. Keeping your elbows high and shoulders depressed, pull the rope until your hands are directly over your shoulders at ear height (*b*). Your upper arms should be parallel to the floor.
4. Return the rope to the starting position by extending your arms. Repeat for reps.

Complete Workout

Complete 4 rounds of the following circuit.

Wide-grip pull-up (#117)
- 8 reps
- 60 seconds of rest

Face pull
- 12 reps
- 60 seconds of rest

Seated cable row with hip flexion (#174)
- 15 reps
- 60 seconds of rest

OPTIONS

Easy Option   Complete 3 sets of the circuit.

Step It Up   Increase wide-grip pull-up to 10 reps.

Cool-Down   Double lat stretch, cross-body stretch, hamstring stretch.

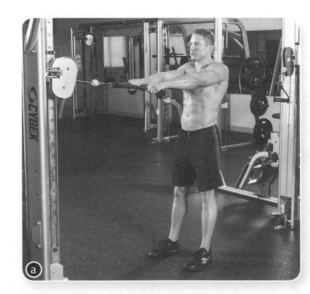

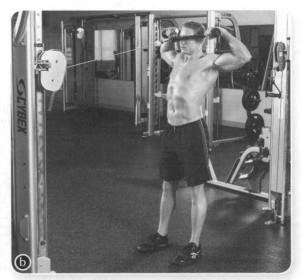

Lots of Squats

Besides being a great leg developer, squats are one of the most metabolically demanding exercises around. So why not combine different squat variations in all their glory for a killer workout? That's exactly what this workout provides, combining explosive, strength, and unilateral versions of this essential movement pattern.

Warm-Up

5 reps of squat to stand; 6 reps per side of kneeling adductor stretch, hip rocker, and quadruped T-spine rotation

● Featured Exercise

Prisoner Jump Squat

1. Place your hands behind your head with your fingers intertwined. Do not pull your neck down or forward (a).
2. Bring your hips back, and bend your knees until you are in a full squat position (b).

3. Reverse the motion and jump off the ground (c). Land with knees slightly flexed, and proceed directly to the next rep. Repeat for reps.

Complete Workout

Complete 4 rounds of the following circuit.

Prisoner jump squat
- 10 reps

Barbell back squat (#63)
- 10 reps

Barbell front-foot elevated split squat (#140)
- 10 reps

Prisoner jump squat
- 10 reps
- 3 minutes of rest

OPTIONS

Easy Option Perform only 5 reps of each of the squat variations.

Step It Up Place an unloaded barbell on your back for the jump squats.

Cool-Down Standing quad stretch, 90-degree stretch, cross-body stretch.

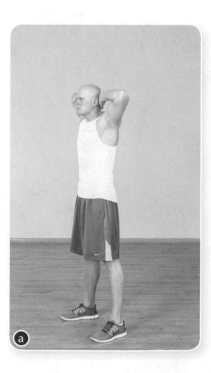

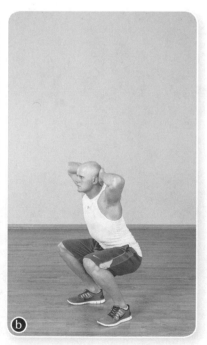

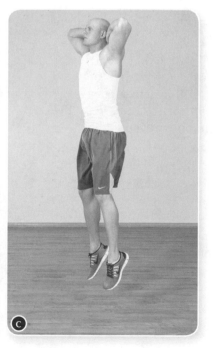

The Ahnold

Named after legendary bodybuilder Arnold Schwarzenegger, the Arnold press increases the range of motion of the dumbbell overhead shoulder press by placing the dumbbells in front of your shoulders in the starting position, placing more emphasis on the anterior (front) head of the deltoid and upper chest. Given that Arnold is considered to have the best chest and shoulder development in the history of bodybuilding, this is definitely a move worth incorporating into your workouts.

Warm-Up

4 reps per side of the world's greatest stretch, 5 reps of inchworm, 8 reps per side of shoulder sweeps

Complete Workout

A. Incline dumbbell chest press (#210)
- 4 sets × 6 reps
- 90 seconds of rest

B1. Seated Arnold press
- 3 sets × 10 reps
- 60 seconds of rest

B2. Lateral raise (#147)
- 3 sets × 10 reps
- 60 seconds of rest

OPTIONS

Easy Option   Perform 3 sets of the incline dumbbell chest press.

Step It Up   Add 1 set to the lateral raise and seated Arnold press.

Cool-Down   Pec stretch, double lat stretch, 90-degree stretch.

⬤ Featured Exercise

Seated Arnold Press

1. Sit on an adjustable bench at a 90-degree angle. Grab a pair of dumbbells, and start with them directly in front of your shoulders, with your palms facing you (*a*).

2. Rotate your hands outward (until they are facing away from you), and press the dumbbells overhead (*b*).

3. Drive the dumbbells completely overhead until your elbows are locked out. Your biceps should be adjacent to your ears in the top position.

4. Lower the dumbbells to the bottom position (making sure to rotate your hands at the bottom). Repeat for reps.

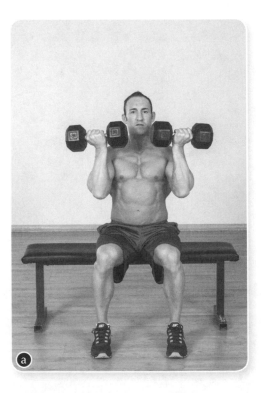
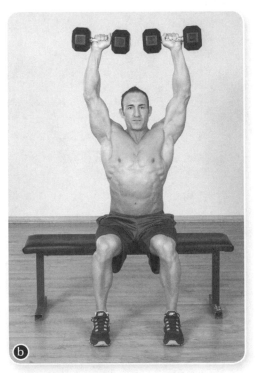

Step It Up

Although step-ups are a knee extension exercise (you start with a bent knee and straighten it), which may look similar to a leg extension or leg press, they should actually be treated as a hip extension exercise. So instead of focusing on straightening your knee, focus on driving your hip forward so you get more out of your posterior chain. Will your quads do some of the work? Certainly. But don't discount how much your hamstrings and glutes should be contributing to the movement.

Warm-Up

4 reps per side of the world's greatest stretch, 5 reps each of inchworm and inverted hamstring stretch, 10 reps of glute bridge

● Featured Exercise

Barbell Lateral Step-Up

1. With a barbell across your traps, stand directly to the right of a bench or box, and place your left foot on top of the step (*a*).

2. Keeping your chest tall, drive your left foot into the box, fully extending your knee (your right foot should remain off the side of the box) (*b*).

3. Lower your body under control until your right foot reaches the ground (your left foot remains on top of the box). Complete all reps for one leg before switching to the other.

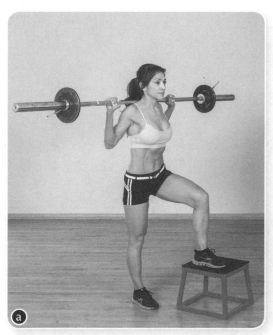

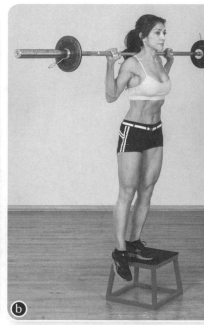

Complete Workout

A. Barbell front squat (#44)
- 4 sets × 3 reps
- 90 seconds of rest

B1. Barbell lateral step-up
- 3 sets × 6 reps/side
- 30 seconds of rest

B2. Leg extension (#124)
- 3 sets × 10 reps
- 30 seconds of rest

B3. Reverse hyperextension (#263)
- 3 sets × 12 reps
- 30 seconds of rest

OPTIONS

Easy Option Reduce the number of sets of the barbell lateral step-up, leg extension, and reverse hyperextension to 2.

Step It Up Add one set to each of the exercises.

Cool-Down Double lat stretch, cross-body stretch, hamstring stretch.

Armed Forces

For some reason, in today's functional fitness world, training your arms has gotten a bad rap. However, arm strength and size can be useful in all manner of sports (think of a lineman in American football), other lifts (Who couldn't use a stronger grip on their deadlift?), and daily tasks (Have you ever tried carrying your suitcase through an airport?). This workout combines compound movements such as chin-ups and a close-grip bench press with isolation moves to deliver a true arm blaster.

Warm-Up

4 reps per side of the world's greatest stretch, 5 reps of inchworm, 8 reps per side of shoulder sweeps

● Featured Exercise

Close-Grip Bench Press

1. Load a barbell at a bench press station. Lie back with your eyes directly under the bar, your feet, glutes, upper back, and head on the bench.
2. Grab the bar at slightly inside shoulder width (a).
3. Lower the bar to the middle of your chest, keeping your elbows tucked toward your sides (b).
4. Forcefully return the bar to the starting position and repeat for reps.

Complete Workout

A1. Chin-up (#73)
- 3 sets × 8 reps
- 60 seconds of rest

A2. Close-grip bench press
- 3 sets × 8 reps
- 60 seconds of rest

B1. Three-position EZ-bar curl (#151)
- 3 sets × 10 reps
- 60 seconds of rest

B2. Decline EZ-bar triceps extension (#145)
- 3 sets × 10 reps
- 60 seconds of rest

OPTIONS

Easy Option   Use a kneeling lat pull-down (#120) or pull-up assistance machine to replace the chin-ups.

Step It Up   Add additional weight to the chin-ups by using a weighted vest or dip belt.

Cool-Down   Double lat stretch, cross-body stretch, hamstring stretch.

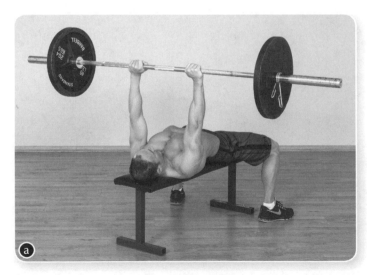

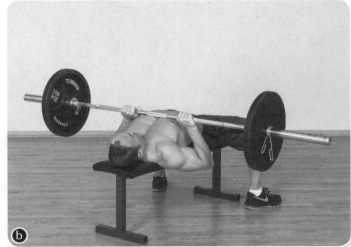

Dead Start

By eliminating the stretch–shortening cycle (the active stretch of a muscle followed by an immediate shortening of that same muscle), usually associated with jumps and other plyometrics, the dead-start jump featured in this workout relies solely on stored muscle tension to express force. Although this can help you develop power, it will limit the height and distance of your jump. So plan accordingly, and use a lower box than you otherwise might choose for box jumps.

Warm-Up

5 reps of squat to stand; 6 reps per side of kneeling adductor stretch, hip rocker, and quadruped T-spine rotation

● Featured Exercise

Dead-Start Jump

1. Place two boxes of varying heights approximately 3 feet (1 m) away from each other (distance will vary based on your height).

2. Sit on the edge of the smaller box, with your chest tall, feet flat in front of you, and knees bent at 90 degrees (*a*).

3. Without generating any momentum by rocking your body forward, drive your feet into the ground and jump onto the higher box (*b*).

4. Land with knees flexed (*c*). Step off the box and repeat for reps.

Complete Workout

A. Dead-start jump
 • 4 sets × 6 reps

B1. Barbell front squat (#44)
 • 3 sets × 4 to 6 reps
 • 90 seconds of rest

B2. Barbell front-foot elevated split squat (#140)
 • 3 sets × 6 to 8 reps/leg
 • 90 seconds of rest

B3. Leg press (#114)
 • 3 sets × 8 to 10 reps
 • 90 seconds of rest

OPTIONS

Easy Option Perform 2 sets of the barbell front squat, leg press, and barbell front-foot elevated split squat.

Step It Up Perform 4 sets of the barbell front squat, leg press, and barbell front-foot elevated split squat.

Cool-Down Standing quad stretch, 90-degree stretch, cross-body stretch.

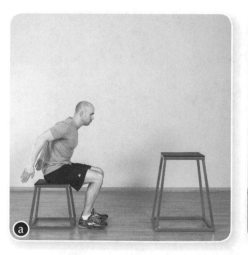

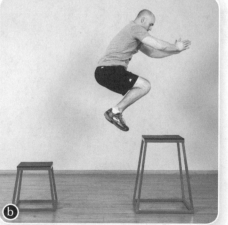

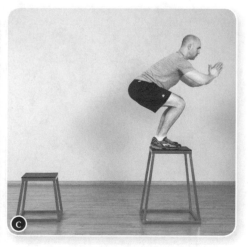

Chest Pain

When it comes to hypertrophy (building muscle), volume—the total amount of work done—is the name of the game. Blasting the same muscle group with different movements repeatedly in the same session is not optimal for building strength, but if getting bigger is the goal, you can't beat multiple exercises for the same muscle group.

Warm-Up

4 reps per side of the world's greatest stretch, 5 reps of inchworm, 8 reps per side of shoulder sweeps

● **Featured Exercise**

Decline Dumbbell Chest Fly

1. Grab a pair of dumbbells, and lie faceup on a decline bench.
2. Hold the dumbbells over your chest with the palms facing each other. Your elbows should be slightly bent (a).
3. Slowly lower the dumbbells down and slightly back toward your shoulders until the dumbbells are directly in line with your shoulders (b). Keep the bend in your elbows static throughout the entire lift.
4. Lift the dumbbells back up to the starting position and repeat for reps.

Complete Workout

A. Barbell bench press (#54)
   - 4 sets × 8 reps
   - 90 seconds of rest

B1. High-to-low cable fly (#62)
   - 2 sets × 10 reps
   - 30 seconds of rest

B2. Decline dumbbell chest fly
   - 2 sets × 12 reps
   - 30 seconds of rest

B3. Banded push-up (#3)
   - 2 sets × 20 reps
   - 30 seconds of rest

OPTIONS

Easy Option   Substitute push-ups (#12) for the banded push-ups.

Step It Up   Add 2 reps per set to the lying cable chest fly and 5 reps to the banded push-ups.

Cool-Down   Pec stretch, double lat stretch, 90-degree stretch.

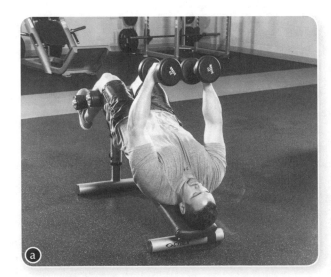

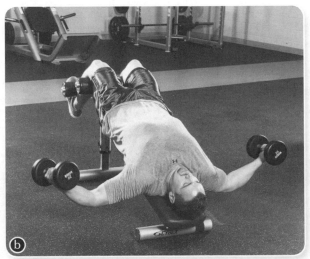

Lean Away

One of the keys to overall upper body strength is developing the smaller muscles of the midback. Although the lats and upper traps tend to get much of the glory, the rhomboids, posterior delts, and middle and lower traps are critical for achieving full range of motion on your pulling exercises and creating a good "shelf" on your pressing exercises. The lean away chin-up featured in this workout is a great way to begin working these typically weaker muscles in the eccentric (lowering) phase.

Warm-Up

5 reps of inchworm, 6 reps per side of quadruped T-spine rotation, 10 reps of cat–cow

● Featured Exercise

Lean-Away Chin-Up

1. Grab a pull-up bar with a supinated grip (palms facing you) at shoulder width (a).
2. Depress your shoulder blades and pull yourself up to the bar, trying to touch the bar with your chest.
3. Once you reach the top of the range of motion, lean back to achieve a more horizontal position in relation to the bar (b).
4. Maintain that position as you lower yourself back to the starting position (c). Repeat for reps.

Complete Workout

Complete 4 rounds of the following circuit.

Lean-away chin-up
- 8 reps
- 60 seconds of rest

Seated cable row with hip flexion (#174)
- 10 reps
- 90 seconds of rest

Straight-arm cable pull-down (#139)
- 12 reps
- 90 seconds of rest

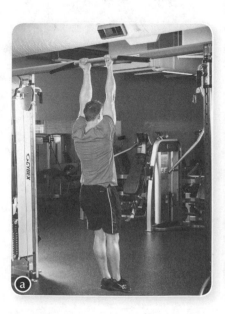
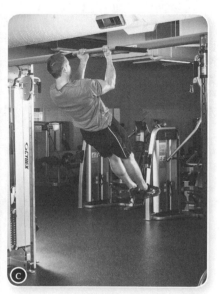
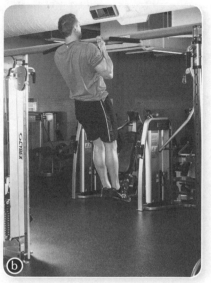

OPTIONS

Easy Option Replace the lean-away chin-up with the chin-up (#73) or kneeling lat pull-down (#120).

Step It Up Add additional load to the lean-away chin-up.

Cool-Down Double lat stretch, cross-body stretch, hamstring stretch.

Tri This

When it comes to fat-loss nutrition, for most people the issue is not about what types of foods to eat, it's about preparing those foods and having them available to you during meal times. Taking a couple of evenings out of your week (say, Sunday and Wednesday) to prepare meals to have with you at work or school will pay off hugely if you are looking to lose weight. In fact, if fat loss is your main goal, preparing and eating quality meals is probably more important than working out those two times per week. So take a couple of nights off from the gym and prepare some meals that will help you reach your goals.

Warm-Up

5 reps of inchworm, 6 reps per side of quadruped T-spine rotation, 10 reps of cat–cow

Complete Workout

A. Barbell floor press (#166)
- 4 sets × 6 reps
- 90 seconds of rest

B1. Single-arm cable press-down
- 3 sets × 10 reps/side
- 45 seconds of rest

B2. Decline EZ-bar triceps extension (#145)
- 3 sets × 10 reps
- 45 seconds of rest

● Featured Exercise

Single-Arm Cable Press-Down

OPTIONS

Easy Option   Perform 2 sets of the single-arm cable press-down and decline EZ-bar triceps extension.

Step It Up   Add one more set to the single-arm cable press-down and decline EZ-bar triceps extension.

Cool-Down   Double lat stretch, cross-body stretch, hamstring stretch.

1. Attach a D handle to the high pulley of a cable station. Grab the handle with a pronated grip (palm facing the floor). Lean your torso slightly forward, and bend at your knees (a).

2. Keeping your upper arm locked to your rib cage, extend at the elbow until your arm is straight (b). Squeeze your triceps at the end position.

3. Bring your forearm back up until it is parallel to the floor. Repeat for reps on one side before switching to the other.

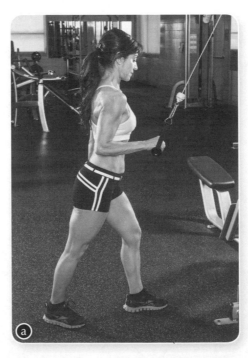
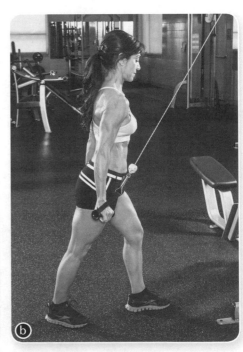

The Calf Jumped Over the Moon

Although it's very important to adhere to the safety precautions listed on training equipment, occasionally you will find that some machines can serve multiple purposes. In the leg press calf raise featured in this workout, you'll be using the leg press machine to overload your calves and really stress the gastrocnemius. So, although you don't want to get too creative with your exercise selection and equipment use, it can be an advantage to think outside the box in order to tax your muscles in a new way.

Warm-Up

4 reps per side of the world's greatest stretch, 5 reps each of inchworm and inverted hamstring stretch, 10 reps of glute bridge

Featured Exercise

Leg Press Calf Raise

1. Sit in a leg press machine with just your forefoot on the bottom of the platform (the heel of your foot should be off the bottom). Straighten your legs to unrack, and keep them locked out (a).

2. Without bending your knees, point your toes away to extend your calves (b). Pause for 2 seconds.

3. Slowly allow the platform to lower until you feel a big stretch in your calves. Pause for 2 seconds.

4. Continue to flex and extend for all reps before reracking the platform.

Complete Workout

A. Barbell front squat (#44)
- 4 sets × 6 reps
- 90 seconds of rest

B1. Leg press calf raise
- 3 sets × 10 reps
- 45 seconds of rest

B2. Seated calf raise (#154)
- 3 sets × 10 reps
- 45 seconds of rest

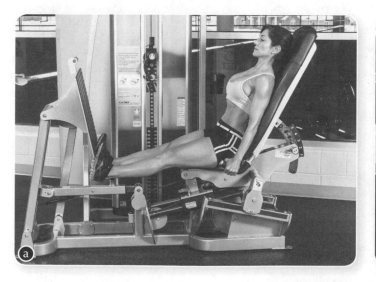
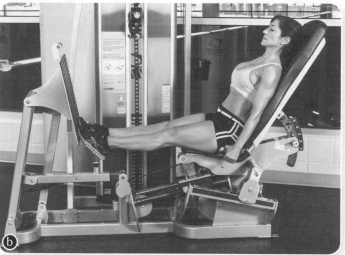

OPTIONS

Easy Option Perform 2 sets of the leg press calf raise and seated calf raise.

Step It Up Add 1 set to the leg press calf raise and seated calf raise.

Cool-Down Standing quad stretch, 90-degree stretch, cross-body stretch.

Shoulder the Burden

One of the most controversial and often-debated exercises is the upright row. Proponents believe it is a great shoulder builder and precursor to the pulls required in the Olympic lifts. Others believe that upright rows put you on the fast track to shoulder injury. So, who's right? Turns out, both arguments have validity (except for the part about the Olympic lifts, which are completely different). Different people have different acromion types (a specific bone formation in the shoulder); some people can handle upright rows with no problem, while others risk shoulder impingement with this movement pattern. Because two-thirds of the population have disadvantageous acromia to perform this exercise pain free, it's better to be safe than sorry. There are plenty of other movements that can help strengthen and build your shoulders, such as the cable diagonal raise.

Warm-Up

4 reps per side of the world's greatest stretch, 5 reps of inchworm, 8 reps per side of shoulder sweeps

● Featured Exercise

OPTIONS

Easy Option Perform 2 sets of the seated dumbbell shoulder press, cable diagonal raise, and face pull.

Step It Up Reduce rest on the seated dumbbell shoulder press, cable diagonal raise, and face pull to 30 seconds.

Cool-Down Pec stretch, double lat stretch, 90-degree stretch.

Cable Diagonal Raise

1. Attach a D handle to the low pulley of a cable station. Standing with your left side toward the weight stack, grab the handle with your right hand just in front of your left hip (a).

2. With a slight bend in your elbow, pull the handle up and across your body until you have externally rotated your shoulder as far as possible (b).

3. Return the cable to the starting position. Repeat all reps for one side before switching to the other.

Complete Workout

A. Push press (#16)
- 4 sets × 4 reps
- 90 seconds of rest

B1. Seated dumbbell shoulder press (#209)
- 3 sets × 8 reps
- 45 seconds of rest

B2. Cable diagonal raise
- 3 sets × 8 reps/side
- 45 seconds of rest

B3. Face pull (#127)
- 3 sets × 10 reps
- 45 seconds of rest

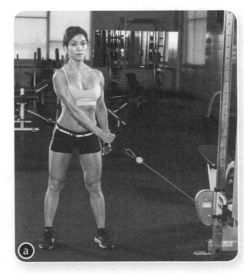
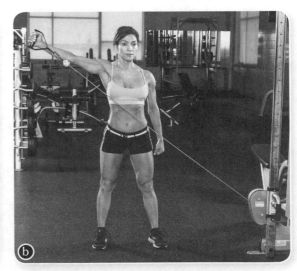

2-Minute Leg Press

Can you get a great workout in 2 minutes? Well, not if you work out for only 2 minutes per day, every day. However, I guarantee if you put an all-out effort into this drill, you will have a hard time getting in and out of your easy chair for the next 2 days. The 2-minute leg press was designed as a way for downhill skiers to mimic the demands of a full run down the slopes. For you, the 2-minute leg press is one of the ultimate tests of strength, endurance, mental toughness, and guts. The goal is to get at least 50 reps with approximately 60 percent of your 1RM. Do so, and I guarantee it will take a lot more than 2 minutes to recover. This exercise also makes for a great finisher at the end of a leg day.

Warm-Up

5 reps of squat to stand; 6 reps per side of kneeling adductor stretch, hip rocker, and quadruped T-spine rotation

● Featured Exercise

Leg Press

1. Sit in the chair of a leg press station. Keep your chest tall and your head against the pad, and maintain a slight arch in your lower back.

2. Unlock the safety mechanism, and lower the sled until you have achieved a full range of motion (a). Drive it back up to the starting position to complete 1 rep (b).

3. Your foot position on this movement will determine the muscles that are emphasized. Keeping your feet narrow and low on the pad will make the movement more quad dominant, while a wider stance with feet toward the top edge of the pad will make the leg press more of a glutes exercise.

Complete Workout

Load a leg press with approximately 60 percent of your 1RM, and perform as many reps as possible for 2 minutes.

Leg press
- 2 minutes × as many reps as possible

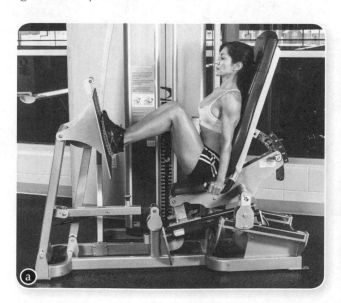
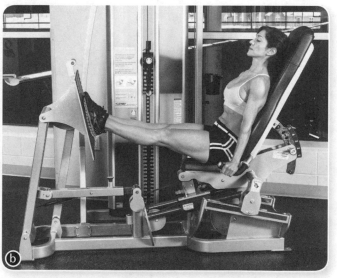

OPTIONS

Easy Option Use 50 percent of your 1RM.

Step It Up Use 70 percent of your 1RM.

Cool-Down Standing quad stretch, 90-degree stretch, cross-body stretch.

6-12-25 Back

Your posterior chain (those muscles you cannot see in the mirror) is truly the most responsible for delivering world-class athletic performance. This workout combines a strength, size, and endurance component of all the major muscle groups in your back—so you'll be prepared for whatever happens on the court, field, pool, or track.

Warm-Up

5 reps of inchworm, 6 reps per side of quadruped T-spine rotation, 10 reps of cat–cow

● Featured Exercise

Straight-Arm Cable Pull-Down

1. Attach a straight bar to a high cable station.
2. Grab the bar with a shoulder-width overhand grip. Your knees should be slightly bent, and your torso should be leaning slightly forward (*a*).
3. Start the motion with your arms at shoulder height. Keeping your arms straight, pull the bar down until it reaches your midthighs (*b*). Contract your lats and return the bar to the starting position. Repeat for reps.

OPTIONS

Easy Option Replace the pull-up with a kneeling lat pull-down (#120), and perform 15 reps of the cable straight-arm cable pull-down.

Step It Up Add an additional round, bringing the total to 5 circuits.

Cool-Down Double lat stretch, cross-body stretch, hamstring stretch.

Complete Workout

Perform the following three exercises as a circuit, resting 10 seconds between exercises and 100 seconds between rounds. Repeat the circuit a total of 4 times.

Pull-up (#231)
- 6 reps
- 10 seconds of rest

Seated cable row with hip flexion (#174)
- 12 reps
- 10 seconds of rest

Straight-arm cable pull-down
- 25 reps
- 100 seconds of rest

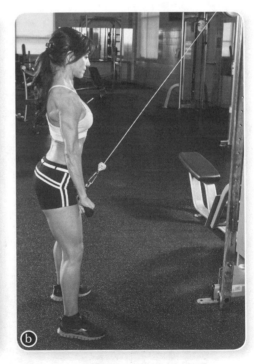

Deadlift Max

For almost every lifter—experienced or newbie, male or female—the most weight they will ever put on the bar occurs when attempting a maximal deadlift. The deadlift requires the coordination of several major muscle groups including the calves, hamstrings, glutes, lower back, upper back and traps, and forearms. And although getting all these major movers to work accurately as a group is not simple, the ability to recruit this much muscle mass allows you to pull big weight. Therefore, once you feel confident in the movement pattern, don't be afraid to load up the bar and rip some serious load off the floor.

Warm-Up

4 reps per side of the world's greatest stretch, 5 reps each of inchworm and inverted hamstring stretch, 10 reps of glute bridge

Featured Exercise

Barbell Front-Foot Elevated Split Squat

1. Begin with a barbell resting on your upper traps as it would in a barbell back squat.
2. Assume a split stance, placing your front foot on a 3-inch (8 cm) box or step (a).
3. Keeping a tall chest and your elbows under the bar, bend both knees and lower yourself until your back knee touches or is 1 inch (2.5 cm) above the floor (b). Your front shin should remain vertical during the entire movement.

4. Drive your front foot into the box to stand up and return to the starting position. Complete all reps for one side before switching to the other.

Complete Workout

Increase the weight used on each set of the deadlift until you reach your maximum weight on the final set.

A. Conventional deadlift (#5)
- 5 sets × 5, 3, 1, 1, 1 reps
- 90 seconds

B1. Leg press (#114)
- 2 sets × 10 reps
- 60 seconds

B2. Barbell front-foot elevated split squat
- 2 sets × 10 reps (5 per leg)
- 60 seconds

B3. Seated calf raise (#154)
- 2 sets × 10 reps
- 60 seconds

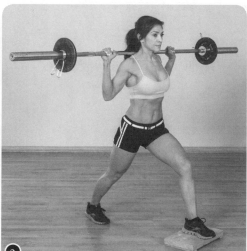
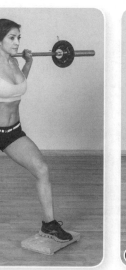
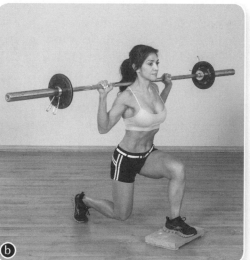

OPTIONS

Easy Option Eliminate the last single rep of the deadlift.

Step It Up Add two more singles with your max weight for the deadlift.

Cool-Down Double lat stretch, hamstring stretch, calf stretch.

Lucky 7s

Sure, seeing three 7s line up across a slot machine during a trip to Vegas may be lucky, but the only winnings you'll walk away with from this workout are sore pecs and triceps. By continually overloading the same muscle groups—in this case the pecs and triceps—you'll accumulate a lot of local fatigue even though the number of reps per set is not particularly high.

Warm-Up

4 reps per side of the world's greatest stretch, 5 reps of inchworm, 8 reps per side of shoulder sweeps

Complete Workout

This workout is performed as a descending ladder. Perform 7 reps of dips, followed by 7 reps of push-ups. Without rest, perform 6 reps of dips, followed by 6 reps of push-ups. Continue with this descending pattern until you reach 1 rep of each.

Dip
- 7 sets × 7, 6, 5, 4, 3, 2, 1 reps

Push-up (#12)
- 7 sets × 7, 6, 5, 4, 3, 2, 1 reps

● Featured Exercise

Dip

1. Your hands should be at shoulder width as you use the dip bar.

2. Jump up so your arms are straight, with your torso tall and head facing forward (*a*).

3. Lower your body by allowing your elbows to come back behind you. Keep your eyes facing forward. You have reached the bottom position when your biceps come in contact with your forearms (you should be able to secure a pencil in the crook of your elbow at the bottom position) (*b*).

4. Press up to return to the starting position and repeat for reps.

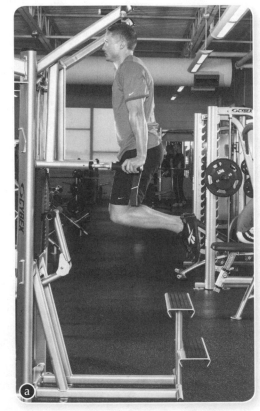
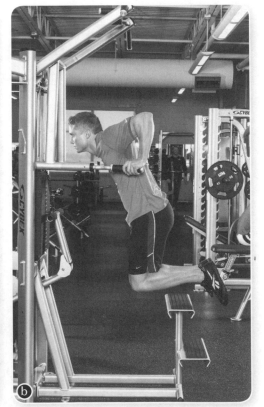

OPTIONS

Easy Option   Start the ladder at 5 reps for each movement.

Step It Up   Start the ladder at 10 reps for each movement.

Cool-Down   Pec stretch, double lat stretch, 90-degree stretch.

Ready, Set, Row

When performing movements such as the seated cable row, face pull, or push-up, avoid the dreaded chin poke—the tendency to jut your chin forward. Because your eyes are the key to all spatial relations, many people will jut their chin forward in an effort to reduce the range of motion of an exercise (i.e., they'll drive their face closer to the floor in a push-up because it seems they are getting closer to full range of motion). This not only restricts full range of motion but also overworks the muscles in your neck and promotes poor posture and stability. Focus on keeping a straight, neutral spine during these exercises, and you will get much more benefit from them.

Warm-Up

5 reps of inchworm, 6 reps per side of quadruped T-spine rotation, 10 reps of cat–cow

● Featured Exercise

Alternating-Arm Seated Cable Row

1. Attach handles to the cable at a seated row machine. Grab the handles with a neutral grip. Brace your feet against the support, with your knees slightly bent, shoulder blades down, and chest tall (*a*).

2. Pull the cable to the side of your rib cage with your right arm, making sure not to extend at the hips or rotate your torso (*b*).

3. Pause at the end position, and contract your lat before returning the handle to the starting position (do not flex at the hips when returning the bar). Complete a rep on the opposite side (*c*).

Complete Workout

A. Chin-up (#73)
- 4 sets × as many reps as possible
- 90 seconds of rest

B1. Straight-arm cable pull-down (#139)
- 4 sets × 10 reps
- 45 seconds of rest

B2. Alternating-arm seated cable row
- 4 sets × 10 reps/side
- 45 seconds of rest

C. Rower (#212)
- 500 meters

OPTIONS

Easy Option   Perform 3 sets of the B exercises.

Step It Up   Rest 90 seconds and repeat the 500-meter row.

Cool-Down   Double lat stretch, cross-body stretch, hamstring stretch.

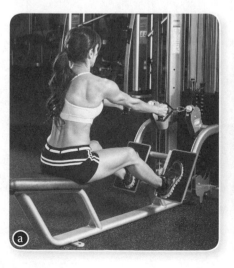
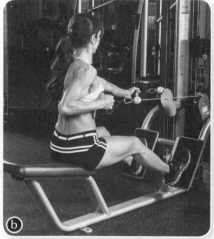
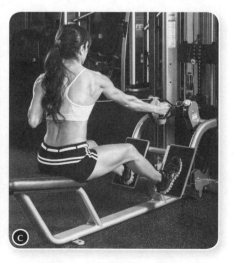

Leg Blaster

If you are fortunate enough to train at a facility that has non-standard, alternative equipment, you'll be well served to use them to add some variety to your training. Things like safety bars, fat grip handles, atlas stones, and sleds can provide a unique stimulus as well as add an element of variety into your workout. Don't be afraid to grab a unique piece of equipment and occasionally incorporate it into your workouts.

Warm-Up

5 reps of squat to stand; 6 reps per side of kneeling adductor stretch, hip rocker, and quadruped T-spine rotation

● Featured Exercise

Lateral Lunge

1. Begin standing tall with your feet at hip-width (a).
2. Step your right foot out to the side (to double hip-width), bend your right knee and sit back into your right hip. Your left leg should remain straight and both feet should point forward (b).
3. Drive off your right foot to return to the start position.
4. Complete all reps for right side before switching to the left.

Complete Workout

Perform 1 rep of the barbell back squat. Rest as long as needed, and then perform 2 reps. Rest as long as needed, and then perform 3 reps. Continue in this fashion until you reach 10 reps. Once you reach the top of this ladder, come back down, starting with 10 reps. Rest as long as needed, and then perform 9 reps. Continue in this fashion until you reach 1 rep. Use approximately 60 percent of your 1RM for all sets.

A. Barbell back squat (#63)
- 1 to 10 reps and back down, as described
- Rest as needed

B. Lateral lunge
- 2 sets × 8 reps/side
- 60 seconds rest

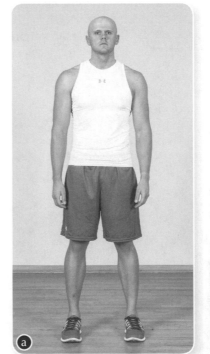
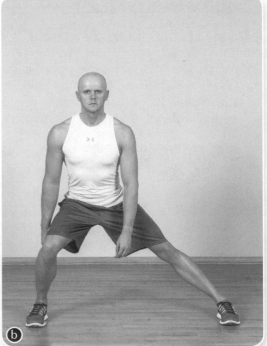

OPTIONS

Easy Option   Perform the ladder up to 6 reps and then back down.

Step It Up   Take 3 seconds to lower the bar with each rep.

Cool-Down   Standing quad stretch, 90-degree stretch, cross-body stretch.

Deltoid Force

It's safe to say the shoulder joint is one of the most crucial yet delicate joints involved in upper body movements. It's therefore critical to take care of your shoulders by incorporating plenty of mobility work, performing as many warm-up sets as necessary, and strengthening both the smaller muscles of the rotator cuff along with the larger deltoids. Finding the proper balance between shoulder mobility and stability is the key to staying injury free.

Warm-Up

4 reps per side of the world's greatest stretch, 5 reps of inchworm, 8 reps per side of shoulder sweeps

Complete Workout

A. Barbell overhead press (#36)
- 5 sets × 4 reps
- 2 minutes of rest

B1. Half-kneeling single-arm kettlebell overhead press
- 3 sets × 8 reps/side
- 60 seconds of rest

B2. Lateral raise (#147)
- 3 sets × 8 reps
- 60 seconds of rest

● Featured Exercise

Half-Kneeling Single-Arm Kettlebell Overhead Press

1. Take a half-kneeling stance, with your left foot and right knee on the floor (you may need to use a pad). Your left knee should be at a 90-degree angle and your left foot directly in front of your left hip.

2. Place a kettlebell in your right hand, directly on the outside of your shoulder (a).

3. Keeping your elbow tucked in, brace your abs and drive the kettlebell straight overhead (b).

4. Return the kettlebell to the starting position. Complete all reps for the right side before switching your stance (left knee on the floor) and pressing with the left arm.

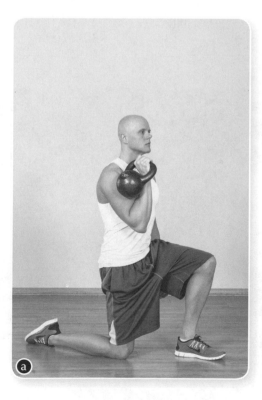

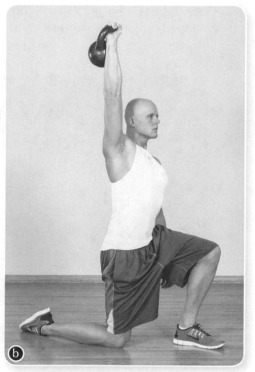

OPTIONS

Easy Option   Perform 3 sets of the half-kneeling single-arm kettlebell overhead press and lateral raise.

Step It Up   Add a 2-second pause at the top of the lateral raises.

Cool-Down   Pec stretch, double lat stretch, 90-degree stretch.

Armed and Dangerous

Let's face the facts: When you first stepped into a gym, one of your main goals was to get a nice set of thick, ripped arms. By supersetting (alternating between two exercises, with a short rest in between) some of the most effective biceps and triceps movements on the planet, this workout will help you put some size onto those pipes, while the short rest periods should deliver a massive pump.

Warm-Up

4 reps per side of the world's greatest stretch, 5 reps of inchworm, 8 reps per side of shoulder sweeps

Featured Exercise

Decline EZ-Bar Triceps Extension

1. Lie back on a decline bench, and have a training partner hand you a loaded EZ bar.
2. Grab the bar with a shoulder-width grip, arms fully extended directly above your chest (a).

3. Keeping your upper arms in place, bend at the elbows, lowering the bar toward your forehead.
4. Once you reach the bottom position (b), reverse the motion, returning the bar to lockout. Repeat for reps.

Complete Workout

A1. Chin-up (#73)
- 3 sets × 8 reps
- 30 seconds of rest

A2. Alternating dumbbell hammer curl (#230)
- 3 sets × 12 reps/side
- 30 seconds of rest

B1. Dip (#141)
- 3 sets × 8 reps
- 30 seconds of rest

B2. Decline EZ-bar triceps extension
- 3 sets × 12 reps
- 30 seconds of rest

OPTIONS

Easy Option   Use a kneeling lat pull-down (#120) or pull-up assistance machine to replace the chin-ups.

Step It Up   Add additional weight to the chin-ups and dips by using a weighted vest or dip belt.

Cool-Down   Pec stretch, double lat stretch, 90-degree stretch.

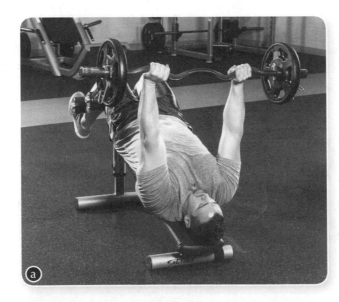

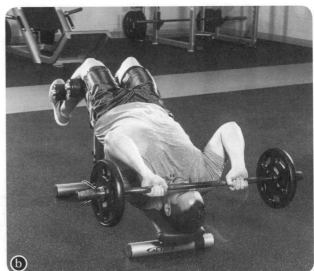

Band on the Run

Mini bands (small elastic bands) can be a great addition to either your warm-up or as part of an exercise circuit. Movements such as the bent-knee lateral mini-band walk (featured in this workout) are great for targeting muscles such as the gluteus medius that are difficult to fire up in more traditional compound movements. If you feel as if the side of your butt is on fire by the time you are at the end of your set, you're doing something right!

Warm-Up

5 reps of squat to stand; 6 reps per side of kneeling adductor stretch, hip rocker, and quadruped T-spine rotation

● Featured Exercise

Bent-Knee Lateral Mini-Band Walk

1. Place a mini band around both legs so it sits right above your kneecaps.
2. Squat halfway down, and drive both knees out. Keep your chest tall and feet facing forward (a).

3. While minimizing any movement in your upper body, begin taking steps directly to your right by pressing off the floor with your left foot (b). Do not let your hips rise up as you step.
4. Once you complete all reps to the right, take an equal number of steps to the left.

Complete Workout

A. Barbell front squat (#44)
- 6 sets × 4 reps
- 90 seconds of rest

B1. Russian step-up (#9)
- 2 sets × 8 reps/side
- 60 seconds of rest

B2. Sliding hip adduction (#156)
- 2 sets × 10 reps
- 60 seconds of rest

B3. Bent-knee lateral mini-band walk
- 2 sets × 10 reps/side
- 60 seconds of rest

OPTIONS

Easy Option   Perform 4 sets of the barbell front squat.

Step It Up   Add an extra set to the Russian step-up, sliding hip adduction, and bent-knee lateral mini-band walk.

Cool-Down   Standing quad stretch, 90-degree stretch, cross-body stretch.

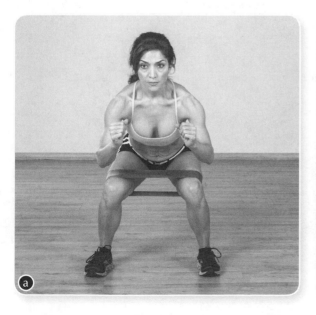

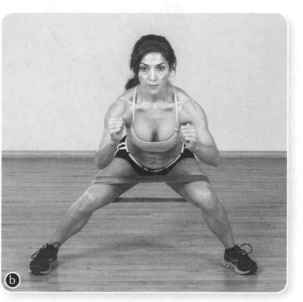

Shoulder the Load

As opposed to many other muscle groups, the deltoids (muscles of the shoulder) consist of a mix of muscle fiber types. What this means is they respond well to both lower-rep power and strength movements as well as higher-rep sets usually associated with hypertrophy and strength-endurance qualities. So if you want big, strong shoulders, make sure you vary your rep ranges.

Warm-Up

4 reps per side of the world's greatest stretch, 5 reps of inchworm, 8 reps per side of shoulder sweeps

Complete Workout

Barbell overhead press (#36)
- 4 sets × 4 reps
- 60 seconds of rest

Lateral raise
- 4 sets × 12 reps
- 2 minutes of rest

● **Featured Exercise**

Lateral Raise

1. Grab a pair of dumbbells with your arms straight at your sides and palms facing each other (*a*).
2. Keep your arms straight and raise the dumbbells out to your sides until they reach shoulder height (*b*).
3. Return dumbbells to start position and repeat for reps.

OPTIONS

Easy Option   Complete 3 sets of each exercise.

Step It Up   Complete 5 sets of each exercise.

Cool-Down   Pec stretch, double lat stretch, 90-degree stretch.

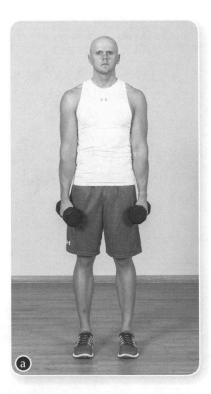

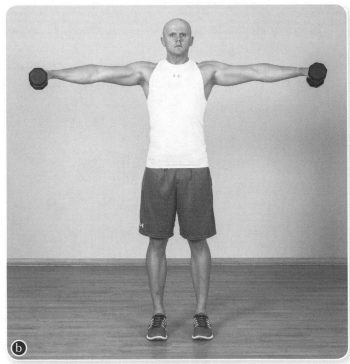

HAM

The reverse bent-knee hip raise is a close relative to the reverse hyperextension (#263). And, like the reverse hyper, it does a great job of working the glutes and hamstrings. If you feel stress in your lower back as opposed to the glutes during movements such as the reverse hyper or glute ham raise, the reverse bent-knee hip raise may be a great substitution because it keeps your back in a locked position, allowing you to focus more on the muscles you are trying to train. And, by the way, the HAM stands for "Hard As a Mother." So just because this exercise makes it easier to isolate your hamstrings, don't fall into the trap of thinking it's an easy exercise.

Warm-Up

4 reps per side of the world's greatest stretch, 5 reps each of inchworm and inverted hamstring stretch, 10 reps of glute bridge

Featured Exercise

Reverse Bent-Knee Hip Raise

1. Lie facedown over the edge of a Roman chair or bench. Your torso should be in contact with the bench, but your hips should be hanging off the edge (a).

2. Hold onto the bench and extend your legs straight behind you (b).

3. Keeping your back locked into place, bend your knees to 90 degrees.

4. Extend your legs back to the starting position and repeat for reps.

Complete Workout

A. Sumo deadlift (#82)
  - 4 sets × 3 reps
  - 90 seconds of rest

B1. Lying hamstring curl (#168)
  - 3 sets × 8 reps
  - 30 seconds of rest

B2. Dumbbell step-up (#121)
  - 3 sets × 8 reps/side
  - 30 seconds of rest

B3. Reverse bent-knee hip raise
  - 3 sets × 12 reps
  - 30 seconds of rest

OPTIONS

Easy Option   Perform 2 sets of the lying hamstring curl, dumbbell step-up, and reverse bent-knee hip raise.

Step It Up   Add 2 reps to the lying hamstring curl, dumbbell step-up, and reverse bent-knee hip raise.

Cool-Down   Double lat stretch, hamstring stretch, calf stretch.

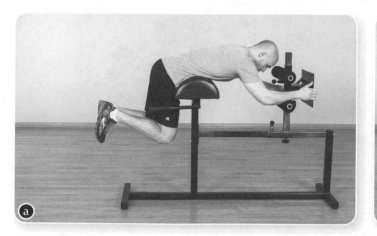

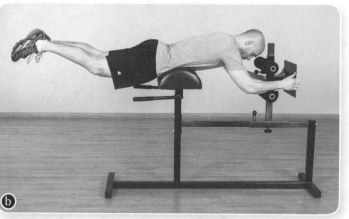

Bi Builder

By allowing you to overload the eccentric (lowering portion) of the lift with more weight than you could usually use for a full reverse or pronated-grip curl, the Zottman curl (featured in this workout) is a great variation for building up not only your biceps but your forearm strength and size as well.

Warm-Up

4 reps per side of the world's greatest stretch, 5 reps of inchworm, 8 reps per side of shoulder sweeps

● Featured Exercise

Standing Zottman Curl

1. Begin in a standing position, feet at hip width, with a pair of dumbbells at your sides. Arms should be straight and palms facing away from you (supinated) (*a*).
2. Curl the dumbbells up to your shoulders (*b*).
3. At the top position, turn your hands over so your palms are facing away from you (pronated).
4. Lower the dumbbells back to the original position (*c*). Repeat for reps.

Complete Workout

A. Chin-up (#73)
  • 4 sets × 6 reps
  • 90 seconds of rest

B1. Standing Zottman curl
  • 3 sets × 10 reps
  • 60 seconds of rest

B2. Single-arm cable curl (#183)
  • 3 sets × 10 reps
  • 60 seconds of rest

OPTIONS

Easy Option Use a kneeling lat pull-down (#120) or pull-up assistance machine in place of the chin-up.

Step It Up Perform 5 sets of the chin-up and 4 sets of the standing Zottman curls and single-arm cable curl.

Cool-Down Pec stretch, double lat stretch, 90-degree stretch.

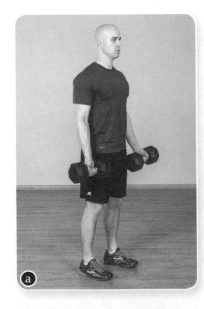
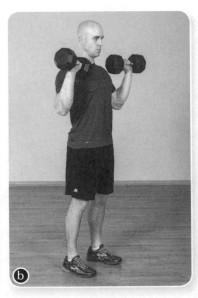
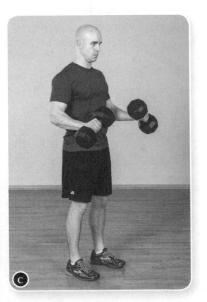

Squat Ladder

Have you always been afraid of performing back squats because of the risk of injuring your lower back? Here's a great tip on how to keep a neutral or slightly arched spine that will keep you injury free. Unrack the bar and take one step back with each foot. Now, picture someone touching your lower back with an ice cube. That thought should instantly make you arch your lower back and stick out your chest. Maintaining this upper body posture throughout the entire movement should keep you out of harm's way.

Warm-Up

5 reps of squat to stand; 6 reps per side of kneeling adductor stretch, hip rocker, and quadruped T-spine rotation

● Featured Exercise

Barbell Back Squat

1. Utilizing a shoulder-width stance, step under a bar in a squat rack, with the barbell resting on your upper traps. Take one step back with each foot (a).

2. Maintaining a neutral or slightly arched lower back, unlock your hips and begin bringing them back. Almost instantaneously, bend at your knees.

3. Keeping your entire foot on the ground, continue to lower yourself to as deep a level as possible (you want your hip crease to be at least below your knee) (b).

4. When you reach your full range of motion, forcefully drive your feet into the ground and stand up, returning to the starting position.

Complete Workout

Complete 10 sets of the barbell back squat as a descending ladder. Perform 10 reps for the first set, 9 reps for the second set, 8 reps for the third set, until you get down to 1 rep. Rest 1 minute between each set, and try to utilize around 70 percent of your 1RM.

Barbell back squat
- 10 sets × 10, 9, 8, 7, 6, 5, 4, 3, 2, 1 reps
- 60 seconds of rest between sets

OPTIONS

Easy Option   Begin the ladder at 7 reps and work down to 1.

Step It Up   After you complete the descending ladder, work your way back up the ladder, starting with 1 rep and ending with 10.

Cool-Down   Standing quad stretch, 90-degree stretch, cross-body stretch.

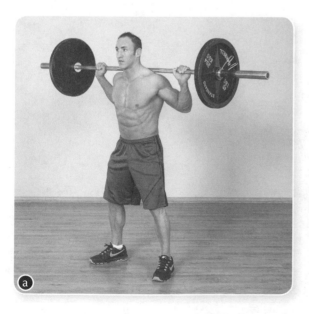

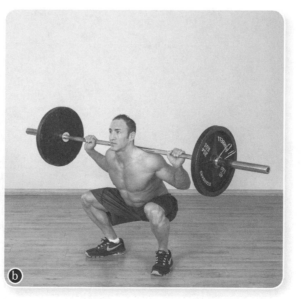

Tank

In today's functional fitness world, isolation exercises (such as the biceps curl and leg extension) have been put on the back burner. And although squats, deadlifts, presses, and pull-ups should make up the bulk of your training program, there is nothing wrong with isolation movements if your goal is to get bigger and stronger. In fact, if you want bigger biceps, calves, or hamstrings, some isolation training is the most efficient and effective way to go about achieving your goal.

Warm-Up

4 reps per side of the world's greatest stretch, 5 reps of inchworm, 8 reps per side of shoulder sweeps

Featured Exercise

Three-Position EZ-Bar Curl

1. Grab an EZ bar with a shoulder-width grip. Keep your chest tall, and allow your arms to hang straight down (*a*).

2. Curl the bar halfway until your forearms are parallel to the floor (*b*). Return the bar to the starting position.

3. Curl the bar all the way up until it is under your chin (*c*). Return the bar halfway down until your forearms are parallel to the floor.

4. Curl the bar back to the top position.

5. Lower the bar back to the starting position. That counts as 1 rep.

Complete Workout

Complete 3 rounds of the following circuit.

Narrow-grip chin-up (#1)
- 8 reps
- 60 seconds of rest

Three-position EZ-bar curl
- 10 reps
- 60 seconds of rest

Offset-grip incline dumbbell biceps curl (#243)
- 12 reps
- 60 seconds of rest

OPTIONS

Easy Option   Replace the narrow-grip chin-up with a kneeling lat pull-down (#120).

Step It Up   Add one more round of the circuit.

Cool-Down   Pec stretch, double lat stretch, 90-degree stretch.

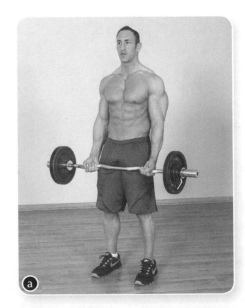

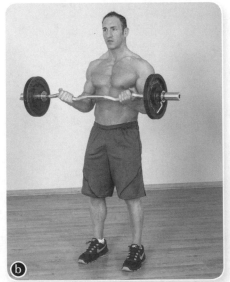

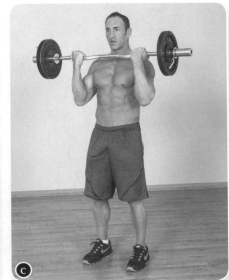

Special Forces

Performing movements explosively is certainly appropriate when utilizing exercises such as medicine ball throws or Olympic lifts. However, there is also benefit to controlling the tempo of your lifts, especially in the eccentric, or lowering, phase. Doing so can lead to greater hypertrophy (muscle gain) and injury prevention. So focus on lowering your barbell, dumbbell, kettlebell, or body with control.

Warm-Up

6 reps of squat to stand, 6 reps per side of quadruped T-spine rotation, 8 reps of glute bridge, 10 reps of cat–cow

● Featured Exercise

Dumbbell Alternating Step-Back Lunge

1. Grab a pair of dumbbells, with your chest tall and feet together (a).
2. Keeping an upright posture in your upper body, take a long step back with your right leg.

3. Lower until your right knee is just above, or touching, the floor (b).
4. Drive off your front (left) foot, and return to the starting position. Repeat the process, with your left leg stepping back (c). Continue to alternate until all reps are completed.

Complete Workout

A. Barbell front squat (#44)
- 4 sets × 4 reps
- 2 minutes of rest

B1. Dumbbell alternating step-back lunge
- 3 sets × 8 reps/side
- 60 seconds of rest

B2. Leg press (#114)
- 3 sets × 8 reps
- 60 seconds of rest

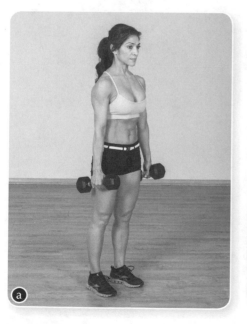
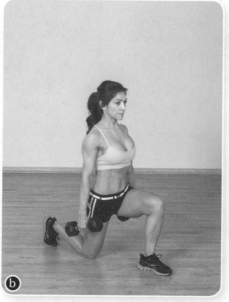
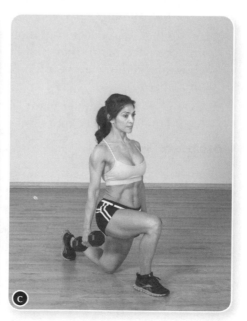

OPTIONS

Easy Option Perform 2 sets of the dumbbell alternating step-back lunge and leg press.

Step It Up Add a 2-second pause at the bottom of each rep of the dumbbell alternating step-back lunge.

Cool-Down Standing quad stretch, 90-degree stretch, double lat stretch.

Bench Death

There is a bit of an art and a science to testing your 1RM in any lift. There is a fine balance between working up to your heaviest lift with appropriate warm-up sets without overdoing it so you are overly taxed when attempting your max sets. Try erring on the side of doing more sets with fewer reps (think sets of 3 or fewer) in the lead-up to your max attempts, even if the early sets feel rather light. This will ensure your muscles and nervous system are primed but not shot.

Warm-Up

4 reps per side of the world's greatest stretch, 5 reps of inchworm, 8 reps per side of shoulder sweeps

● **Featured Exercise**

Barbell Bench Press

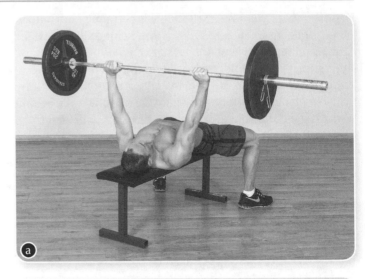

1. At a flat bench press station, lie back so your head, the area between your shoulder blades, and your butt are in contact with the bench and your feet are flat on the floor. Position your head so your eyes are directly under the bar (a).

2. Unrack the bar, squeeze your shoulder blades together, and lower the bar to midchest height (b). Keep your elbows tucked toward your rib cage during the lowering phase.

3. As the bar touches your chest, drive it up and back toward the starting lockout position. Repeat for reps.

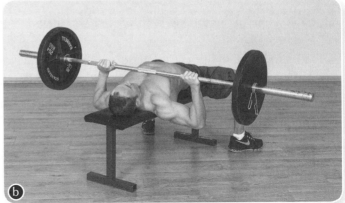

OPTIONS

Easy Option Reduce the percentage of your 1RM by 5 percent for each set.

Step It Up Before set 1, work up to your 1RM barbell bench press.

Cool-Down Double lat stretch, cross-body stretch, hamstring stretch.

Complete Workout

Barbell bench press
- Set 1: 85 percent of your 1RM for 5 reps
- Set 2: 75 percent of your 1RM for 6 reps
- Set 3: 65 percent of your 1RM for 8 reps
- Set 4: 55 percent of your 1RM for as many reps as possible

Donkey Kick

Although genetic factors affect the potential of all muscle growth, no muscle gets singled out for being genetically "stubborn" as much as the calves. Do not let this excuse stop you from trying to develop the calves you want. Instead, hit the calves frequently with a variety of straight-leg and bent-knee exercises in a wide variety of rep ranges.

Warm-Up

4 reps per side of the world's greatest stretch, 5 reps each of inchworm and inverted hamstring stretch, 10 reps of glute bridge

Featured Exercise

Seated Calf Raise

1. Sit in a seated calf raise machine with the balls of your feet on the foot rest, back straight, and chest tall.

2. Unlock the machine and lower your heels to the ground as far as your range of motion will allow, getting a stretch in your calves (a).

3. Drive up on your toes as high as possible, maximally contracting your calf muscles (b). Note: While you can keep your hands on the handles, do not use your arms to pull the weight up. Repeat for reps.

Complete Workout

A. Conventional deadlift (#5)
   - 5 sets × 4 reps
   - 90 seconds of rest

B1. Barbell walking lunge (#112)
   - 3 sets × 8 reps/side
   - 60 seconds of rest

B2. Leg press (#114)
   - 3 sets × 10 reps
   - 60 seconds of rest

B3. Seated calf raise
   - 3 sets × 25 reps
   - 60 seconds of rest

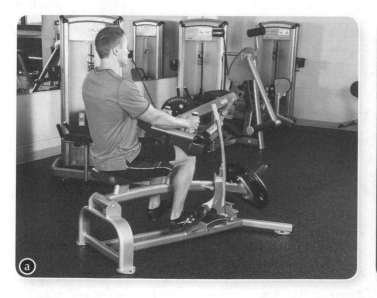
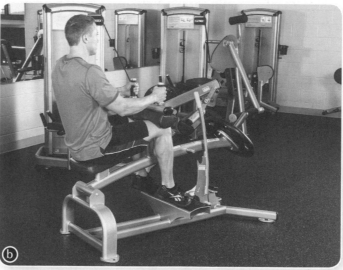

OPTIONS

Easy Option   Perform 2 sets of the barbell walking lunge, leg press, and seated calf raise.

Step It Up   Perform 4 sets of the barbell walking lunge, leg press, and seated calf raise.

Cool-Down   Double lat stretch, hamstring stretch, calf stretch.

The Twist

Looking to increase core activation during your workouts? Simply have less of your body supported by seats, benches, pads, machines, and even the floor. The closer you come to standing on your two feet (or one foot, when appropriate), the more core activation you will get, regardless of which lift you are performing. Want a great example? Try doing a seated shoulder press on a bench with back support and then try it on a bench without support. You'll notice your core has to do a lot more work stabilizing your body during the movement without the back rest.

Warm-Up

4 reps per side of the world's greatest stretch, 5 reps of inchworm, 8 reps per side of shoulder sweeps

● Featured Exercise

Alternating Dumbbell Shoulder Press With Twist

1. Stand tall with two dumbbells at shoulder height. Your elbows should be tucked into your rib cage (a).

2. In one motion, rotate your torso to the left, pivot on the ball of your right foot, and press the dumbbell overhead (b).

3. Rotate back to the starting position, and lower the dumbbell back to your shoulder.

4. Repeat for the other side. Continue to alternate until you have completed all reps.

OPTIONS

Easy Option   Reduce to 3 sets of the push press.

Step It Up   Add 1 set to the alternating dumbbell shoulder press with twist, dive-bomber push-up, and cable diagonal raise.

Cool-Down   Pec stretch, double lat stretch, 90-degree stretch.

Complete Workout

A. Push press (#16)
- 5 sets × 3 reps
- 90 seconds of rest

B1. Alternating dumbbell shoulder press with twist
- 2 sets × 8 reps/side
- 30 seconds of rest

B2. Dive-bomber push-up (#190)
- 2 sets × 10 reps
- 30 seconds of rest

B3. Cable diagonal raise (#137)
- 2 × 12 reps
- 30 seconds of rest

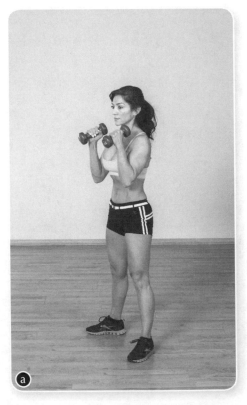
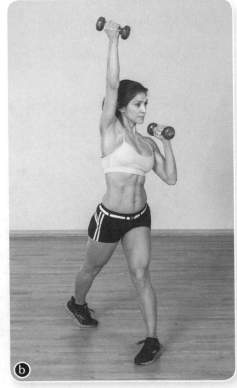

Adductor Madness

Your adductors (the muscles that run on the inside of your upper legs) may be one of the most overlooked and underappreciated muscle groups in your entire body. The adductor group works at both the hip and the knee and comes into play directly in lateral (side to side) movements as well as synergistically in exercises such as the squat and deadlift. It pays to train these muscles in both compound and isolation exercises—such as the barbell back squat and sliding hip adduction, respectively—as featured in this workout.

Warm-Up

6 reps of squat to stand, 6 reps per side of quadruped T-spine rotation, 8 reps of glute bridge, 10 reps of cat–cow

Featured Exercise

Sliding Hip Adduction

1. Kneel on the floor and place a Valslide, paper plate, or towel under each knee (a).
2. Keeping your torso upright and your hips directly under you, push your knees out as far as you can (b).
3. After a brief pause, pull your knees back together. Repeat for reps.

Complete Workout

A. Barbell back squat (#63)
  - 5 sets × 3 reps
  - 90 seconds of rest

B1. Lateral lunge (#143)
  - 2 sets × 8 reps/side
  - 60 seconds of rest

B2. Sliding hip adduction
  - 2 sets × 10 reps
  - 60 seconds of rest

B3. Dumbbell Romanian deadlift (#267)
  - 2 sets × 12 reps
  - 60 seconds of rest

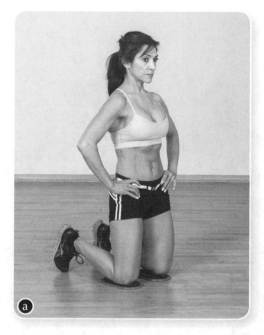

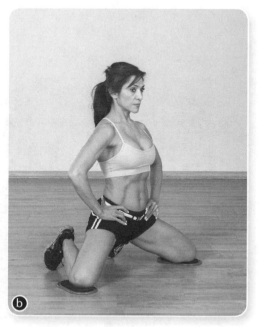

OPTIONS

Easy Option Perform 3 sets of the barbell back squat.

Step It Up Add an extra set to the lateral lunge, sliding hip adduction, and dumbbell Romanian deadlift.

Cool-Down Standing quad stretch, 90-degree stretch, double lat stretch.

Chest Bump

Nothing says "Yeah, I work out" like a set of strong-looking pecs. Though, truth be told, most gym-goers do tend to work on pressing movements such as the bench press much more than pulling movements such as pull-ups or seated rows, which can cause an imbalance and that dreaded "caveman" look. So make sure you balance out your pressing and pulling movements.

Warm-Up

4 reps per side of the world's greatest stretch, 5 reps of inchworm, 8 reps per side of shoulder sweeps

⬤ Featured Exercise

Low-to-High Cable Chest Fly

1. Start by attaching D handles to both ends of a cable station. Set the cables to just below hip height.
2. Stand directly between the two cables, grabbing each D handle; your arms should be extended out from your sides (*a*).

3. With a slight bend in your elbows, bring your arms up and together. At the end of the movement, your hands should be out in front of your chest (*b*).
4. Return to the starting position and repeat for reps.

Complete Workout

A. Barbell bench press (#54)
  - 4 sets × 6 reps
  - 90 seconds of rest between sets

B1. Low-to-high cable chest fly
  - 2 sets × 10 to 12 reps
  - Proceed to the next exercise without rest

B2. Incline dumbbell chest press (#210)
  - 2 sets × 10 to 12 reps
  - 45 seconds of rest, return to cable fly

C. Push-up (#12)
  - 1 set × as many reps as possible

OPTIONS

Easy Option   Perform 3 sets of the barbell bench press.

Step It Up   Perform 3 sets of the low-to-high cable chest fly and the incline dumbbell bench press and 2 sets of the max-reps push-ups.

Cool-Down   Pec stretch, double lat stretch, 90-degree stretch.

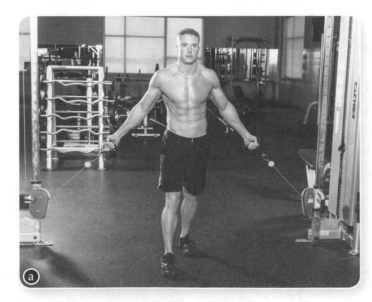
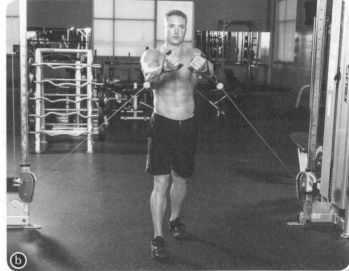

Pumped

Resist the urge to let a business trip or other trip derail your normal fitness routine. In fact, maintaining your regular training schedule while on the road can help you adapt and acclimate to your new environment much more quickly—particularly if you are traveling to another time zone. So find a local gym, hit the hotel fitness center, or just go for a run outside. Doing so will help you feel much more productive, relaxed, and normal when traveling from home.

Warm-Up

5 reps of inchworm, 6 reps per side of quadruped T-spine rotation, 10 reps of cat–cow

⬤ Featured Exercise

Hercules Curl

1. Set up two D handles at the top pulleys of a cable crossover station. Stand directly between both handles, and grab them with your arms extended and palms facing up (a).

2. Keeping your upper arms parallel to the floor, curl both handles toward your ears (b). Do not let your elbows come forward.

3. Squeeze both biceps and return to the starting position. Repeat for reps.

Complete Workout

A. Narrow-grip chin-up (#1)
   - 4 sets × 8 reps
   - 60 seconds of rest
B1. Alternating dumbbell hammer curl (#230)
   - 3 sets × 12 reps
   - 30 seconds of rest
B2. Hercules curl
   - 3 sets × 12 reps
   - 30 seconds of rest

OPTIONS

Easy Option   Perform 3 sets of the narrow-grip chin-up.

Step It Up   Increase the number of reps per set of the narrow-grip chin-up to 12 reps.

Cool-Down   Double lat stretch, cross-body stretch, hamstring stretch.

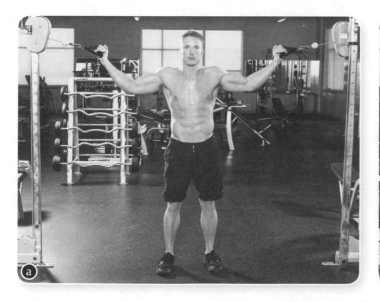

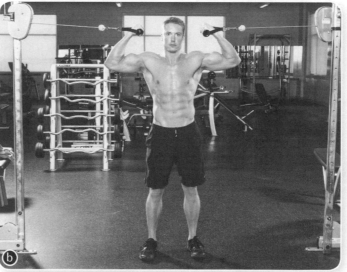

Split Ends

You can have the perfect gym, the perfect program, and the perfect workout partner, but if you don't put the right effort into your training, you'll never get anywhere. In fact, someone putting everything he has into a terrible training program in a rundown gym will get further than someone half-stepping the perfect workout. So don't worry about the brand of the barbells, the music that's playing, or how crowded the gym may be. Just focus on putting everything you have into every rep of every set, and you'll get much further than you could ever believe.

Warm-Up

5 reps of inchworm, 6 reps per side of quadruped T-spine rotation, 10 reps of cat–cow

● Featured Exercise

Low Cable Split Squat

1. Grab the D handle attached to the low pulley of a cable station with your left hand. Assume a split stance, with your right foot forward and torso tall. Make sure there is tension in the cable (a).

2. Drive your right knee forward to lower yourself toward the floor. Keep your back leg straight (b).

3. Once your hamstring touches your calf, drive off your front foot to return to the starting position.

4. Complete all reps for one side before switching.

Complete Workout

A. Barbell front squat (#44)
   • 5 sets × 3 reps
   • 90 seconds of rest

B1. Low cable split squat
   • 3 sets × 8 reps/side
   • 60 seconds of rest

B2. Lying hamstring curl (#168)
   • 3 sets × 8 reps/side
   • 60 seconds of rest

OPTIONS

Easy Option   Perform 2 sets of the low cable split squat and lying hamstring curl.

Step It Up   Increase to 4 sets for the low cable split squat and lying hamstring curl.

Cool-Down   Double lat stretch, cross-body stretch, hamstring stretch.

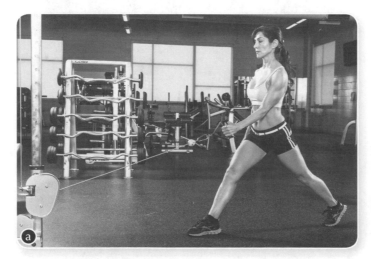
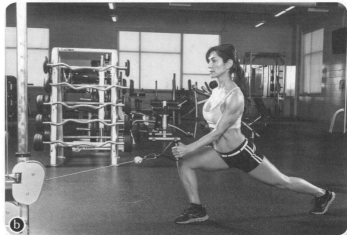

Big Pull

Although developing pull-up and chin-up strength is difficult for many, doing multiple reps is something you should aspire to and work toward. If you are having difficulty, begin with a chin-up (palms facing you) because that is the easiest variation. You can also jump up to the bar and perform slow eccentrics (lowering phases), which can build up your pulling strength. Finally, although the lat pull-down is a reasonable substitution for muscle development, it does not require the same strength as actually pulling your body up to the bar for pull-up variations. So don't rely on this exercise substitution indefinitely. Get yourself up to the bar!

Warm-Up

5 reps of inchworm, 6 reps per side of quadruped T-spine rotation, 10 reps of cat–cow

● Featured Exercise

Weighted Chin-Up

1. Use a dip belt or place a dumbbell between your knees or ankles to add weight.
2. Grab a pull-up bar with a supinated grip (palms facing you) at shoulder width.
3. Start in a dead hang (your arms should be straight) (a), and begin the movement by depressing your shoulder blades.
4. Drive your elbows down and behind you, bending at the elbows in order to pull your chest up toward the bar (b).
5. Once your chin clears the bar, return to the starting position under control. Repeat for reps.

Complete Workout

For the weighted wide-grip pull-up, begin with a weight you can comfortably complete for 3 or 4 reps. Perform 1 rep. Rest for 60 seconds, and add weight for set number 2. Continue in this manner (adding weight each set when possible) until you have completed 5 singles. Using the same weights you used for the 5 sets of the wide-grip pull-up, perform

4 reps per set of the weighted neutral-grip chin-up. When you have completed those 5 sets, use the same weights to complete all 5 sets of 6 reps of the weighted chin-up. For example, if you used 35 lb, 55 lb, 65 lb, 75 lb, and 80 lb for the weighted wide-grip pull-up singles, use those same weights for the sets of weighted neutral-grip chin-ups and weighted chin-ups (but with the increased number of reps).

Wide-grip pull-up (#117)
- Use weights as in the weighted chin-up
- 5 sets × 1, 1, 1, 1, 1 reps
- 60 seconds of rest

Neutral-grip pull-up (#237)
- Use weights as in the weighted chin-up
- 5 sets × 4, 4, 4, 4, 4 reps
- 60 seconds of rest

Weighted chin-up
- 5 sets × 6, 6, 6, 6, 6 reps
- 60 seconds of rest

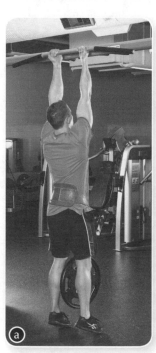 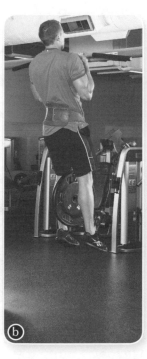

OPTIONS

Easy Option   Perform all sets and reps without additional weight.

Step It Up   Add 2 reps per set to the neutral-grip chin-up and weighted chin-up.

Cool-Down   Double lat stretch, cross-body stretch, hamstring stretch.

The Gauntlet

Many people lack the mobility to maintain a proper rack position (see step 1 of the featured exercise for a description) during a front squat. This is often misdiagnosed as a lack of wrist flexibility, when often the issue is tight lats. If you are having a hard time getting your upper arms parallel to the floor, try foam-rolling your lats, and see if your rack position improves.

Warm-Up

5 reps of squat to stand; 6 reps per side of kneeling adductor stretch, hip rocker, and quadruped T-spine rotation

● Featured Exercise

Paused Front Squat

1. Grab a barbell set up in a squat rack just outside shoulder width. Allow the bar to sit on the front of your shoulders, and rotate your arms around the bar until your upper arms are parallel to the ground (often referred to as the rack position) (*a*).

2. Unlock your hips, and slowly descend into a squat by bringing your hips back and bending your knees.

3. Once you reach full range of motion (you are attempting to get the crease of your hips below the height of your knees), pause for 3 full seconds (*b*).

4. After the pause, drive your feet into the ground, keeping your elbows high and chest tall, and return to the starting position. Repeat for reps.

Complete Workout

Begin with 3 reps of the paused front squat at 50 percent of your 1RM. Add 5 lb (2.5 kg), and complete 3 reps. Continue to add 5 lb until you can no longer complete 3 reps. Rest no longer than 60 seconds between sets.

Paused front squat

- Sets of 3 reps, as described

OPTIONS

Easy Option   Perform 2 reps per minute.

Step It Up   Increase the pause to 4 seconds.

Cool-Down   Standing quad stretch, 90-degree stretch, cross-body stretch.

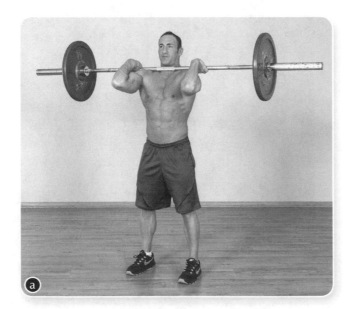

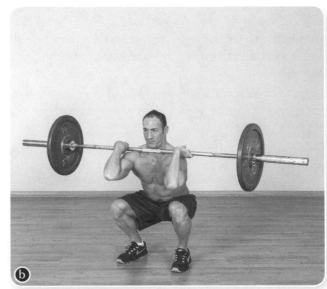

There is a tendency to strictly adhere to rest periods only during metabolic phases of training where you are trying to keep your heart rate elevated. This is a mistake. Making sure you are abiding by the prescribed rest periods during mass building and strength phases is just as critical to ensure that you are getting the desired training effect of the workout. Bottom line: Keep your eye on the clock and obey your rest periods, no matter what strength quality you are training.

Warm-Up

4 reps per side of the world's greatest stretch, 5 reps of inchworm, 8 reps per side of shoulder sweeps

● Featured Exercise

Incline Alternating Dumbbell Chest Press

1. Set a bench at a 30-degree incline. Grab a pair of dumbbells, and lie back on the bench.
2. Press both dumbbells directly above your shoulders, utilizing a neutral grip (palms facing each other) (a).

3. Lower the left dumbbell, keeping your elbow tucked toward your rib cage, while keeping the right dumbbell fully extended (b).
4. Drive the left dumbbell up to the starting position. Lower the right dumbbell, keeping your left arm extended (c). Continue to alternate until all reps are completed.

Complete Workout

A. Barbell bench press (#54)
- 5 sets × 4 reps
- 2 minutes of rest

B1. Incline alternating dumbbell chest press
- 3 sets × 8 reps/side
- 60 seconds of rest

B2. Cable chest fly (#181)
- 3 sets × 8 reps
- 60 seconds of rest

OPTIONS

Easy Option   Perform 2 sets of the incline alternating dumbbell chest press and cable chest fly.

Step It Up   Add a 1-second pause at the bottom of each rep of the alternating dumbbell chest press.

Cool-Down   Pec stretch, double lat stretch, 90-degree stretch.

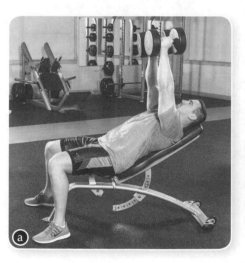
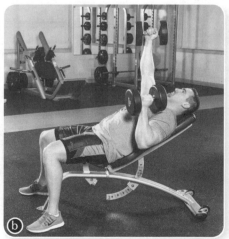
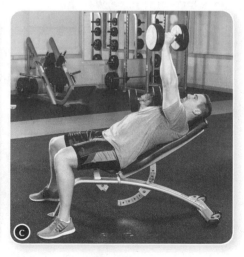

Carry On

Carries are a fantastic exercise because they can be loaded in various positions (at your sides, at your shoulders, overhead, single arm, double arm) and can drive up core activation and the metabolic demands of your workout. This workout combines heavy bilateral farmer's walks with core-crushing single-arm dumbbell overhead carries that will challenge your obliques and shoulder stability.

Warm-Up

5 reps of squat to stand; 6 reps per side of kneeling adductor stretch, hip rocker, and quadruped T-spine rotation

● Featured Exercise

Single-Arm Overhead Dumbbell Carry

1. Using your left arm, press a dumbbell until it is locked out overhead. Make sure the dumbbell is directly over your shoulder and your biceps is in line with your ear.

2. Keeping your chest tall and your arm in that locked-out position, walk forward, resisting the urge to lean to the side.

3. Once you have walked for the prescribed distance, lower the dumbbell, switch hands, and repeat on the other side.

OPTIONS

Easy Option   Use 75 percent (or less) of your body weight for the farmer's walk.

Step It Up   Use 50 percent of your body weight for the single-arm overhead dumbbell carry.

Cool-Down   Standing quad stretch, 90-degree stretch, cross-body stretch.

Complete Workout

You can use dumbbells, kettlebells, or farmer's walk handles for the farmer's walk. Use a load that is equal to your body weight. For the single-arm overhead dumbbell carry, use a dumbbell that is 25 percent of your body weight.

Farmer's walk (#187)
- 8 sets × 40 yards (40 m)
- 60 seconds of rest

Single-arm overhead dumbbell carry
- 8 sets × 20 yards (20 m)/side
- 60 seconds of rest

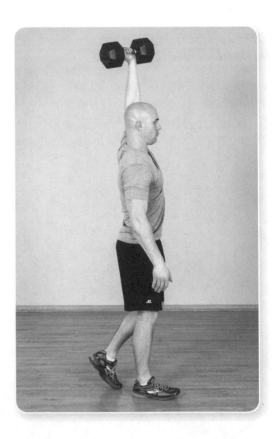

Elevation

Rather than seeking more weight, more reps, or shorter rest, you can look for other tweaks to increase the challenge of an exercise. Factors such as changing hand position, raising your feet, working one side at a time, or adding instability can test your muscles in a completely different way and force some positive adaptations. Once you have a solid handle on the basic movement, experiment with some variations that can add more demand to your training.

Warm-Up

5 reps of inchworm, 6 reps per side of quadruped T-spine rotation, 10 reps of cat–cow

● Featured Exercise

Single-Leg Hip Raise With Foot Elevation

1. Lie faceup on the floor, with your left knee bent and your left foot on a bench or step or foam roller. Your right leg should be bent with your hands interlocked around the knee (a).

2. Maintain this position as you push your hips upward until your body forms a straight line from your shoulders to your knees (b).

3. Squeeze your glutes at the top of the range of motion, and then lower slowly to the starting position. Repeat all reps for one side before switching to the other.

Complete Workout

A. Trap bar deadlift (#8)
- 6 sets × 6 reps
- 90 seconds of rest

B. Lateral lunge (#143)
- 2 sets × 8 reps/side
- 60 seconds of rest

B2. Heel-elevated back squat (#96)
- 2 sets × 10 reps
- 60 seconds of rest

B3. Single-leg hip raise with foot elevation
- 2 sets × 12 reps/side
- 60 seconds of rest

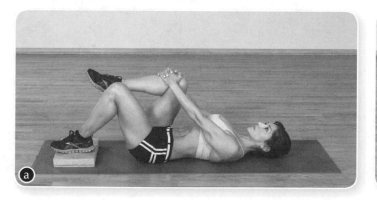
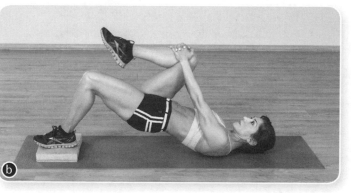

OPTIONS

Easy Option Perform 4 sets of the trap bar deadlift.

Step It Up Add an extra set to the lateral lunge, heel-elevated back squat, and single-leg hip raise with foot elevation.

Cool-Down Double lat stretch, cross-body stretch, hamstring stretch.

Plyo Press

Upper body plyometric exercise selections are difficult to come by. One of the main exceptions is the plyo push-up, which allows you to train upper body explosive power. Make the most of this movement by really driving off the floor and getting as much hang time as possible. But also remember to train smart. Minimize the number of repetitions, and be sure to utilize excellent technique in order to maximize training effect and reduce the risk of injury.

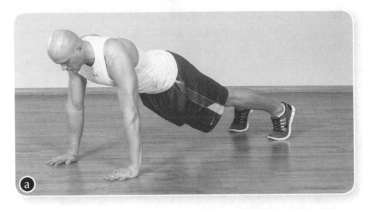

Warm-Up

4 reps per side of the world's greatest stretch, 5 reps of inchworm, 8 reps per side of shoulder sweeps

● Featured Exercise

Plyo Push-Up

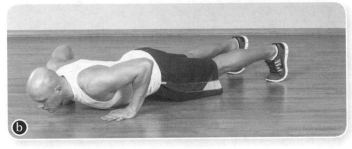

1. Begin in a push-up position, with your hands on the floor directly under your shoulders and your body forming a straight line from your head to your heels (a).

2. Lower your body toward the ground, keeping your elbows tucked at your sides.

3. When your chest is approximately 2 inches (5 cm) off the ground (b), reverse directions and forcefully and explosively launch yourself off the floor (c).

4. Catch yourself with your elbows slightly bent, and immediately begin the next rep.

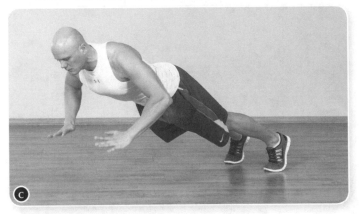

Complete Workout

Complete 6 rounds of the following exercise pairing.

Plyo push-up
- 3 reps
- 30 seconds of rest

Incline barbell bench press (#179)
- 8 reps
- 2 minutes of rest

OPTIONS

Easy Option Reduce the number of reps of the incline barbell bench press to 6 per set.

Step It Up Increase to 8 total rounds.

Cool-Down Pec stretch, double lat stretch, 90-degree stretch.

The Gun Show

Looking for a nice pair of sleeve stretchers to poke out of your T-shirt this summer? Well you may as well punch your ticket to the gun show once you are done with this biceps and triceps workout. The variety of biceps and triceps work will force a lot of blood into your arms, giving you such a massive pump that you may find it hard to bend your elbows for the rest of the day.

Warm-Up

5 reps of inchworm, 6 reps per side of quadruped T-spine rotation, 10 reps of cat–cow

● Featured Exercise

Barbell Floor Press

1. Set up a barbell in a squat rack that is slightly below knee level.

2. Lie on the floor with your eyes directly under the bar (*a*).

3. Unrack the bar and lower until both triceps touch the ground (*b*). Pause and drive the weight back up to lockout. Repeat for reps.

Complete Workout

A1. Barbell floor press
- 3 sets × 10 reps
- 60 seconds of rest

A2. Decline EZ-bar triceps extension (#145)
- 3 sets × 10 reps
- 60 seconds of rest

B1. Single-arm cable curl (#183)
- 2 sets × 10 reps
- 60 seconds of rest

B2. Alternating dumbbell hammer curl (#230)
- 2 sets × 10 reps
- 60 seconds of rest

C1. Single-arm cable curl (#183)
- 1 set × 50 reps
- 60 seconds of rest

C2. Triceps rope press down (#64)
- 1 × 50 reps

OPTIONS

Easy Option Reduce the number of reps on the single-arm cable curl and triceps rope press-down to 25.

Step It Up Increase the number of reps on the single-arm cable curl and triceps rope press-down to 75.

Cool-Down Double lat stretch, cross-body stretch, hamstring stretch.

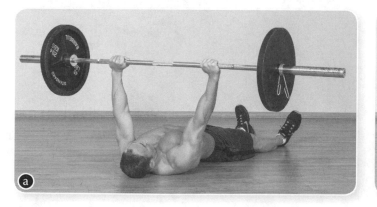

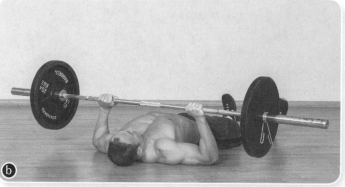

Mechanical Squat Drop

Most drop sets require you to perform an exercise for a set amount of reps, reduce the weight, and complete more reps in order to get in more total work. A mechanical drop set uses a similar principle, but instead of reducing the amount of weight, it combines three variations of an exercise, starting with the most technically demanding and ending with the least challenging.

Warm-Up

5 reps of squat to stand; 6 reps per side of kneeling adductor stretch, hip rocker, and quadruped T-spine rotation

● Featured Exercise

Overhead Squat

1. Begin with the barbell on your back, your hands in a snatch-grip position (outside shoulder width). Press the bar straight up, locking out your elbows at the top (*a*).

2. Keeping your chest tall, bring your hips back and bend at the knees to descend into a squat (*b*).

3. Keep the bar directly over or slightly behind your head for the entire movement.

4. Once you reach the bottom position, return to standing. Repeat for reps.

Complete Workout

Perform 5 rounds of the following circuit, keeping the same weight on the bar for each movement.

Overhead squat
- 6 reps
- 15 seconds of rest

Barbell front squat (#44)
- 6 reps
- 15 seconds of rest

Barbell back squat (#63)
- 12 reps
- 2 minutes of rest

OPTIONS

Easy Option   Reduce to 4 rounds of the circuit.

Step It Up   Increase reps to 8 for both the overhead squat and front squat.

Cool-Down   Standing quad stretch, 90-degree stretch, cross-body stretch.

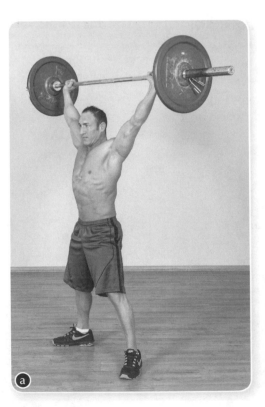
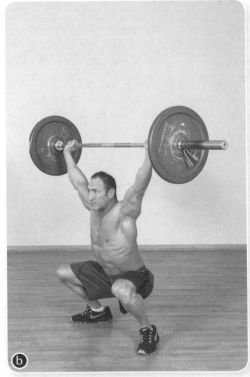

The Hammer

The lying hamstring curl is a machine-based movement that works the muscles on the posterior (back) side of the upper leg. This exercise works the hamstrings in knee flexion, a difficult movement to train under load otherwise. Proper hamstring strength is critical because it reduces the risk of quad dominance, which can lead to knee and other lower body injuries.

Warm-Up

4 reps per side of the world's greatest stretch, 5 reps each of inchworm and inverted hamstring stretch, 10 reps of glute bridge

● Featured Exercise

Lying Hamstring Curl

1. Lie down in a hamstring curl machine, with your knees positioned off the edge of the bench (a).

2. With your heels under the pad, press your hips into the bench and curl the weight all the way up until the pad touches the back of your legs (b).

3. Slowly control the weight back down to the starting position. Repeat for reps.

Complete Workout

Perform 4 rounds of the following circuit.

Conventional deadlift (#5)
- 4 reps
- 60 seconds of rest

Lying hamstring curl
- 4 reps
- 60 seconds of rest

Back extension (#116)
- 12 reps
- 2 minutes of rest

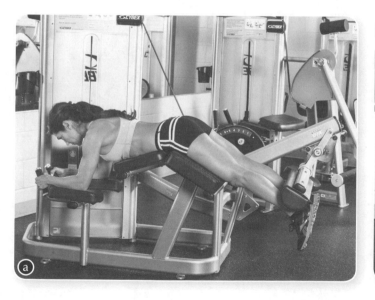

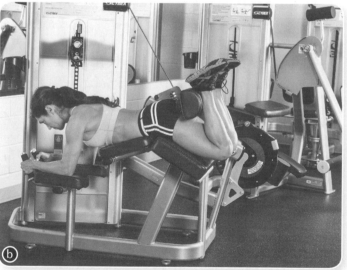

OPTIONS

Easy Option Complete 3 rounds of the circuit.

Step It Up Complete 5 rounds of the circuit.

Cool-Down Double lat stretch, hamstring stretch, calf stretch.

169 Im-pec-cable

There is a lot of debate on whether certain exercises can work the upper pecs versus lower pecs. Truth be told, there is no upper or lower pec—the pecs are one muscle group. However, certain exercises can target muscle fibers of the upper pecs, such as the incline bench press and low-to-high cable flys, and certain movements will bring more focus to the lower pecs, such as decline bench press and dips. This workout hits the fibers of the upper pecs, driving more development around the collarbones and shoulders.

Warm-Up

4 reps per side of the world's greatest stretch, 5 reps of inchworm, 8 reps per side of shoulder sweeps

● Featured Exercise

Crossover Push-Up

1. Get in a push-up position (hands on floor slightly wider than shoulder width, straight line from head to heels). Place your left hand on the floor and your right hand on a 3-inch (8 cm) box or a 45 lb (20 kg) weight plate.

2. Lower your torso to the floor, keeping your elbows tucked toward your rib cage (a).

3. Explosively push up so both hands leave the floor.

4. Land with your right hand on the floor and left hand on the box or weight plate (b).

5. Repeat (c), this time with your left hand landing on the floor and your right hand on the box. Continue to alternate until all reps are complete.

Complete Workout

A. Barbell bench press (#54)
   - 5 sets × 3 reps
   - 90 seconds of rest

B1. Incline dumbbell chest press (#210)
   - 4 sets × 8 reps
   - 30 seconds of rest

B2. Crossover push-up
   - 4 sets × 8 reps
   - 30 seconds of rest

B3. Low-to-high cable chest fly (#157)
   - 4 sets × 12 reps
   - 30 seconds of rest

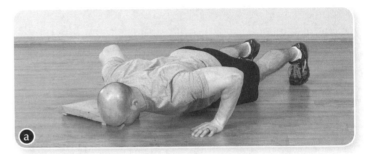

a

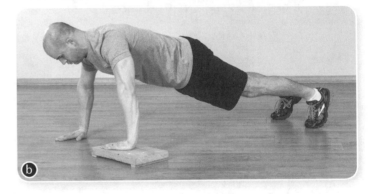

b

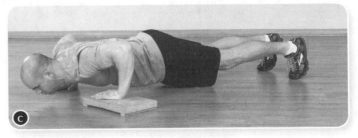

c

OPTIONS

Easy Option Reduce the incline nest bench press, crossover push-up, and low-to-high cable chest fly to 3 sets.

Step It Up Add 2 reps to the incline dumbbell nest press, crossover push-up, and low-to-high cable chest fly.

Cool-Down Pec stretch, double lat stretch, 90-degree stretch.

Speedskater

The jumps in this workout are named after Eric Heiden, an Olympic gold-medal speedskater from the United States. The jumps themselves are a plyometric version of the side-to-side motion used by skaters to propel themselves forward. Since we tend to minimize lateral (side to side) movement in both everyday life and training, these jumps can be quite challenging yet very effective in developing lower body power. Begin by sticking the landing on each jump before moving to the more continuous landing-in-to-jumping technique as you advance.

Warm-Up

5 reps of squat to stand; 6 reps per side of kneeling adductor stretch, hip rocker, and quadruped T-spine rotation

● Featured Exercise

Heiden Jump

1. Standing tall with flexed knees, lift your right foot slightly off the ground (a).
2. Jump off your left forefoot to propel yourself laterally (sideways) to the right, jumping as high up and as far over as possible (b).

3. Land on your right forefoot with your right knee flexed (c). Without touching your left foot to the floor, propel yourself to the left, jumping as high and as far over as possible.
4. Continue to alternate in this manner until you have completed all reps for each side.

Complete Workout

A. Heiden jump
   - 5 sets × 6 reps/leg

B1. Barbell back squat (#63)
   - 3 sets × 4 to 6 reps
   - 90 seconds of rest

B2. Bulgarian split squat (#200)
   - 3 sets × 6 to 8 reps/leg
   - 90 seconds of rest

B3. Leg press (#114)
   - 3 sets × 8 to 10 reps
   - 90 seconds of rest

OPTIONS

Easy Option   Perform 2 sets of the barbell back squats, Bulgarian split squats, and leg press.

Step It Up   Perform 4 sets of the barbell back squats, Bulgarian split squats, and leg press.

Cool-Down   Standing quad stretch, 90-degree stretch, double lat stretch.

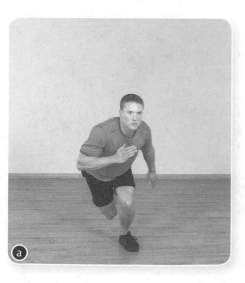
(a)

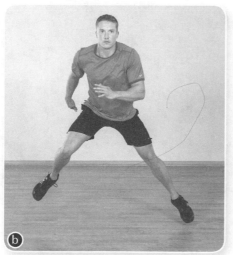
(b)

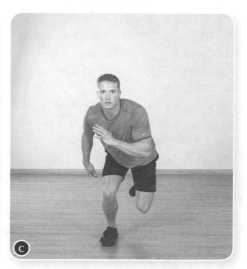
(c)

Scared Straight

When performing the concentric (lifting) portion of movements such as the Romanian deadlift or the single-leg barbell straight-leg deadlift, featured in this workout, it is very easy to overuse your lower back to lift the weight. To prevent this, think about squeezing your glutes before driving your hips forward to get back to the starting position. If your glutes are doing the work, they will take the stress off your lower back, allowing you to be safer and stronger for the entire set.

Warm-Up

5 reps of inchworm, 6 reps per side of quadruped T-spine rotation, 10 reps of cat–cow

Complete Workout

A. Trap bar deadlift (#8)
- 4 sets × 8 reps

B1. Single-leg barbell straight-leg deadlift
- 3 sets × 8 reps/side

B2. Glute–ham raise (#70)
- 3 sets × 8 reps

● **Featured Exercise**

Single-Leg Barbell Straight-Leg Deadlift

1. Grab a barbell with an overhand grip just outside shoulder width. Your arms should be straight, with your elbow locked out.

2. Keeping a slight bend in your knees, reach your left leg back (a) and lower your torso toward the floor (b). Think about driving your left heel back and up toward the ceiling throughout the entire movement.

3. Once the barbell reaches mid-shin, reverse the motion to return to the starting position.

4. Complete all reps for one side before switching to the other.

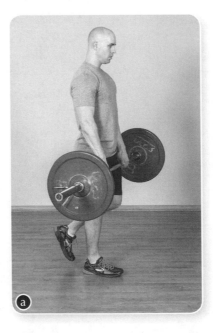
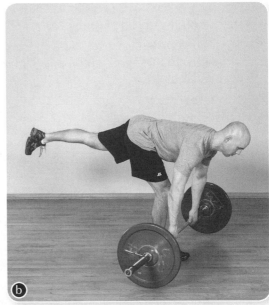

OPTIONS

Easy Option   Perform 3 sets of the trap bar deadlift.

Step It Up   Add 1 set to the single-leg barbell straight-leg deadlift and glute–ham raise.

Cool-Down   Double lat stretch, cross-body stretch, hamstring stretch.

Fly Away

The cable chest fly is a great exercise to include during a chest-focused workout. It does a better job of isolating the pecs than most pressing movements and is usually safer on both your shoulder and elbow joints. The cable fly also lets you use a variety of angles, including low-to-high, high-to-low, parallel, and lying.

Warm-Up

4 reps per side of the world's greatest stretch, 5 reps of inchworm, 8 reps per side of shoulder sweeps

 Featured Exercise

Lying Cable Chest Fly

1. Place a flat bench directly in the middle and slightly in front of both weight stacks. Lower the cables to the bottom setting, and attach a D handle to each.

2. Grab a handle in each hand, sit on the far end of the bench, and lie back (resist the force of the cables sliding you back on the bench).

3. Extend your arms overhead into a giant V (*a*). With a very slight bend in your elbows, pull your arms up and over until your hands are above your belly button (*b*).

4. Return to the starting position and repeat for reps.

Complete Workout

Incline dumbbell chest press (#210)
- 5 sets × 8 reps
- 60 seconds of rest

Lying cable chest fly
- 5 sets × 15 reps
- 60 seconds of rest

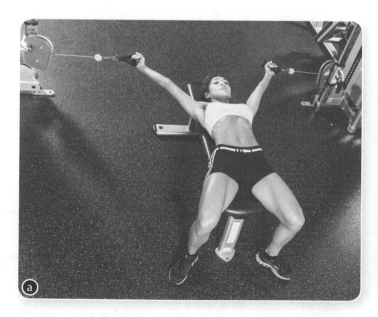

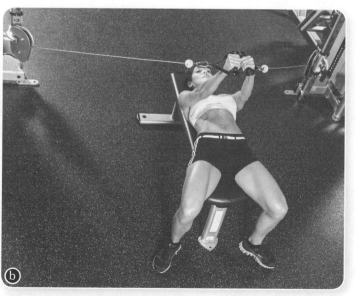

OPTIONS

Easy Option   Perform 3 sets of each exercise.

Step It Up   Add a third exercise of 20 push-ups (#12), resting 60 seconds before returning to the incline dumbbell chest press.

Cool-Down   Pec stretch, double lat stretch, 90-degree stretch.

Front Loaded

Fitness fads come and go. And although some of them can be effective, many more are strictly gimmicky and full of marketing hype. There is some benefit to trying different exercise modalities and nutrition plans from time to time, but the bedrock of your fitness plan should be the tried and true exercises and programs that have proven to work for years. Get great at the basics and make them the foundation of everything you do, and you'll get better results in the long run.

Warm-Up

5 reps of squat to stand; 6 reps per side of kneeling adductor stretch, hip rocker, and quadruped T-spine rotation

● Featured Exercise

Barbell Front Squat

1. Set up a barbell just below collarbone height in a squat rack.
2. Step under the bar so it sits on your front deltoids (shoulders), and grab the bar with a clean grip, with your elbows high and your upper arms parallel to the ground. Unrack the bar, and take one step back with each foot (*a*).
3. Tighten up your upper body, unlock your hips, bend your knees, and lower your body toward the ground, trying to sit as low as possible while keeping the bar over the center of your foot (for more on proper squat technique, see chapter 1, Ramping Up) (*b*).
4. Once you reach the bottom of your range, reverse the motion and stand up. Repeat for reps.

Complete Workout

This is a tonnage workout featuring the barbell front squat; you are trying to lift a total of 9,000 lb (4,100 kg) throughout the entire workout. You can use whatever weight you wish throughout the workout and perform as many reps per set as you'd like. For example, if you performed 10 sets of 9 reps with 100 lb (45 kg) on the barbell, you would reach the 9,000 lb ($10 \times 9 \times 100 = 9,000$). The goal is to lift a total of 9,000 lb in as little time as possible.

Barbell front squat
- 9,000 lb (4,100 kg) total in as little time as possible

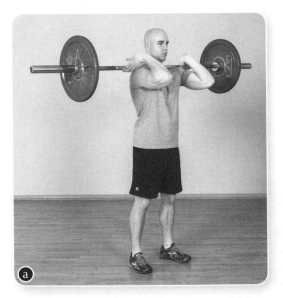

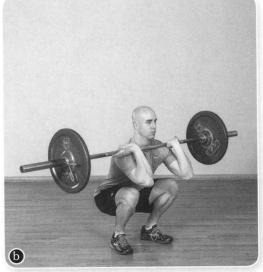

OPTIONS

Easy Option Lift a total of 7,000 lb (3,200 kg) for the entire workout.

Step It Up Get to 9,000 lb in fewer than 50 reps.

Cool-Down Standing quad stretch, 90-degree stretch, cross-body stretch.

Lean and Mean

Although it's human nature to put yourself in the most advantageous position possible to complete a task, when it comes to building muscle, putting yourself at a disadvantage can be a more powerful strategy for recruiting more motor units or different muscle groups. In this workout, you'll be performing a seated row with hip flexion, which is opposite to your natural tendency to extend at the hips while pulling in order to gain some momentum during your pull. By reversing this tendency, you'll get a great contraction from the muscles of your midback. Just beware that this mechanical disadvantage comes at the cost of the amount of load you can use, so adjust the weights accordingly.

Warm-Up

5 reps of inchworm, 6 reps per side of quadruped T-spine rotation, 10 reps of cat–cow

Featured Exercise

Seated Cable Row With Hip Flexion

1. Attach your favorite bar or handle to a seated cable row machine, and grab it with a neutral grip.
2. Keeping your chest tall, your knees slightly bent, and your upper traps depressed, begin pulling the handle toward your sternum.
3. As you pull, flex forward slightly at your hips, bringing your torso closer to the handle.
4. At the end of the pull, your torso should be flexed at approximately 20 degrees, the handle should be at the bottom of your rib cage, and your elbows should be behind you.
5. Reverse the motion by extending your arms and bringing your torso back to a neutral position. Repeat for reps.

Complete Workout

Perform 4 rounds of the following circuit.

Wide-grip pull-up (#117)
- 4 sets × 8 reps
- 60 seconds of rest

Seated cable row with hip flexion
- 4 sets × 10 reps
- 90 seconds of rest

TRX Y (#75)
- 4 sets × 12 reps
- 90 seconds of rest

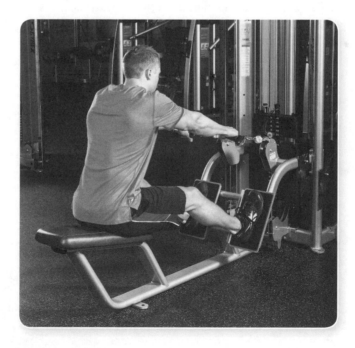

OPTIONS

Easy Option   Substitute a kneeling lat pull-down (#120) for the wide-grip pull-up.

Step It Up   Add external load to the wide-grip pull-up.

Cool-Down   Double lat stretch, cross-body stretch, hamstring stretch.

Catch the Wave

Wave loading is a protocol that allows you to increase weights used from set to set while still keeping volume (total amount of work being done) fairly high. There are many ways to utilize wave loading, but the scheme in the following workout tends to be most effective for developing strength and size.

Warm-Up

5 reps of squat to stand; 6 reps per side of kneeling adductor stretch, hip rocker, and quadruped T-spine rotation

Featured Exercise

Side Plank

1. Lie on the ground on your right side.
2. Place your elbow directly under your shoulder and your left foot in front of your right (your left heel should be touching or just in front of your right toes).
3. Press yourself up so that you are creating a straight line from head to heels, with only your elbow, forearm, and feet touching the ground.
4. Hold this position for the prescribed amount of time, and then repeat for the other side.

OPTIONS

Easy Option   Perform the side plank for 15 seconds per side, and reduce the number of reps on the reverse crunch to 12 per set.

Step It Up   Perform the side plank for 40 seconds per side, and increase the number of reps on the toes to bar to 25 per set.

Cool-Down   Standing quad stretch, 90-degree stretch, cross-body stretch.

Complete Workout

As the number of reps decreases for the front squat, increase the load used. The second time through the wave (sets 4, 5, and 6), attempt more weight than you used for the corresponding number of reps on sets 1, 2, and 3. For example, your second set of 6 reps (set 5) should be heavier than your first set of 6 (set 2).

A. Barbell front squat (#44)
   - 6 sets × 8, 6, 4, 8, 6, 4 reps
   - 75 seconds of rest

B1. Side plank
   - 2 sets × 30 seconds/side
   - 60 seconds of rest

B2. Toes to bar (#28)
   - 2 sets × 20 reps
   - 60 seconds of rest

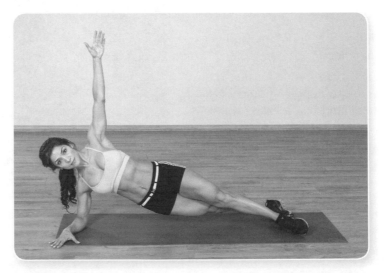

Atlas

A great way to maintain shoulder integrity and health when doing push-ups and push-up variations (such as the inverted shoulder press featured in this workout) is to externally rotate your shoulders as you lower your body to the floor. This can be accomplished by thinking about "screwing your hands" (your right hand clockwise, your left hand counterclockwise) into the floor. Your hands shouldn't actually move, you are just putting some rotational force into your hands. This creation of torque can lead to a more stable joint position, helping you perform push-ups more effectively and with less risk of injury.

Warm-Up

4 reps per side of the world's greatest stretch, 5 reps of inchworm, 8 reps per side of shoulder sweeps

● Featured Exercise

Inverted Shoulder Press

1. Assume a push-up position, with your feet on a bench or box.
2. Walk your hands back toward the bench, and push your hips up toward the ceiling until your torso is nearly perpendicular to the floor.
3. Bend your elbows, lowering your body until your head nearly touches the floor (a).
4. Push your hands into the floor, straightening your arms until you reach lockout (b). Repeat for reps.

Complete Workout

A1. Push press (#16)
- 3 sets × 6 reps
- 60 seconds of rest

A2. Cable diagonal raise (#137)
- 12 reps/side
- 60 seconds of rest

B1. Seated dumbbell shoulder press (#209)
- 3 sets × 6 reps
- 60 seconds of rest

B2. Inverted shoulder press
- 3 sets × 12 reps
- 60 seconds of rest

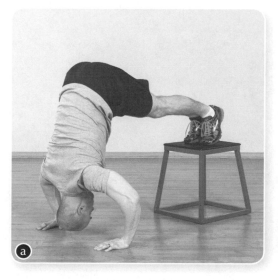
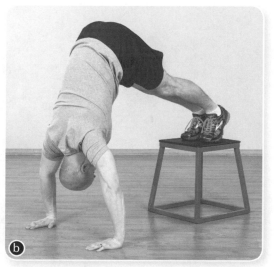

OPTIONS

Easy Option Perform 8 reps of the cable diagonal raise and inverted shoulder press.

Step It Up Increase the number of sets to 4 for each movement.

Cool-Down Pec stretch, double lat stretch, 90-degree stretch.

Squat 'til You Drop

The squat is often referred to as the king of all exercises, and with good reason. It's very hard to find another movement that challenges the calves, quads, glutes, abdominals, lower back, and midback with the same intensity as the back squat. And major compound movements such as the squat create the perfect anabolic hormonal environment for growth. So, by including squats in your program, you'll see more muscle gain over your entire body.

Warm-Up

5 reps of squat to stand; 6 reps per side of kneeling adductor stretch, hip rocker, and quadruped T-spine rotation

● Featured Exercise

Barbell Back Squat

1. Set up a barbell just below collarbone height in a squat rack.
2. Step under the bar so it sits on your upper traps, and take one step back with each foot (*a*).
3. Tighten up your upper body, unlock your hips, bend your knees, and lower your body toward the ground, trying to sit as low as possible while keeping the bar over the center of your foot (for more on proper squat technique, see chapter 1, Ramping Up) (*b*).
4. Once you reach the bottom of your range, reverse the motion and stand up. Repeat for reps.

Complete Workout

Perform 5 rounds of the following drop set, reducing the load for each set as prescribed.

Barbell back squat
- 8 reps
- 30 seconds of rest

Barbell back squat (reduce load by 20 percent)
- 8 reps
- 30 seconds of rest

Barbell back squat (reduce load by an additional 20 percent)
- 8 reps
- 2 minutes of rest

OPTIONS

Easy Option   Perform 4 rounds of the drop set.

Step It Up   Reduce the weight only 10 percent between sets.

Cool-Down   Standing quad stretch, 90-degree stretch, cross-body stretch.

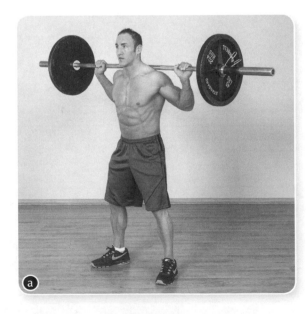

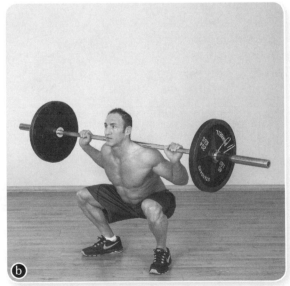

The Savage

There will come a time in certain lifts where your grip strength will be the limiting factor in how much load you can use. The deadlift is a great example of this. There are two ways to approach this issue. The first is to continue working on improving your grip strength so you can maintain a double overhand grip for as many sets as possible. However, when working closer to maximal loads, you can employ a mixed grip where one hand is pronated (palm facing you) while the other is supinated (palm facing away from you). Utilizing the mixed grip will certainly make grip strength less of a factor and allow you to add more weight to the bar.

Warm-Up

4 reps per side of the world's greatest stretch, 5 reps each of inchworm and inverted hamstring stretch, 10 reps of glute bridge

● **Featured Exercise**

Single-Leg Back Extension

1. Position yourself in a back extension station, and hook one foot under the foot pads.
2. Keeping your back flat and tight, hinge at the hips to lower your torso toward the floor (you want to create approximately a 90-degree angle between your upper and lower body) (a).
3. Contract your hamstrings and lift your torso back up to a flat position; be sure to fire your glutes at the top of the movement (this will take stress off your lower back) (b).
4. Complete all reps for one leg before switching to the other.

Complete Workout

A. Conventional deadlift (#5)
- 5 sets × 3 reps
- 90 seconds of rest

B1. Dumbbell step-up (#121)
- 2 sets × 8 reps/side
- 30 seconds of rest

B2. Lying hamstring curl (#168)
- 2 sets × 10 reps
- 30 seconds of rest

B3. Single-leg back extension
- 2 sets × 6 reps/side
- 30 seconds of rest

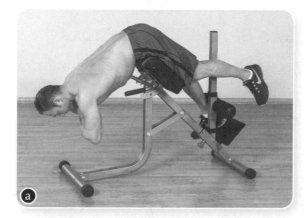

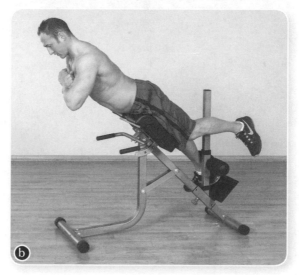

OPTIONS

Easy Option   Complete 3 sets of the conventional deadlift.

Step It Up   Add 1 set to each of the exercises.

Cool-Down   Double lat stretch, hamstring stretch, calf stretch.

Chest Thumper

When performing any barbell version of the bench press (flat, incline, decline), always start with your eyes under the bar. Doing so will allow you to pull the bar off the catches and set your shoulders and lats into a good pressing position. It will also ensure that you don't hit the barbell catches or bench supports at the top of your press.

Warm-Up

4 reps per side of the world's greatest stretch, 5 reps of inchworm, 8 reps per side of shoulder sweeps

● Featured Exercise

Incline Barbell Bench Press

1. At an incline bench press station, grab the bar just outside shoulder width, and unrack it from the barbell catches (a).

2. Keeping a slight natural arch in your lower back, lower the bar until it touches your torso at midchest level (b). Keep your elbows tucked toward your side as you lower the bar.

3. Forcefully drive the weight back up until you achieve lockout of your elbows. Repeat for reps.

Complete Workout

Incline barbell bench press
- 4 sets × 4 reps
- 60 seconds of rest

Flat dumbbell bench press (#109)
- 4 sets × 4 reps
- 60 seconds of rest

Low-to-high cable chest fly (#157)
- 4 sets × 12 reps
- 2 minutes of rest

OPTIONS

Easy Option   Complete 3 sets of each exercise.

Step It Up   Complete 5 sets of each exercise.

Cool-Down   Pec stretch, double lat stretch, 90-degree stretch.

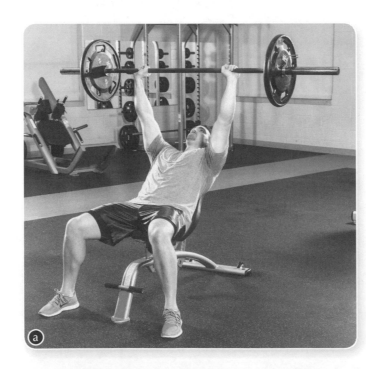

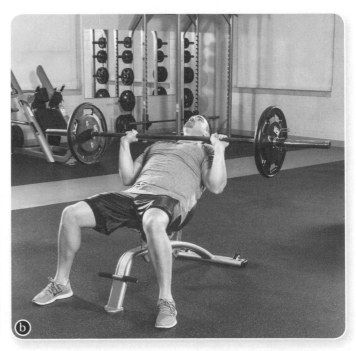

Toss 'n Turn

Do you need to train more rotational movements? Yes. Do you need to train for power more often? Yes. Do you need to have fun throwing a medicine ball at a wall or your training partner? Yes. The rotational medicine ball throw (featured in this workout) provides all these things and can help improve sport-specific skills such as throwing a punch, putting a golf ball, and swinging a bat.

Warm-Up

5 reps of inchworm, 6 reps per side of quadruped T-spine rotation, 10 reps of cat–cow

Featured Exercise

Rotational Medicine Ball Throw

1. Grab a medicine ball and stand 3 feet (1 m) away from a padded wall or workout partner, with your left shoulder facing whichever you choose.

2. Hold the ball at mid-torso level, with your arms straight. Rotate the ball to your left by pivoting your hips, left foot, and shoulders and give the ball to your partner (a).

3. Quickly rotate back to the right and take the ball from your partner (b).

4. Complete all reps for one side before switching to the other.

Complete Workout

A1. Barbell front squat (#44)
- 4 sets × 6 reps
- 75 seconds of rest

A2. Dumbbell step-up (#121)
- 4 sets × 6 reps/side
- 75 seconds of rest

B1. Foam roller reverse crunch (#229)
- 3 sets × 10 reps
- 60 seconds of rest

B2. Rotational medicine ball throw (#180)
- 3 sets × 10 reps
- 60 seconds of rest

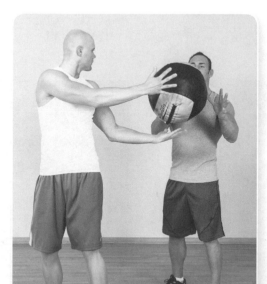

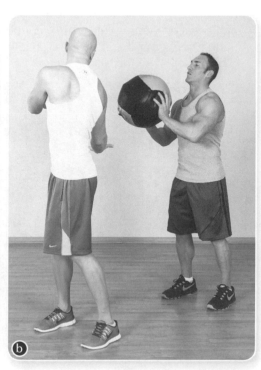

OPTIONS

Easy Option   Perform 3 sets of the barbell front squat and dumbbell step-up.

Step It Up   Add 2 reps to each exercise.

Cool-Down   Double lat stretch, cross-body stretch, hamstring stretch.

6-12-25 Chest

The first time you ever walked into a gym, you probably sat down on a bench press and worked your chest. But I promise you, you've never worked your pecs this way before. By combining several different strength qualities (strength, hypertrophy, and endurance) in one workout, you'll get a pump that will have you walking around looking like a superhero for days.

Warm-Up

4 reps per side of the world's greatest stretch, 5 reps of inchworm, 8 reps per side of shoulder sweeps

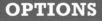 **Featured Exercise**

Cable Chest Fly

1. Stand between two cable crossover stations. The cables should be set at midchest height and have D-ring attachments
2. Utilizing a split stance (one foot in front of the other), grab each handle with arms extended to your sides and a slight bend at the elbow (a).

3. Without bending your elbows further, bring your hands together in front of your chest, squeezing your pecs as you come to the end range of motion (it should look as if you are hugging an invisible barrel as hard as you can) (b).
4. Return to the starting position and repeat for reps.

Complete Workout

Perform the following three exercises as a circuit, resting 10 seconds between exercises and 100 seconds between rounds. Repeat the circuit a total of 4 times.

Barbell bench press (#54)
- 6 reps
- 10 seconds of rest

Incline dumbbell chest press (#210)
- 12 reps
- 10 seconds of rest

Cable chest fly
- 25 reps
- 100 seconds of rest

OPTIONS

Easy Option   Reduce the number of reps of the cable chest fly to 15.

Step It Up   Add an additional round, bringing the total number of circuits to 5.

Cool-Down   Pec stretch, double lat stretch, 90-degree stretch.

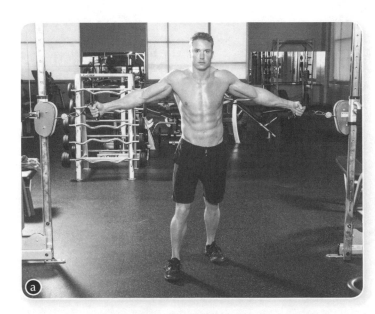

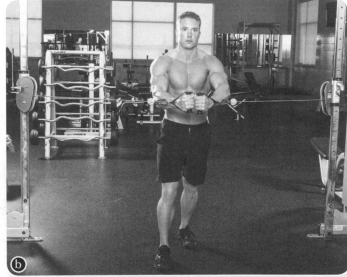

Well Suited

You've just gotten off a long flight. You're waiting at the baggage carousel. Finally, you spot your overstuffed, oversized suitcase coming your way. But instead of struggling to grab your bag like everyone else, you rip it off the conveyor belt and get on your way. The barbell suitcase deadlift, featured in this workout, can help you prepare for moments like this by training your grip, glutes, hamstrings, and core in a way that clearly has carryover to real-world activities.

Warm-Up

4 reps per side of the world's greatest stretch, 5 reps each of inchworm and inverted hamstring stretch, 10 reps of glute bridge

● Featured Exercise

Barbell Suitcase Deadlift

1. Place a loaded barbell next to your right ankle.

2. Keeping your spine in a neutral position, chest tall and eyes forward, bring your hips back and bend at the knees until you are able to grasp the center of the barbell (a).

3. Extend at the knees and hips until you are in a standing position (b).

4. Return the barbell to the starting position and repeat for reps, completing all reps on one side before switching to the other.

Complete Workout

A. Barbell suitcase deadlift
- • 4 sets × 6 reps/side
- • 90 seconds of rest

B1. Goblet squat (#2)
- • 3 sets × 10 reps
- • 60 seconds of rest

B2. Leg press (#114)
- • 3 sets × 10 reps
- • 60 seconds of rest

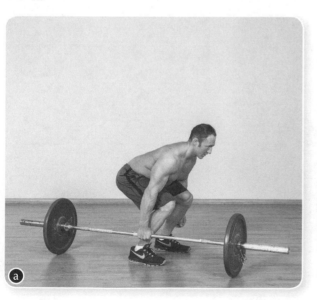
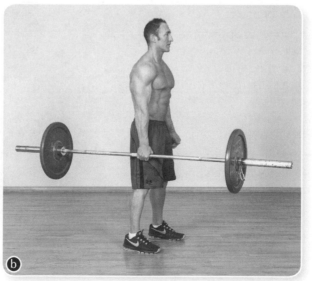

OPTIONS

Easy Option   Reduce the goblet squat and leg press to 2 sets.

Step It Up   Add 2 reps per side to the barbell suitcase deadlift.

Cool-Down   Double lat stretch, hamstring stretch, calf stretch.

Bi This

If larger arms are your goal, it would definitely be valuable to train your arms directly once or twice per week. Although you should not abandon squats, deadlifts, and other full-body movements, training a muscle group directly is still a critical component for most efficiently gaining size in that muscle group. In other words, squatting might help you get bigger overall, but you'd be much better off adding in some biceps curls if you are looking for a serious pair of guns.

Warm-Up

5 reps of inchworm, 6 reps per side of quadruped T-spine rotation, 10 reps of cat–cow

Complete Workout

A. Narrow-grip chin-up (#1)
- 4 sets × 6 reps
- 90 seconds of rest

B1. Single-arm cable curl
- 3 sets × 10 reps/side
- 45 seconds of rest

B2. Offset-grip incline dumbbell curl (#243)
- 3 sets × 10 reps
- 45 seconds of rest

● **Featured Exercise**

Single-Arm Cable Curl

1. Attach a D handle to the low pulley of a cable station. Grab the handle with a supinated grip (palm facing the ceiling). Stand tall with your arm extended and knees slightly bent (*a*).

2. Keeping your upper arm locked to your rib cage, flex at the elbow until your fist is directly in front of your shoulder (*b*). Squeeze your biceps at the end position.

3. Straighten your arm to return to the starting position. Repeat for reps on one side before switching to the other.

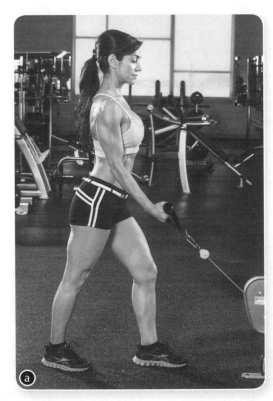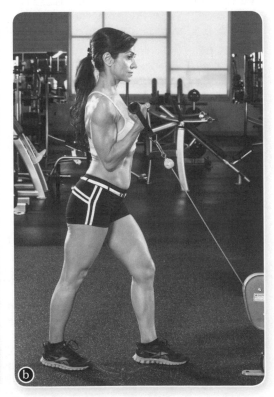

OPTIONS

Easy Option Perform 2 sets of the single-arm cable curl and offset-grip incline dumbbell curl.

Step It Up Add 1 set to the single-arm cable curl and offset-grip incline dumbbell curl.

Cool-Down Double lat stretch, cross-body stretch, hamstring stretch.

CHAPTER 5

Last (Wo)Man Standing

This chapter is all about conditioning, or the ability to perform movements or skills while under fatigue. At this point you should be familiar and skilled in all the major exercise patterns, so it's time to up the challenge and see how well you can perform them when your muscles are tired, your lungs are on fire, and the sweat is pouring into your eyes. These workouts require precision, determination, and guts, which is why you will notice that many of them have military-inspired names. Besides transferring directly to your abilities on the court or field, this type of training is excellent for improving body composition, particularly stripping off body fat in a hurry.

Clean the Plate

Your mother always told you that you couldn't leave the dinner table until you cleaned your plate. Using a bit of Mom's wisdom, you're not allowed to leave the lifting platform until you've "cleaned the plate" for the entire length of this workout. This, I can promise you, is a bit tougher than finishing your broccoli.

Warm-Up

4 reps per side of the world's greatest stretch, 6 reps per side of hip rocker and inverted hamstring stretch, 8 reps per side of shoulder sweeps

● Featured Exercise

Full Clean

1. Start by grabbing the barbell with an overhand grip, placing your hands and feet slightly wider than shoulder-width apart (*a*).

2. Keeping the bar close to your shins, slowly pull your knees back while lifting the bar off the ground.

3. Once the bar gets to your midthighs, explosively jump upward, extending at the ankles, knees, and hips (*b*).

4. Aggressively pull your body under the bar, rotating your elbows around the bar.

5. You should time the lift so you are catching the bar at the bottom position of a squat (*c*).

6. A rep is completed when you stand up with the bar (*d*). Repeat for reps.

Complete Workout

Complete the workout by loading one plate (a 45 lb or 20 kg weight plate) on each side of a barbell, and set a timer for 20 minutes.

Full clean
  • Complete 1 rep every minute for 20 minutes (20 total reps)

OPTIONS

Easy Option   Perform 1 rep every minute for 15 minutes.

Step It Up   Perform 2 reps each minute for the entire 20 minutes.

Cool-Down   Standing quad stretch, 90-degree stretch, double lat stretch.

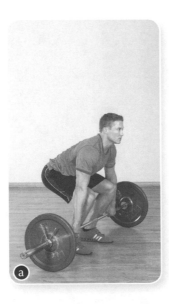

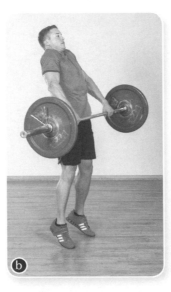

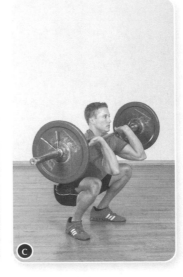

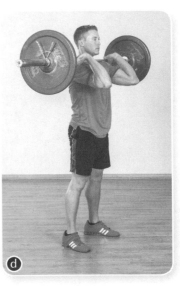

Go Hard

Sport psychologists have known for a long time that visualization can help with performance and achieving goals. So next time you are stuck at a plateau and find yourself not able to improve your time or hit a rep, take a few minutes to visualize yourself reaching your goal. This can actually be most effectively done when you are nowhere near the gym, field, or court. At night, before you go to sleep, envision yourself hitting that 400 lb deadlift, completing that circuit 15 seconds faster, or scoring the game-winning free throw. It could just help you blast through a sticking point.

Warm-Up

6 reps of squat to stand, 6 reps per side of quadruped T-spine rotation, 8 reps of glute bridge, 10 reps of cat–cow

● Featured Exercise

Glute–Ham Raise Sit-Up

1. Set up a glute–ham raise machine so the pads are directly under the bottom of your glutes when your legs are straight.

2. Enter the machine facing the ceiling, with your legs straight (this is the opposite of how you would enter the machine to do a glute–ham raise).

3. Lean back until your upper body reaches below parallel to the ground (a). As you lean back, allow your knees to bend slightly.

4. Once you've reached the end of your range of motion, forcefully sit up and extend your knees (b). Reach out and touch your toes. Repeat for reps.

Complete Workout

Perform 3 rounds of the following circuit. In the first round perform 20 reps per exercise. In the second round perform 15 reps per exercise. In the third round perform 10 reps per exercise. Complete all three rounds as quickly as possible, resting only when needed.

Goblet squat (#2)

Neutral-grip pull-up (#237)

Glute–ham raise sit-up

 Warning: The glute–ham raise sit-up can be difficult for people with lower back issues. If that is the case, use a traditional sit-up. Also, be sure to use extreme caution when entering and exiting the machine.

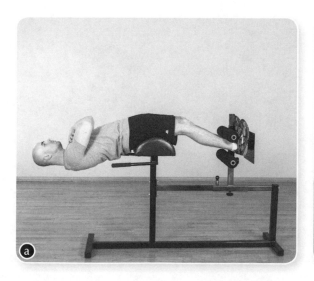

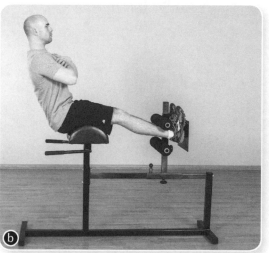

OPTIONS

Easy Option Reduce the number of reps per round to 12, 10, and 8.

Step It Up Add an additional round of 8 reps per exercise to the end of the circuit.

Cool-Down Standing quad stretch, 90-degree stretch, double lat stretch.

Push-Pull-Jump

Performing circuits for time requires not only strength and endurance but also strategy. Is it best to do as many reps as possible before taking a break? Is it smarter to have a few reps in the tank so you don't redline before taking a breather? Try utilizing different strategies during your timed circuit workouts to determine which works best for you.

Warm-Up

4 reps per side of the world's greatest stretch, 6 reps per side of hip rocker and inverted hamstring stretch, 8 reps per side of shoulder sweeps

● Featured Exercise

Feet-Elevated Push-Up

1. Begin with your feet elevated on a box or bench (the higher the box, the more difficult the exercise), your hands just outside shoulder width and arms straight. You should be forming a straight line from your shoulders to your heels (*a*).

2. Lower your body to the ground, keeping your elbows tucked toward your sides. Do not let your hips sag or stick up as you perform the movement (*b*).

3. Once you reach the bottom position, forcefully drive up until your arms reach lockout. Repeat for reps.

OPTIONS

Easy Option Perform 20 foot-elevated push-ups and 10 pull-ups.

Step It Up Perform as many rounds as possible for 12 minutes.

Cool-Down Hamstring stretch, calf stretch, pec stretch.

Complete Workout

Perform as many rounds of this circuit as possible in 10 minutes.

Feet-elevated push-up
- 30 reps

Pull-up (#231)
- 15 reps

Box jump (#198)
- 10 reps

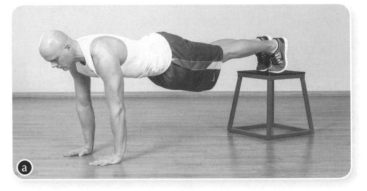

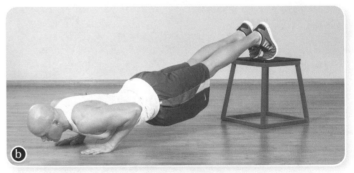

E-I-E-I-Ouch

The farmer's walk (named as such because it replicates the type of carry often performed by farmers) is a simple yet very effective total-body conditioning tool. It's great for taxing the grip as well as developing total-body strength that has significant carryover to many day-to-day activities (such as carrying heavy grocery bags or suitcases).

Warm-Up

6 reps of squat to stand, 6 reps per side of quadruped T-spine rotation, 8 reps of glute bridge, 10 reps of cat–cow

Featured Exercise

Farmer's Walk

1. This exercise can be completed using dumbbells, kettlebells, or farmer's handles.
2. Grab a pair of dumbbells, one in each hand.
3. Stand with your arms hanging at your sides, chest tall, shoulders down and back.
4. Maintain this posture and, at a moderate pace, complete a forward walk for the distance prescribed.

Complete Workout

Perform 4 rounds of the following circuit, resting as little as possible between exercises.

Farmer's walk
- 40 yards (40 m)

Goblet squat (#2)
- 10 reps

Farmer's walk
- 40 yards (40 m)

Incline dumbbell chest press (#210)
- 10 reps

Farmer's walk
- 4 sets × 40 yards (40 m)

Double-arm kettlebell swing (#13)
- 20 reps
- 2 minutes of rest

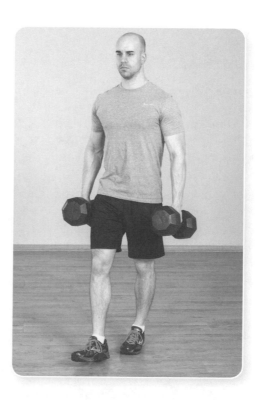

OPTIONS

Easy Option   Reduce the distance of the farmer's walk to 20 yards (20 m).

Step It Up   Increase the distance of the farmer's walk to 60 yards (60 m).

Cool-Down   Hamstring stretch, calf stretch, pec stretch.

The Perfect 10

It's the score given to a flawless performance. The number used to describe Bo Derek's beauty in the famous 1970s movie. The number of years in a decade. However, in the case of this workout, 10 describes the number of gut-wrenching rounds and number of reps per set that you will have to survive in order to make it to the finish line. And if those 10s aren't enough of a challenge for you, try completing this metabolically grueling workout in under 10 minutes. Do so and you'll earn the title of a perfect 10.

Warm-Up

6 reps of squat to stand, 6 reps per side of quadruped T-spine rotation, 8 reps of glute bridge, 10 reps of cat–cow

Complete Workout

Complete 10 rounds of the following circuit, resting as little as possible.

Dumbbell thruster (#208)
- 10 reps

Frog sit-up (#27)
- 10 reps

Prisoner squat
- 10 reps

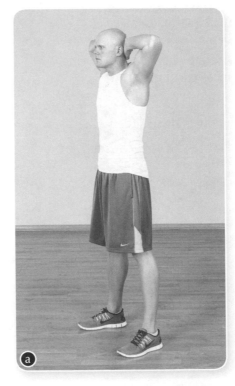
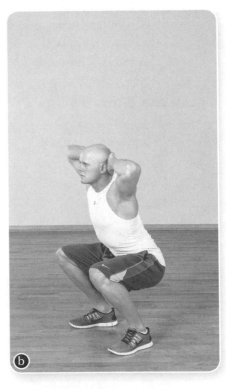

Featured Exercise

Prisoner Squat

1. Stand with your feet between hip- and shoulder-width apart and place your hands behind your head with your elbows directly out to the side (a).

2. Unlock your knees and your hips and lower yourself into as deep a squat as possible (b). Be sure to keep your chest tall and do not pull your head forward with your hands.

3. When you reach the bottom position, return to standing. Repeat for reps.

OPTIONS

Easy Option Perform 5 reps per round of the dumbbell thrusters.

Step It Up Perform an additional 2 rounds (12 total) of the entire circuit.

Cool-Down Standing quad stretch, 90-degree stretch, double lat stretch.

Row and Press

Trying to complete as many sets as possible in a certain amount of time (often referred to as density training) is a great way to shed fat and challenge yourself. This density circuit featuring the leg press and a chest-supported DB row works noncompeting muscle groups, which should leave you just fresh enough after each set to work as hard as possible on each rep.

Warm-Up

4 reps per side of the world's greatest stretch, 6 reps per side of hip rocker and inverted hamstring stretch, 8 reps per side of shoulder sweeps

Featured Exercise

Chest-Supported Dumbbell Row

1. Set an adjustable bench to a 30-degree angle.
2. Grab a set of dumbbells and lie on the bench. Your head should be higher than your feet. Allow the dumbbells to hang straight down from your shoulders (*a*).
3. Keeping your arms close to your sides, row the dumbbells up as high as possible by driving your elbows behind you (*b*).
4. Lower to the starting position and repeat for reps.

Complete Workout

Complete the following exercises, alternating between the two movements for 20 minutes with as little rest as possible between sets and rounds. Use 60 percent of your usual 6RM (repetition maximum) for each exercise.

Leg press (#114)
- 6 reps

Chest-supported dumbbell row
- 6 reps

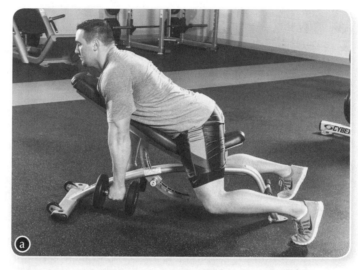

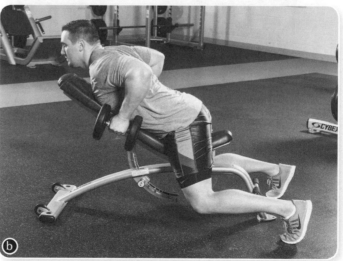

OPTIONS

Easy Option Perform the circuit for 15 minutes.

Step It Up Use 75 percent of your 6RM for both movements.

Cool-Down Standing quad stretch, double lat stretch, 90-degree stretch.

Nifty 50

To complete the Nifty 50, you'll need to get through 5 rounds of 10 reps of each exercise (50 reps total per exercise, hence the name). And although you won't be using any load outside your body weight, the combination of pushing, pulling, squatting, and jumping should leave your muscles fatigued and your lungs burning by the time you make it to the end. Don't let this workout, or any other using only body weight, fool you into a false sense of security. When a workout is designed just right, moving your body through space can be more demanding than you may have imagined.

Warm-Up

6 reps of squat to stand, 6 reps per side of quadruped T-spine rotation, 8 reps of glute bridge, 10 reps of cat–cow

● Featured Exercise

Dive-Bomber Push-Up

1. Begin in push-up position, with your hands just outside shoulder width and your body forming a straight line from your head to your heels.

2. Press your hands down into the floor and rock your hips back, bringing your butt into the air. Your arms and legs should remain straight, and your hands should be beyond your head (*a*).

3. Bend your elbows, bring your chest down toward the floor, and rock your body forward (*b*).

4. Drive your head through your arms, lifting your chest up and keeping your legs just above the floor (*c*).

5. Reverse this motion to get back to the starting position. Repeat for reps.

Complete Workout

Complete 5 rounds of the following circuit, resting as little as possible.

Prisoner squat (#188)
- 10 reps

Dive-bomber push-up
- 10 reps

Split jump (#14)
- 10 reps (5 per leg)

Chin-up (#73)
- 10 reps

OPTIONS

Easy Option Complete 3 rounds of the circuit.

Step It Up Add a weighted vest during the entire workout.

Cool-Down Standing quad stretch, 90-degree stretch, double lat stretch.

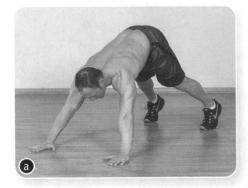
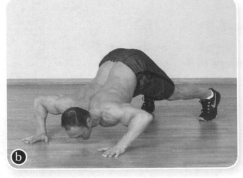
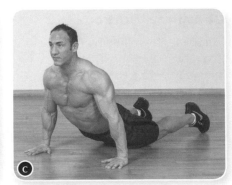

Hardcore

Although there is nothing wrong with trying to improve your flexibility, there is also little value in just trying to get more flexible for flexibility's sake. You should be trying to accomplish the range of motion you need to perform in the gym, your sport, and your life. Beyond that, getting your legs behind your head may be a great party trick, but it's not going to do much for you.

Warm-Up

5 reps of squat to stand; 6 reps per side of kneeling adductor stretch, hip rocker, and quadruped T-spine rotation

● Featured Exercise

Wide-Hands Push-Up

1. Begin with your hands and toes on the floor, in a straight plank position from your head to your heels. Your hands should be twice shoulder-width apart (a).

2. Lower your torso toward the ground by bending your elbows, keeping them tucked toward your rib cage.

3. When you reach the bottom position (b), press the floor away with your hands, straightening your elbows until you reach lockout. Your hips, thighs, and torso should all rise simultaneously. Repeat for reps.

Complete Workout

Complete the following circuit as quickly as possible. Take as little rest between exercises and within sets as necessary.

Barbell back squat (#63)
- 25 reps

Wide-hands push-up
- 50 reps

Double-arm kettlebell swing (#13)
- 75 reps

Wide-hands push-up
- 50 reps

Barbell back squat (#63)
- 25 reps

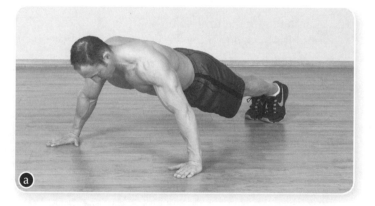

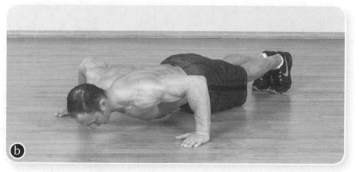

OPTIONS

Easy Option Reduce the number of reps to 15 for the barbell back squat, 25 for the wide-hands push-up, and 50 for the kettlebell swing.

Step It Up Increase the number of reps of the kettlebell swing to 100.

Cool-Down Standing quad stretch, 90-degree stretch, cross-body stretch.

Sucker Punch

Why is this workout called Sucker Punch? Because you'll be cruising along for a round or two, thinking to yourself, *This isn't too bad*. Then, out of nowhere, it'll feel as if you just took a right hook to body. Your abs will be sore. You'll be gasping for air. You'll wonder how you'll make it to the end of the round. But keep fighting, make it to the end, and you'll feel as if you just won the championship belt.

Warm-Up

6 reps of squat to stand, 6 reps per side of quadruped T-spine rotation, 8 reps of glute bridge, 10 reps of cat–cow

● Featured Exercise

Double Kettlebell Snatch

1. Stand tall, holding a kettlebell in each hand. Your arms should be at your sides.

2. Maintaining a neutral spine and braced core, bring your hips back and bring the kettlebells behind you (*a*).

3. Forcefully extend at the hips and allow your arms to extend overhead, keeping your arms locked out (*b*).

4. The kettlebells should flip over the top of your hands and come to rest on the back of your wrists (be sure to snake the kettlebell around your hands—don't let it crash onto your wrists) (*c*).

5. Pop the kettlebells over your hands as you bring your arms back down toward your sides, and immediately begin the next rep.

Complete Workout

Perform 10 rounds of the following circuit in as little time as possible, resting as needed.

Double kettlebell snatch
- 5 reps

Banded push-up (#3)
- 10 reps

Toes to bar (#28)
- 10 reps

OPTIONS

Easy Option   Perform the circuit for 6 rounds.

Step It Up   Add 5 reps to the toes to bar.

Cool-Down   Standing quad stretch, 90-degree stretch, double lat stretch.

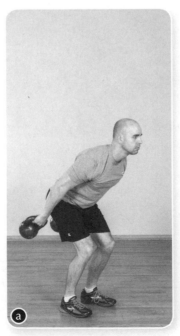
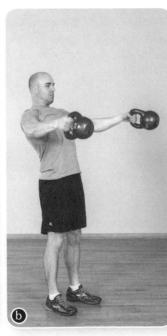
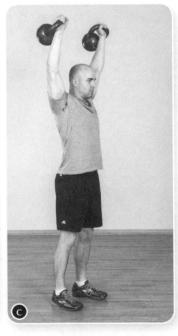

Jack of All Trades

Jumping jacks, which are featured in this workout, are a great entry point to plyometric training. They are fairly low impact and can easily be performed for higher repetitions. If you do not have a lot of experience with box jumps, bounding, hops, and vertical leaps, the jumping jack (and jumping rope) is a great place to start.

Warm-Up

6 reps of squat to stand, 6 reps per side of quadruped T-spine rotation, 8 reps of glute bridge, 10 reps of cat–cow

● Featured Exercise

Jumping Jack

1. Begin in a tall standing position (*a*). As you shuffle your feet out to the side, swing both arms laterally up and overhead (*b*).

2. Reverse the motion by simultaneously bringing your arms back down to your sides and your feet together. Repeat for reps.

Complete Workout

Complete 1 round of the following circuit, resting as little as possible.

Jumping jack
- 100 reps

Prisoner squat (#188)
- 75 reps

Push-up (#12)
- 50 reps

Chin-up (#73)
- 25 reps

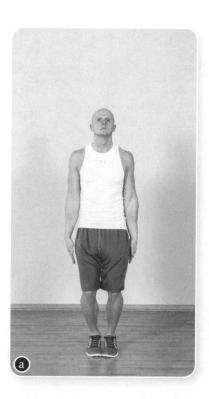

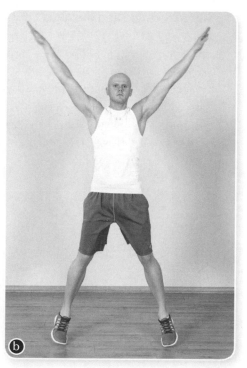

OPTIONS

Easy Option   Reduce the number of chin-ups to 10.

Step It Up   Perform the circuit twice.

Cool-Down   Hamstring stretch, calf stretch, pec stretch.

Run Devil Run

You'll think a hellhound is on your trail by the end of this workout. By combining sprints with push-ups, you'll never really give your body a full chance to rest—really testing your ability to perform while being fatigued. Get your running shoes on and give it a shot.

Warm-Up

6 reps of squat to stand, 6 reps per side of quadruped T-spine rotation, 8 reps of glute bridge, 10 reps of cat–cow

● Featured Exercise

Push-Up

1. Lie in a prone (facedown) plank position, with your arms extended and hands just outside shoulder width (*a*).

2. Maintaining a straight line from your head to your heels, lower your body until your chest is 2 to 3 inches (5 to 8 cm) from the floor (*b*). Keep your elbows tucked close to your rib cage as you descend.

3. Forcefully reverse the motion, driving yourself back up to the starting position. Repeat for reps.

Complete Workout

Alternate between the following two exercises for a total of 10 sets, resting as little as possible between movements and rounds.

100-yard (100 m) sprint (#41)
- 10 sets

Push-up
- 10 sets of 10, 9, 8, 7, 6, 5, 4, 3, 2, 1 reps

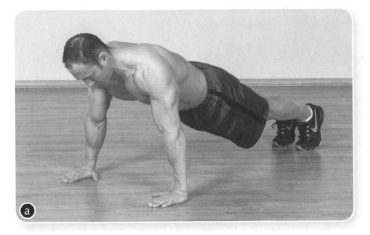

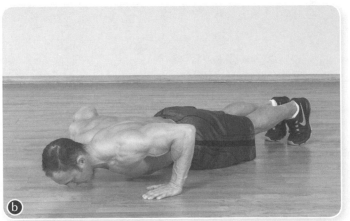

OPTIONS

Easy Option Reduce the sprints to 50 yards.

Step It Up Do 20 push-ups between each of the sprints.

Cool-Down Standing quad stretch, 90-degree stretch, double lat stretch.

On Top

When it comes to pull-ups, chin-ups, and all their variations, most people fail in the top half of the movement. The chin-up featured in this workout adds an isometric hold at the top of the movement (when your chest is up at the bar) in order to increase strength and confidence in that range of motion. You won't be able to bang out many reps, but you should see an increase in your pulling strength when consistently adding this movement to your workouts or warm-ups.

Warm-Up

5 reps of inchworm, 6 reps per side of quadruped T-spine rotation, 10 reps of cat–cow

● Featured Exercise

Chin-Up With Top Hold

1. Grab a pull-up bar with a shoulder-width double underhand grip (palms facing you). Your arms should hang straight down (a).

2. Bring your shoulder blades down to initiate your movement up to the bar. Keeping your knees back, drive your elbows down and behind you to bring your chest up to the bar (b).

3. Hold this top position for 5 seconds before lowering yourself back to a full hang. Repeat for reps.

Complete Workout

A. Chin-up with top hold
- 5 sets × 3 reps (with 5-second hold)
- 60 seconds of rest

B1. Single-arm dumbbell thruster (#199)
- 4 sets × 8 reps per side
- 45 seconds of rest

B2. Push-up (#12)
- 4 sets × 15 reps
- 45 seconds of rest

C. Run (#41)
- 1 mile (1.6 km)

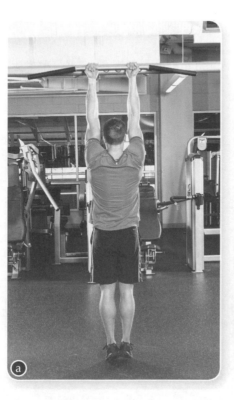
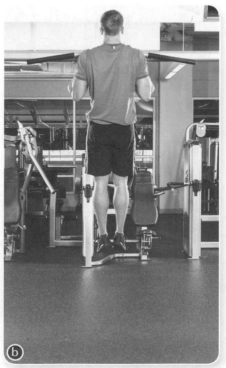

OPTIONS

Easy Option   Perform 3 sets of the single-arm dumbbell thruster and push-up. Reduce the run to .5 mile (.8 km).

Step It Up   Increase the number of reps of the chin-up with top hold to 6 per set.

Cool-Down   Double lat stretch, cross-body stretch, hamstring stretch.

Hang Time

Although performing Olympic-style lifts with a barbell is the ultimate goal for a good number of athletes and training enthusiasts, many people lack the technique, strength, or mobility to accomplish these lifts successfully. That does not mean, however, that you should eliminate snatches, cleans, and presses from your repertoire. Versions of these movements using kettlebells, dumbbells (as in this workout), and even medicine balls mimic these important movement patterns without the demands of the full barbell versions.

Warm-Up

4 reps per side of the world's greatest stretch, 6 reps per side of hip rocker and inverted hamstring stretch, 8 reps per side of shoulder sweeps

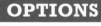 **Featured Exercise**

Dumbbell Hang Clean

1. Grab a dumbbell with your right hand, and assume a shoulder-width stance. Keeping your chest tall, bend at the knees and bring your hips back until the dumbbell is right above knee level (a).

2. Explosively drive your hips forward, shrug your right shoulder, and extend at the ankle, driving the dumbbell up to shoulder height (b). Keep the dumbbell close to your body for the entire movement.

3. Catch the dumbbell by bringing your elbow in tight to your rib cage (c). Lower the dumbbell back to the starting position. Complete all reps for one side before switching.

Complete Workout

A. Dumbbell hang clean
- 5 sets × 3 reps/side
- 90 seconds of rest

B1. Wide-grip pull-up (#117)
- 3 sets × 8 reps
- 60 seconds of rest

B2. Barbell walking lunge (#112)
- 3 sets × 6 reps/side
- 60 seconds of rest

B3. American kettlebell swing (#206)
- 3 sets × 12 reps
- 60 seconds of rest

OPTIONS

Easy Option Perform 2 sets of the wide-grip pull-up, barbell walking lunge, and American kettlebell swing.

Step It Up Add an extra set to the wide-grip pull-up, barbell walking lunge, and American kettlebell swing.

Cool-Down Hamstring stretch, calf stretch, pec stretch.

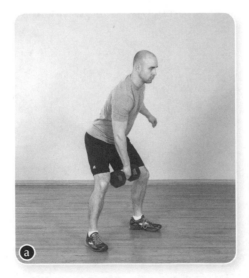

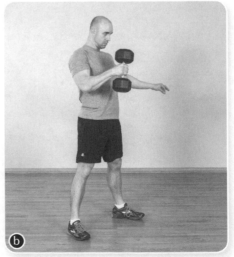

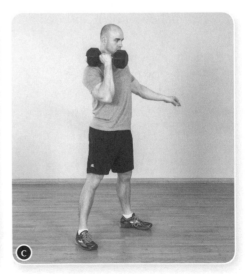

Swing Thing

Doing a circuit for time has its own unique set of challenges and strategies. Do you go all out right from the get-go? Do you pace yourself so you don't run out of gas after a couple of minutes? Regardless of which strategy you use, the one thing to always keep in mind that as your muscles fatigue and your lungs burn, there's a tendency to cheat reps and use bad form. Do your best to fight these bad habits in order to get the most out of your workout while staying in one piece.

Warm-Up

4 reps per side of the world's greatest stretch, 5 reps each of inchworm and inverted hamstring stretch, 10 reps of glute bridge

Featured Exercise

Single-Arm Kettlebell Swing

1. Begin with a kettlebell just beyond your toes. Reach down with your right hand, grab the handle, and pull the kettlebell back between your legs, being sure to hinge at the hips (a).
2. Reverse the momentum of the kettlebell by driving your hips forward, allowing the kettlebell to rise to anywhere between belly button and shoulder height (b). Don't "arm it up"—all the drive should be coming from your lower body.

3. Once the kettlebell reaches its pinnacle, drive your hips backward and pull the kettlebell back between your legs.
4. Complete all reps for the right arm before repeating for the left. If you have experience with single-arm kettlebell swings, switch arms between every rep.

Complete Workout

Perform as many rounds of this circuit as possible in 12 minutes.

Push-up (#12)
* 10 reps

Single-arm kettlebell swing
* 10 reps/side

Rower (#212)
* 300 meters

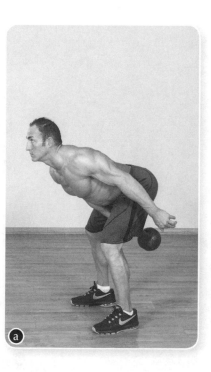
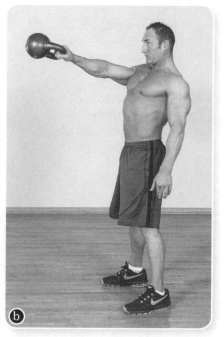

OPTIONS

Easy Option   Perform as many rounds as possible for 9 minutes.

Step It Up   Perform as many rounds as possible for 15 minutes.

Cool-Down   Double lat stretch, hamstring stretch, calf stretch.

The Bucket

In the gym setting, *the bucket* can refer to one of two things. A deep squat is often referred to as "sitting in the bucket," meaning you are getting your glutes as close to the ground as possible with every rep. The vessel in the corner of the gym into which you may lose your breakfast in the middle of a particularly grueling workout is also called the bucket, for obvious reasons. In this workout, you should definitely be aiming to sit in the bucket during your squats. And, if you push hard enough, you just may need that other bucket in the corner as well.

Warm-Up

4 reps per side of the world's greatest stretch, 5 reps each of inchworm and inverted hamstring stretch, 10 reps of glute bridge

● Featured Exercise

Box Jump

1. Stand approximately 12 inches (30 cm) away from a plyo box, feet hip-width apart.
2. In one motion, keep your arms straight and bring them behind you while flexing at the knees (a).

3. Without pausing, drive your arms forward and jump onto the box (b).
4. Land with your knees flexed, and then stand up to lockout (c). Step off the box and repeat for reps.

Complete Workout

Complete as many rounds as possible of the following circuit in 12 minutes. Use 50 percent of your 1RM for the deadlift. Use a 24-inch (60 cm) box for the box jumps.

Box jump
- 5 reps

Conventional deadlift (#5)
- 10 reps

Push-up (#12)
- 15 reps

OPTIONS

Easy Option   Perform 8 reps of the deadlift.

Step It Up   Use 60 percent of your 1RM on the deadlift.

Cool-Down   Double lat stretch, hamstring stretch, calf stretch.

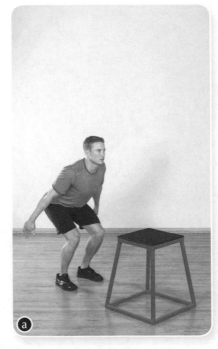
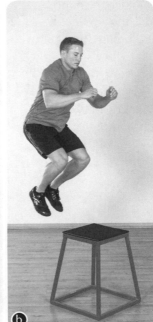
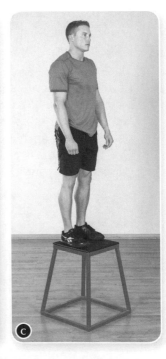

The Rocket

One of the least discussed aspects of exercise is developing a rhythm during combination movements (such as the single-arm dumbbell thruster, featured in this workout) or total-body coordination movements such as the pull-up or kettlebell swing. Being able to seamlessly transition from one phase of a movement to another or from rep to rep means you'll save energy as well as transfer more easily to athletic and sport-specific movements. So do your best to reduce any herky-jerkiness by getting smooth and finding your groove.

Warm-Up

4 reps per side of the world's greatest stretch, 6 reps per side of hip rocker and inverted hamstring stretch, 8 reps per side of shoulder sweeps

Complete Workout

A. Box jump (#198)
- 3 sets × 6 reps
- 60 seconds of rest

B1. Single-arm dumbbell thruster
- 3 sets × 8 reps per side
- 45 seconds of rest

B2. Wide-grip pull-up (#117)
- 3 sets × 8 reps per side
- 45 seconds of rest

C. Rower (#212)
- 2 sets × 500 meters
- 2 minutes of rest

● Featured Exercise

Single-Arm Dumbbell Thruster

1. Grab a dumbbell with your left hand, and assume a slightly wider than shoulder-width stance. Keeping the dumbbell at shoulder height and your chest tall (*a*), squat as low as you can (*b*).

2. Once you hit the bottom position, drive your hips forward and extend your knees. As you near the top position, use the power generated by your lower body to press the dumbbell directly overhead (*c*).

3. Return the dumbbell to the starting position before lowering to the next rep. Repeat all reps for one side before switching to the other.

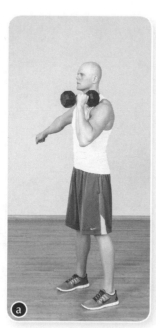
(a)

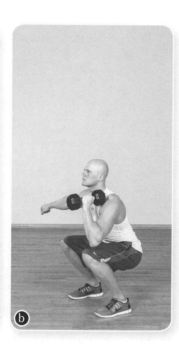
(b)

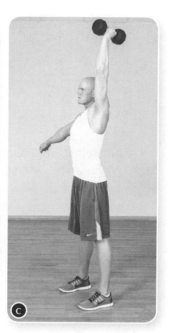
(c)

OPTIONS

Easy Option   Replace the wide-grip pull-up with the kneeling lat pull-down (#120).

Step It Up   Add one more set of the rower.

Cool-Down   Standing quad stretch, 90-degree stretch, double lat stretch.

Time to Split

Different foot elevations and positions will affect the degree of difficulty of every version of the split squat. Although mobility will play a role in which version is the most challenging for you, as a general rule of thumb front-foot elevated is the easiest version, while rear-foot elevated (also known as the Bulgarian split squat) is the most challenging. It's certainly beneficial to get a variety of split squats into your program because training unilaterally (one leg at a time) will help with structural balance and athletic development.

Warm-Up

6 reps of squat to stand, 6 reps per side of quadruped T-spine rotation, 8 reps of glute bridge, 10 reps of cat–cow

Complete Workout

Perform as many rounds as possible of the following exercise pairing in 20 minutes. Rest only as needed between sets and rounds.

Chin-up (#73)
- 6 reps

Bulgarian split squat
- 6 reps per leg

● Featured Exercise

Bulgarian Split Squat

1. Utilizing a split stance (one foot forward), place your back foot on a bench or plyo box (a).
2. Keeping your chest upright, lower your body until your back knee is 1 to 2 inches (2.5 to 5 cm) above the floor (b).
3. Focus on pressing your front foot into the floor to get yourself back to the starting position.
4. Complete all repetitions on one side before switching your stance.

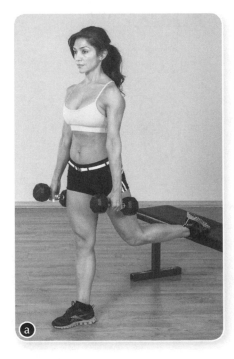
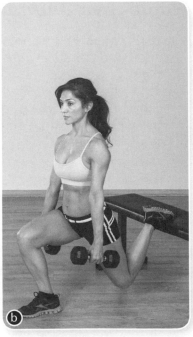

OPTIONS

Easy Option   Replace the chin-up with a kneeling lat pull-down (#120).

Step It Up   Add weight to either or both movements.

Cool-Down   Standing quad stretch, 90-degree stretch, double lat stretch.

The Inferno

A famous saying claims that *what gets measured, gets managed*. In the following workout, what's being measured is how many reps you can perform in a specific time frame. But just because speed is a key component of being successful in a timed workout, resist the temptation to throw form out the window just to get reps completed. Form, technique, and safety should always take precedence over speed or weight. Shaving a couple of reps off your total in order to perform quality reps and stay injury free is always the way to go.

Warm-Up

5 reps of inchworm, 6 reps per side of quadruped T-spine rotation, 10 reps of cat–cow

● Featured Exercise

TRX Jumping Split Squat

1. Grab the handles of a TRX with your arms straight, and legs in a split (lunge) stance, with your left foot forward.

2. Bend both knees to lower yourself toward the floor. With your back knee 1 to 2 inches (2.5 to 5 cm) off the floor (a), explosively jump (b).

3. With both feet in the air, quickly switch positions so your right foot is in front and your left foot is in back (c). Be sure to land on the ball of the back foot.

4. Continue to alternate in this manner until all reps are complete.

Complete Workout

Complete as many rounds of the following circuit as possible in 12 minutes.

Box jump (#198)
- 6 reps

TRX jumping split squat
- 12 reps (6 per leg)

Wall ball (#25)
- 24 reps

Push-up (#12)
- 36 reps

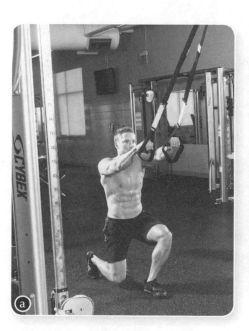 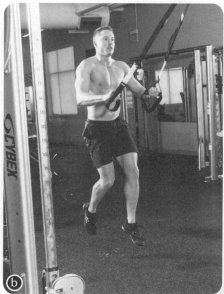 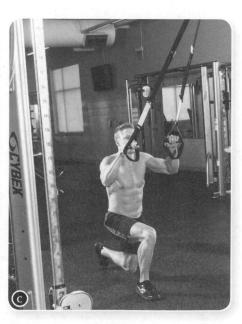

OPTIONS

Easy Option Perform as many reps as possible in 9 minutes.

Step It Up Perform 10 reps of the box jumps and 18 reps of the TRX jumping split squats.

Cool-Down Double lat stretch, cross-body stretch, hamstring stretch.

T-Rex

TRX and other suspension training systems are great tools for body-weight exercises. By either allowing you to support a portion of your body weight (making movements such as split squats and inverted rows easier) or creating a variety of more challenging vector angles, suspension trainers are excellent for varying the degree of difficulty of both traditional and unique exercises. Along with barbells, kettlebells, dumbbells, cables, and sandbags, they are another useful tool to add to your strength training arsenal.

Warm-Up

4 reps per side of the world's greatest stretch, 6 reps per side of hip rocker and inverted hamstring stretch, 8 reps per side of shoulder sweeps

● Featured Exercise

TRX Low Row

1. Grab a TRX or other suspension trainer with a neutral grip (palms facing each other).
2. Walk your feet toward the anchor point to adjust the degree of difficulty of the movement (*a*). The closer your feet are to the anchor point, the more your body will be at a horizontal angle and the more challenging the exercise.
3. Keeping your wrists locked, row your elbows behind you, keeping your forearms close to your rib cage during the entire movement (*b*).
4. Once the handles reach your rib cage, reverse the motion, lowering yourself with control. Keep a straight line between your shoulders and ankles for the entire movement. Repeat for reps.

Complete Workout

Complete 5 rounds of the following circuit.

TRX jumping split squat (#201)
- 15 reps
- 15 seconds of rest

TRX low row
- 15 reps
- 15 seconds of rest

Lateral lunge (#143)
- 8 reps/leg
- 15 seconds of rest

Lying cable chest fly (#172)
- 15 reps
- 90 seconds of rest

OPTIONS

Easy Option   Perform 4 rounds of the circuit.

Step It Up   Decrease rest to 60 seconds between circuits.

Cool-Down   Hamstring stretch, calf stretch, pec stretch.

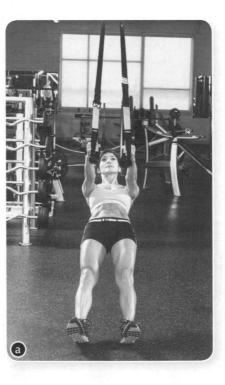
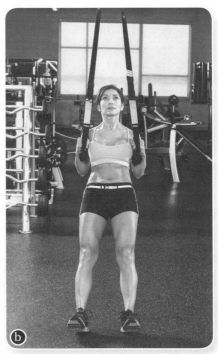

Push and Lunge

Push-ups are a piece of cake. Body-weight lunges? Easy. That's all well and good until you try doing them both. Back to back. With no rest. This workout delivers the muscle-building benefits of two basic movement patterns, and the metabolic demand created by the little to no rest makes it a great fat burner as well.

Warm-Up

4 reps per side of the world's greatest stretch, 6 reps per side of hip rocker and inverted hamstring stretch, 8 reps per side of shoulder sweeps

● Featured Exercise

Alternating Body-Weight Lunge

1. Place your hands on your hips (*a*).
2. Take a long stride forward, bending your knees until your back knee is approximately an inch (2.5 cm) off the ground (both legs should make 90-degree angles) (*b*).

3. Push off the heel of the front foot until you return to the starting position (*c*).
4. Alternate legs until all reps are completed (*d*).

Complete Workout

Perform 10 rounds of the following exercise combination, resting as little as needed between exercises and rounds.

Alternating body-weight lunge
- 10 reps/per leg
- Rest as little as possible

Push-up (#12)
- 10 reps

OPTIONS

Easy Option Perform only 5 reps of the alternating body-weight lunge.

Step It Up Substitute banded push-ups (#3) for the push-ups.

Cool-Down Hamstring stretch, calf stretch, pec stretch.

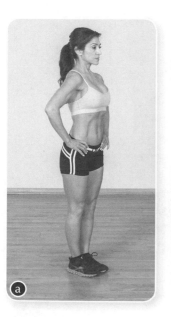
(a)

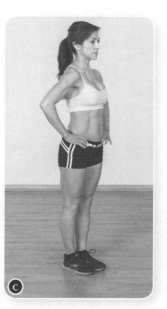
(b)

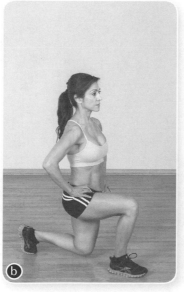
(c)

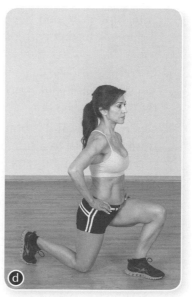
(d)

Committed

To tackle a workout this tough, you have to be committed—either committed enough to your training that you are willing to take on a workout this demanding or committed to an asylum because you are so insane for even attempting it. Whichever the case, be prepared for a brutal test of upper and lower body strength-endurance and mental toughness, which is what it will take to make it to the end.

Warm-Up

6 reps of squat to stand, 6 reps per side of quadruped T-spine rotation, 8 reps of glute bridge, 10 reps of cat–cow

● Featured Exercise

Overhead Squat

1. Begin with the barbell on your back, your hands in a snatch-grip position (outside shoulder width). Press the bar straight up, locking out your elbows at the top (*a*).
2. Keeping your chest tall, bring your hips back and bend at the knees to descend into a squat (*b*).
3. Keep the bar directly over or slightly behind your head for the entire movement.
4. Once you reach the bottom position, return to a standing position. Repeat for reps.

Complete Workout

Load a barbell with 50 percent of your body weight, and complete the following circuit for time, resting as little as necessary within sets and between exercises.

Split jerk (#17)
- 5 reps

Overhead squat
- 10 reps

Barbell overhead press (#36)
- 15 reps

Barbell front squat (#44)
- 20 reps

Push press (#16)
- 25 reps

Barbell back squat (#63)
- 30 reps

Push jerk (#81)
- 35 reps

OPTIONS

Easy Option Use a barbell with 35 to 40 percent of body weight.

Step It Up Use a barbell with 55 to 60 percent of body weight.

Cool-Down Standing quad stretch, 90-degree stretch, cross-body stretch.

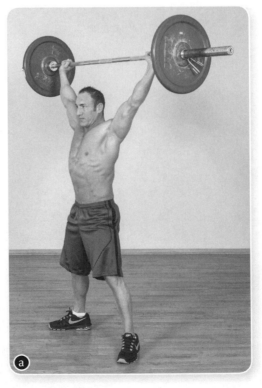
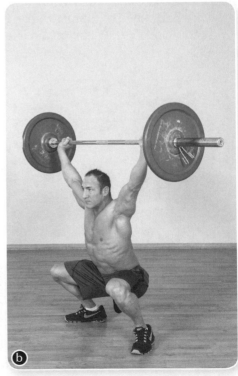

The Captain

There is a huge difference between moving when fresh and unloaded and trying to perform exercises while fatigued or under relatively heavy load. It is only when you can achieve proper movement patterns and mechanics when tired or challenged by weight that you will attain the type of fitness that carries over into sports. A lot of players look great in warm-ups, but it's the athletes who can perform when fatigued in the final stages of the game that are the true difference makers.

Warm-Up

6 reps of squat to stand, 6 reps per side of quadruped T-spine rotation, 8 reps of glute bridge, 10 reps of cat–cow

● Featured Exercise

Hanging Knees to Elbows

1. Grab a pull-up bar with a double underhand grip at shoulder width (*a*).
2. Initiate the motion by retracting your shoulder blades, driving your hips up and forward, and bending your knees to 90 degrees.
3. Continue driving your hips forward until your knees touch your elbows (*b*).
4. Lower under control to the starting position and repeat for reps.

Complete Workout

Complete 2 rounds of the following circuit, resting as little as possible between exercises and between circuits.

Barbell overhead press (#36)
- 5 reps

Hanging knees to elbows
- 10 reps

Push-up (#12)
- 20 reps

Frog sit-up (#27)
- 30 reps

Prisoner squat (#188)
- 40 reps

Jump rope
- 50 reps

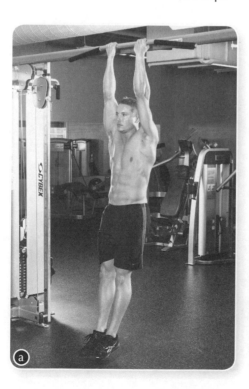
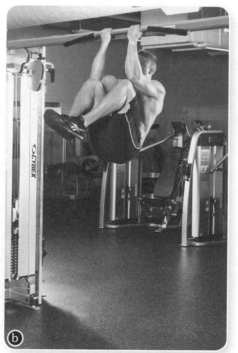

OPTIONS

Easy Option   Perform the circuit once.

Step It Up   Perform the circuit three times.

Cool-Down   Standing quad stretch, 90-degree stretch, double lat stretch.

The American

The American kettlebell swing (featured in this workout) can be considered a hybrid, or combination, movement—half kettlebell swing, half snatch. In fact, if you are new to Olympic weightlifting, the American kettlebell swing can be a good learning tool for the snatch because it teaches how to dynamically drive weight overhead from below your hips in one motion.

Warm-Up

6 reps of squat to stand, 6 reps per side of quadruped T-spine rotation, 8 reps of glute bridge, 10 reps of cat–cow

● Featured Exercise

American Kettlebell Swing

1. Place a kettlebell on the floor in front of you, just beyond your feet. Assume a tall stance, with your feet at or just outside shoulder width.

2. With a slight bend in your knees, reach your hips back and grab the kettlebell with a double overhand grip.

3. Pull the kettlebell between your legs, being sure to keep it high (close to your crotch) (*a*).

4. As you drive your hips forward, bend your elbows slightly to bring the kettlebell up and close to your body.

5. Allow the momentum of the kettlebell to continue upward. As it gets to about shoulder height, punch the kettlebell upward until it is nearly directly overhead (*b*).

6. Reverse the process, allowing the weight of the kettlebell to bring it back down, keeping it close to the body and swinging between your legs. Repeat for reps.

Complete Workout

Complete 4 rounds of the following circuit, resting as little as possible between exercises and resting 1 minute between rounds.

Glute–ham raise (#70)
- 10 reps

Push-up (#12)
- 15 reps

Frog sit-up (#27)
- 20 reps

American kettlebell swing
- 25 reps

OPTIONS

Easy Option   Perform 3 rounds of the circuit.

Step It Up   Add 5 reps to each of the movements.

Cool-Down   Standing quad stretch, 90-degree stretch, double lat stretch.

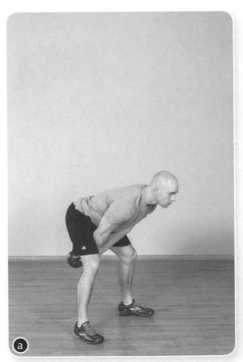
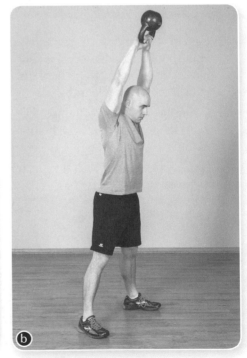

The Brigadier

When practicing new movements, begin by learning the movement positions with loads that do not put you at great risk for injury. Once you can reach the appropriate positions (bottom position of a back squat, launch position of a snatch), you can begin to use these movements in workouts for reps and with loads. Learning proper technique with low loads will not only keep you safe but also reduce the number of bad habits you can develop from learning and performing a movement incorrectly.

Warm-Up

4 reps per side of the world's greatest stretch, 6 reps per side of hip rocker and inverted hamstring stretch, 8 reps per side of shoulder sweeps

● Featured Exercise

Wall Ball

1. Begin with a medicine ball in front of your torso and your hands on either side of it (*a*).

2. Squat down until your hip creases are below your knees (you can put a medicine ball behind you and touch the ball with your glutes as a reference). Keep your chest tall and your spine neutral as you squat (*b*).

3. Once you reach the bottom position, stand up and throw the ball against a target 9 to 12 feet (3 to 4 m) above the floor (*c*). This should be done as one continuous motion.

4. Catch the ball and immediately descend into the squat. Repeat for reps.

Complete Workout

Complete 2 rounds of the following circuit, resting as little as possible between exercises and between circuits.

Overhead squat (#167)
- 15 reps

Push-up (#12)
- 30 reps

Wall ball
- 45 reps

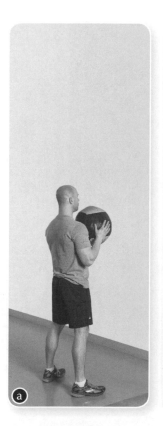

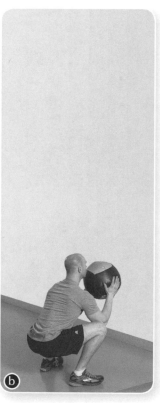

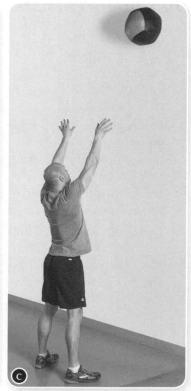

OPTIONS

Easy Option Perform the circuit once.

Step It Up Perform the circuit three times.

Cool-Down Hamstring stretch, calf stretch, pec stretch.

Damage

Improving body composition is probably the most popular fitness goal. And, no doubt, it's a great one. Getting leaner and more muscular will improve your health, strength, mood, and confidence. However, your training session is a time to focus solely on performance. Are you getting stronger? Faster? Better? If you are making sure that you improve every time you step into the gym, you'll end up with the body you want. You can't control how much weight you lose, but you can control how much weight you put on the bar.

Warm-Up

5 reps of inchworm, 6 reps per side of quadruped T-spine rotation, 10 reps of cat–cow

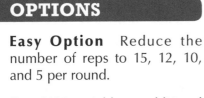
Featured Exercise

Dumbbell Thruster

1. Grab a pair of dumbbells, and hold them with a neutral grip (palms facing each other) at your shoulders (a).

2. Unlock your hips and squat down toward the floor, keeping your chest tall and eyes forward throughout the entire movement (b).

3. Once you've reached the bottom of your range of motion (your upper legs should be at or below parallel to the floor), reverse the motion, driving your hips forward.

4. As you return to the standing position, drive the dumbbells overhead until they reach lockout (c).

5. Bring the dumbbells back to shoulder height and repeat for reps.

Complete Workout

Complete 4 rounds of the following workout as quickly as possible, resting as little as needed within or between sets. Reps decrease with each set as shown.

Dumbbell thruster
- 25, 20, 15, 10 reps

Push-up (#12)
- 25, 20, 15, 10 reps

American kettlebell swing (#206)
- 25, 20, 15, 10 reps

Frog sit-up (#27)
- 25, 20, 15, 10 reps

OPTIONS

Easy Option   Reduce the number of reps to 15, 12, 10, and 5 per round.

Step It Up   Add one additional set of 8 reps to each exercise (so you'll be doing 5 sets × 25, 20, 15, 10, and 8 reps).

Cool-Down   Double lat stretch, cross-body stretch, hamstring stretch.

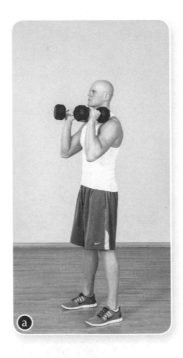

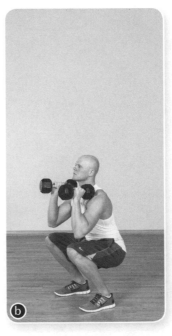

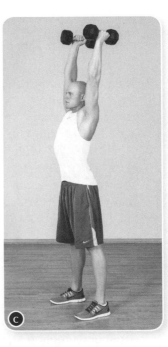

The Walking Dead

What are the typical features of a zombie's walk? Not being able to fully bend your knees and being able to lift your arms only to shoulder height as you waddle down the street in search of human flesh. That distinctive walk is most probably what you'll look like the day after this workout, given the huge demand on your hamstrings, glutes, and shoulders.

Warm-Up

4 reps per side of the world's greatest stretch, 5 reps each of inchworm and inverted hamstring stretch, 10 reps of glute bridge

● Featured Exercise

Seated Dumbbell Shoulder Press

1. Grab a set of dumbbells, and sit on a bench with the back in a 90-degree position.
2. Lift both dumbbells up to your shoulders with a neutral grip. Your palms should be facing your ears (a).
3. Keeping your back pressed against the bench, drive the weight straight up until your elbows are fully locked out (b).
4. Lower to the starting position and repeat for reps.

Complete Workout

Perform the following circuit for 20 minutes, alternating between the two movements with as little rest as possible. Use 60 percent of your usual 6RM for each exercise.

Conventional deadlift (#5)
- 6 reps

Seated dumbbell shoulder press
- 6 reps

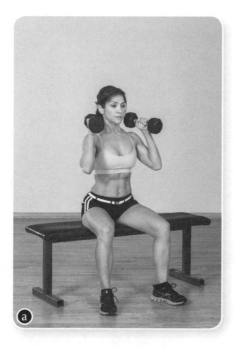

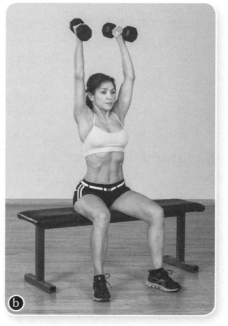

OPTIONS

Easy Option   Use 50 percent of your 6RM for both movements.

Step It Up   Use 75 percent of your 6RM for both movements.

Cool-Down   Double lat stretch, hamstring stretch, calf stretch.

Squat and Press

Two staples of any fitness routine, the squat and the chest press, are like the chocolate and peanut butter of the fitness world—great when they are on their own, even better when combined. This workout has you alternating between these two critical movements in a density circuit, meaning you are trying to get in as many sets as possible in a certain amount of time.

Warm-Up

4 reps each of the world's greatest stretch and inchworm; 8 reps each of the kneeling adductor stretch, hip rocker, and shoulder sweeps

● Featured Exercise

Incline Dumbbell Chest Press

1. Set an adjustable bench to a 30-degree incline.
2. Grab a set of dumbbells, lie back on the bench (a), and extend your arms directly above your shoulders (b).
3. Utilizing a neutral grip (palms facing each other), lower the dumbbells down toward your rib cage, keeping your elbows tucked (do not flare your elbows out).
4. Drive the weight up and repeat for reps.

Complete Workout

Complete as many rounds of the following exercise pairing in 20 minutes, resting as little as possible until time is up. Use 60 percent of your usual 6RM for each exercise.

Barbell back squat (#63)
- 6 reps

Incline dumbbell chest press
- 6 reps per leg

OPTIONS

Easy Option   Complete as many rounds as possible for 15 minutes.

Step It Up   Use 75 percent of your 6RM for both movements.

Cool-Down   Standing quad stretch, hamstring stretch, pec stretch.

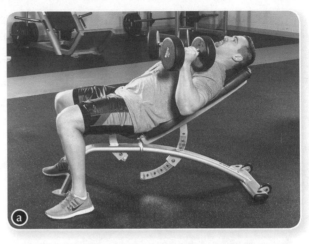

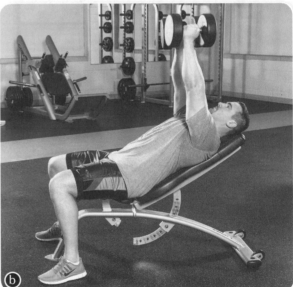

Upended

One often-overlooked aspect of increasing training intensity is the change in vector angles. A vector angle, as applied to strength training, is a biomechanical term that relates to the line of pull between the muscle and the load being used. Suspension trainers, such as the TRX, use these vector angles to increase or decrease the level of difficulty of many movements. The simplest way to adjust vector angles on upper body pulling and pushing movements is to adjust your feet relative to the anchor point of the TRX. Move your feet farther away from the anchor point on pulling movements such as a row, and the movement gets easier because you have to pull less of your body weight.

Warm-Up

4 reps per side of the world's greatest stretch, 6 reps per side of hip rocker and inverted hamstring stretch, 8 reps per side of shoulder sweeps

● Featured Exercise

TRX Incline Push-Up

1. Interlock the two TRX handles so they are in single handle mode.
2. Place one foot in the handle, face the anchor point, and assume a push-up position.
3. Keep your feet together, and walk your hands away from the anchor point as far as possible while being able to complete a push-up (as you walk back your feet will get higher) (a).
4. Once you reach this top position, perform a push-up by keeping a straight line from your head to your heels and your elbows tucked at your sides as you lower toward the floor (b).
5. Forcefully press yourself away from the floor and repeat for reps.

Complete Workout

TRX jumping split squat (#201)
- 12 reps
- 15 seconds of rest

TRX incline push-up
- 12 reps
- 15 seconds of rest

TRX hamstring curl (#65)
- 12 reps
- 15 seconds of rest

TRX low row (#202)
- 12 reps
- 90 seconds of rest

 Warning: The TRX incline push-up is an advanced movement requiring a lot of upper body strength. If you cannot safely perform this exercise, use a push-up or banded push-up as a substitute.

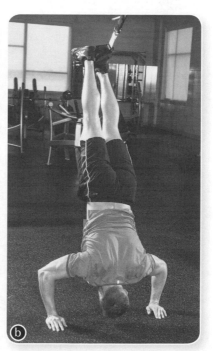
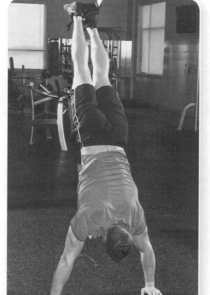

(a) (b)

OPTIONS

Easy Option   Perform 8 reps of each movement.

Step It Up   Increase the number of reps of each exercise to 15. Decrease rest to 60 seconds between circuits.

Cool-Down   Standing quad stretch, 90-degree stretch, double lat stretch.

The Midshipman

Although it appears rather simple, great rowing technique is not easy to accomplish. There are many strategies for developing maximal power, speed, and technique, all of which could make up their own book. However, there are certain quick fixes that will help improve your time, including maintaining good posture in your upper back, driving with your legs, and making sure your strokes are long and powerful. Efficiency in technique is a surefire way to ensure you are hitting your distances as quickly as possible.

Warm-Up

6 reps of squat to stand, 6 reps per side of quadruped T-spine rotation, 8 reps of glute bridge, 10 reps of cat–cow

Featured Exercise

Rower

1. Tightly strap your feet into a rowing machine, and grab the handle with a double overhand grip.
2. Flex at your hips, bend at the knees, and reach your arms forward. Keep your chest tall and your back straight (*a*).
3. Forcefully extend at your knees and hips, and pull the handle to the middle of your torso (*b*). Rely on your legs and back to bring the handle to the torso—your arms shouldn't do that much work beyond guiding the chain and handle along.
4. Quickly reverse positions until you are back at the starting position (knees bent, flexed at the hips, arms straight). Load up and repeat until you have reached your distance.

Complete Workout

Complete 1 round of the circuit, utilizing the same weight on the barbell for all pressing movements.

Barbell overhead press (#36)
- 12 reps

Rower
- 250 meters

Push press (#16)
- 12 reps

Rower
- 250 meters

Push jerk (#81)
- 12 reps

Rower
- 250 meters

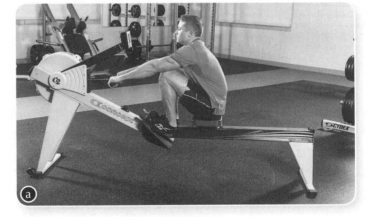

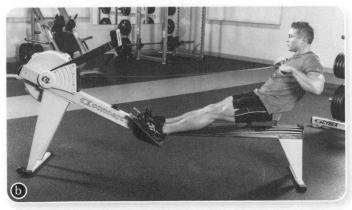

OPTIONS

Easy Option Reduce the distance on the rower to 200 meters per set.

Step It Up Increase the distance on the rower to 300 meters per set.

Cool-Down Standing quad stretch, 90-degree stretch, double lat stretch.

The Patriot

You've performed your dynamic mobility work, done a couple of specific warm-ups of the key exercises in your program, even downloaded a new playlist to get you psyched up to train. So you're all set to go, right? Well, not if you haven't paid attention to your nutrition before, during, and after your workout. And although there is no one blanket solution on how to fuel up for training, there is no shortage of prearranged formulas or simple meals that will help you optimize your performance while you work out. Bottom line: Getting your workout nutrition correct is just as important as any other step you take to prepare for the demands of training.

Warm-Up

6 reps of squat to stand, 6 reps per side of quadruped T-spine rotation, 8 reps of glute bridge, 10 reps of cat–cow

● Featured Exercise

Close-Grip Push-Up

1. Assume a plank position on the floor, with your hands directly under or slightly inside shoulder width (*a*).

2. Lower your body to the floor, keeping a straight line from your head to your heels. Your elbows should stay tucked closely to your sides (*b*)

3. When your chest reaches 3 inches (8 cm) above the floor, press your hands into the floor to drive yourself back up to the starting position. Repeat for reps.

Complete Workout

Perform 4 rounds of the following circuit.

Chin-up (#73)
- 10 reps

Close-grip push-up
- 20 reps

Frog sit-up (#27)
- 30 reps

Prisoner squat (#188)
- 40 reps
- 2 minutes of rest

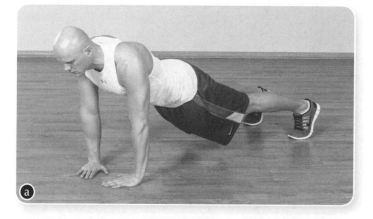

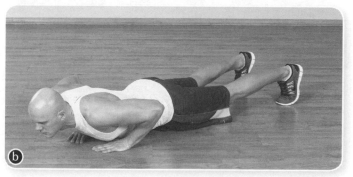

OPTIONS

Easy Option   Perform 3 rounds, and rest 3 minutes between rounds.

Step It Up   Rest 1 minute or less between rounds.

Cool-Down   Standing quad stretch, 90-degree stretch, double lat stretch.

Thrusters On

The barbell thruster is a great combination of the front squat and overhead press. This movement works the calves, glutes, quads, core, shoulders, and triceps, and it is also an incredibly metabolically demanding exercise that will drive your heart rate through the roof after a couple of reps.

Warm-Up

5 reps of squat to stand; 6 reps per side of kneeling adductor stretch, hip rocker, and quadruped T-spine rotation

● Featured Exercise

Power Clean to Barbell Thruster

1. Grab a barbell with a double overhand clean grip, just outside shoulder width. Your feet should be under the bar, with your chest tall and shoulders just above or behind the bar (*a*).
2. Lift the bar until it reaches midthigh position. Explosively drive your hips forward and send the bar upward (*b*), catching it in the front rack (*c*).
3. With the barbell in the rack position, sitting across your anterior (front) deltoids, perform a front squat by unlocking your hips, bending your knees, and lowering toward the ground while keeping your torso in a tall, upright position.
4. Once you reach the bottom position, reverse the motion. Using the momentum generated by standing up, drive the barbell overhead until your arms achieve lockout (*d*).
5. Return the barbell to the starting position and repeat for reps.

Complete Workout

Power clean to barbell thruster
- Perform 1 rep every 30 seconds for up to 20 minutes
- Once you can't complete a rep, end the workout

OPTIONS

Easy Option Perform one power clean to barbell thruster every 60 seconds.

Step It Up Perform two power clean to barbell thrusters every 30 seconds.

Cool-Down Standing quad stretch, 90-degree stretch, cross-body stretch.

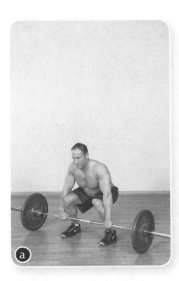
a

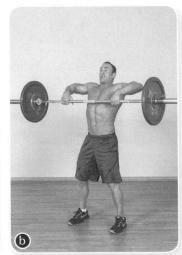
b

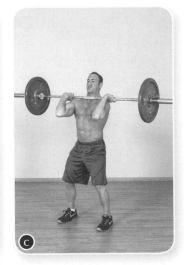
c

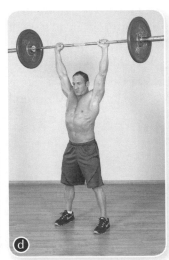
d

Ball Buster

Medicine balls are a great way of training for power without the technical skill required for traditional power movements such as the clean and the snatch. This medicine ball circuit trains the core through a variety of movement patterns for a truly integrated 360-degree approach. Note that you can perform this circuit by throwing the medicine ball to a partner (preferred) or against a padded or reinforced wall.

Warm-Up

4 reps per side of the world's greatest stretch, 6 reps per side of hip rocker and inverted hamstring stretch, 8 reps per side of shoulder sweeps

● Featured Exercise

Medicine Ball Bridge

1. Lie flat on your back with your knees bent 90 degrees and your feet flat on the floor.

2. With your arms slightly bent, simultaneously touch the medicine ball behind your head while bridging up at your hips (*a*).

3. Utilizing the power stored in your hips, forcefully sit up and throw the medicine ball to your partner or against a wall (*b*).

4. Catch the ball off the rebound or have your partner throw it back to you. Repeat for reps.

Complete Workout

Perform 4 rounds of the following circuit, resting as little as possible.

Medicine ball bridge
- 12 reps

Medicine ball slam (#20)
- 12 reps

Rotational medicine ball throw (#180)
- 6 reps/side

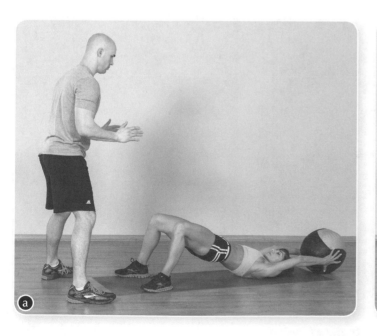

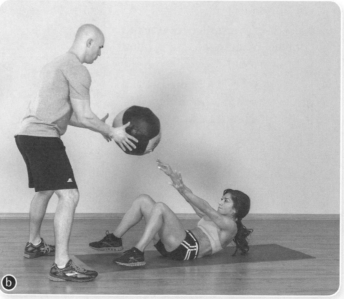

OPTIONS

Easy Option   Perform 3 rounds of the circuit.

Step It Up   Perform 5 rounds of the circuit.

Cool-Down   Hamstring stretch, calf stretch, pec stretch.

The Admiral

Combining various movements that incorporate several strength qualities (power, strength, hypertrophy) is a great way to make sure you are training your body to handle anything that comes your way. This workout focuses on developing the posterior chain—the back side of your body most responsible for athletic performance.

Warm-Up

4 reps per side of the world's greatest stretch; 4 reps of inchworm; 10 reps each of cat–cow and quadruped T-spine rotation

● Featured Exercise

Straight-Arm Cable Pull-Down

1. Attach a straight bar to a high cable station.
2. Grab the bar with straight arms at shoulder height. Stand with your kneed slightly bent and have a small forward bend at your hips (*a*).
3. Pull your arms straight down into your lap, making sure not to bend your arms (*b*).
4. Contract your lats in the bottom position before returning the bar to the starting position. Repeat for reps.

OPTIONS

Easy Option   Perform 4 rounds of the circuit.

Step It Up   Add an additional round to the circuit.

Cool-Down   Double lat stretch, hamstring stretch, calf stretch.

Complete Workout

Perform 5 rounds of the following circuit.

Power clean (#52)
- 3 reps
- 60 seconds of rest

Conventional deadlift (#5)
- 6 reps
- 60 seconds of rest

Seated cable row with hip flexion (#174)
- 8 reps
- 60 seconds of rest

Straight-arm cable pull-down
- 10 reps
- 2 minutes of rest

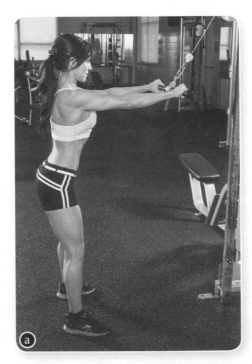
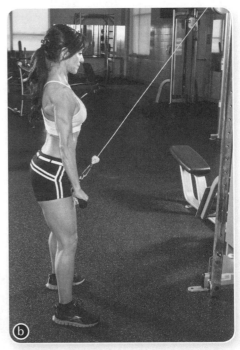

Henry's Ladder

This workout combines power, strength, and strength-endurance in a manner that will challenge your work capacity, exercise technique, and guts. And although your goal is to get as many reps as possible in 12 minutes, make sure your form is solid (particularly on the hang power clean) so you get the most out of the movements and stay in one piece.

Warm-Up

4 reps per side of the world's greatest stretch, 6 reps per side of hip rocker and inverted hamstring stretch, 8 reps per side of shoulder sweeps

● Featured Exercise

Hanging Leg Raise

1. Grab a pull-up bar with a double overhand grip at shoulder width (*a*).

2. Retract your shoulder blades, and raise your legs until they are parallel to the floor (*b*). Keep your legs as straight as possible and your knees and heels together.

3. Return your legs to the starting position, being sure not to swing before beginning the next rep.

Complete Workout

Perform the following circuit for as many rounds as possible in 12 minutes. Increase the reps in each subsequent set as noted. Rest as needed, but keep in mind that the goal is to get as many reps as possible in the 12 minutes.

Hang power clean (#93)
- Begin with 1 rep and then increase by 1 rep each set (1, 2, 3, 4, etc.)

Dip (#141)
- Begin with 2 reps and then increase by 2 reps each set (2, 4, 6, 8, etc.)

Hanging leg raise
- Begin with 3 reps and then increase by 3 reps each set (3, 6, 9, 12, etc.)

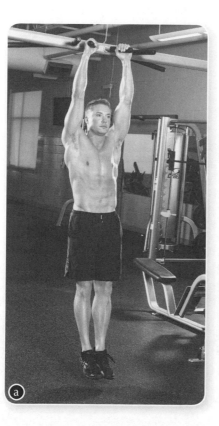

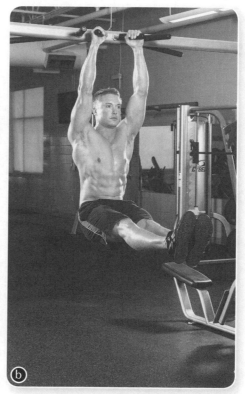

OPTIONS

Easy Option Perform as many reps as possible for 8 minutes.

Step It Up Perform as many reps as possible for 15 minutes.

Cool-Down Hamstring stretch, calf stretch, pec stretch.

The Last Leg

Most often, plyometric training is completed before strength training. This is for good reason—plyos require explosiveness and utilize the stretch-shortening cycle, both of which are trained most effectively when you are not fatigued by strength training. However, in athletics, you are often required to produce explosive movements while fatigued. For example, a basketball player still needs to run and jump in the fourth quarter of a game when he may already be exhausted. Adding some unloaded bounding in the middle of this workout lets you start training for this type of demand. However, you will notice that the bounding is done after the overhead squat, a movement that usually does not sap much leg strength. It is this type of balance that you should keep in mind when combining strength and plyos in the same workout.

Warm-Up

5 reps of inchworm, 6 reps per side of quadruped T-spine rotation, 10 reps of cat–cow

● **Featured Exercise**

Double-Leg Bound

1. Begin with your feet hip-width apart. Flex your knees and bring your arms directly behind you (a).

2. Drive your forefoot into the ground, swing your arms forward, and explosively propel yourself as far forward as possible (b).

3. Land on your full foot with flexed knees (c).

4. Reset and repeat for reps (as you get more advanced, you can complete the bounds in a continuous series).

Complete Workout

Complete 4 rounds of the following circuit.

Overhead squat (#167)
- 3 reps
- 30 seconds of rest

Double-leg bound
- 5 reps
- 30 seconds of rest

Barbell back squat (#63)
- 7 reps
- 2 minutes of rest

OPTIONS

Easy Option Add an additional 30 seconds of rest to each set.

Step It Up Add 2 reps to each exercise.

Cool-Down Double lat stretch, cross-body stretch, hamstring stretch.

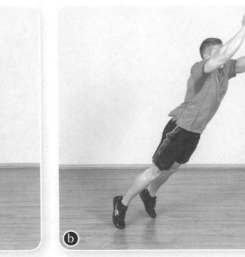

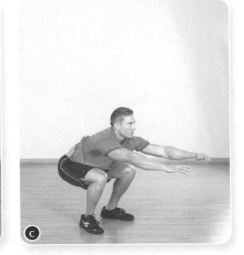

CHAPTER 6

The Core of the Matter

Six-pack abs. Everyone wants them. But there are much better reasons to dedicate a training session or phase to your core. The muscles of your abdomen, lower back, and hips are responsible for posture, stability, and power production. In fact, it's very difficult to perform nearly any movement or exercise without some assistance from the core musculature. Rather than strictly staying with crunches or sit-ups, this chapter utilizes rotational, antirotational, flexion, extension, and static-hold exercises that truly train the core as it was designed—to both produce force and stabilize against it. Dedicate yourself to a full phase of core training (or prioritize it at least once per week), and you'll notice all of your lifts improving. And you may just end up with that six-pack you are looking for.

Center of Attention

All the abdominal work in the world is not going to get you thinner or give you a six-pack you can show off while strutting down the beach. To make your abs pop you need to drop the fat that is surrounding them. The most effective way to do that is to address your nutrition. Make sure you are getting adequate amounts of protein, healthy fats, and plenty of veggies. Combine that with a great training plan and you'll be chiseling out a set of stare-worthy abs in no time.

Warm-Up

5 reps of squat to stand; 6 reps per side of kneeling adductor stretch, hip rocker, and quadruped T-spine rotation

● Featured Exercise

Standing Lateral Cable Rope Chop

1. Attach a rope to a pulley set at midchest height at a cable crossover station.

2. Stand with your right shoulder perpendicular to the pulley. Grab the rope with a double overhand grip (a).

3. Keeping your arms straight, a slight bend in your knees, and your feet facing forward, rotate until the rope is directly in front of your left hip (b).

4. Control the rope back to the starting position. Complete all reps for one side before switching to the other.

OPTIONS

Easy Option   Perform 3 sets of all the exercises.

Step It Up   Add 2 reps to the barbell rollout and 10 reps/side to the side plank.

Cool-Down   Standing quad stretch, 90-degree stretch, cross-body stretch.

Complete Workout

Barbell rollout (#228)
- 4 sets × 8 reps
- 30 seconds of rest

Side plank (#175)
- 4 sets × 20/side
- 30 seconds of rest

Standing lateral cable rope chop
- 4 sets × 12 reps/side
- 30 seconds of rest

Single-contact mountain climber (#281)
- 4 sets × 25 reps/side
- 30 seconds of rest

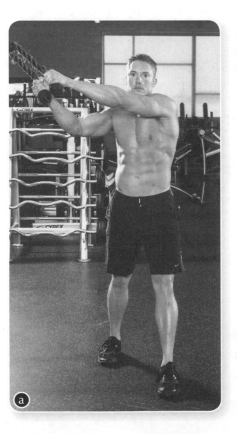
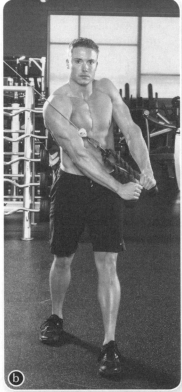

Get Crushed

Although the foam roller is a great tool for self-myofascial release (a type of self-massage designed to improve the quality and texture of tissues within the body), it can also be very useful in your core training. By utilizing it in moves such as the foam roller reverse crunch (#229) or the foam roller crush (featured in this workout), you can deactivate your hip flexors and place more of the emphasis of your crunching-style movements on your abs, where you want them.

Warm-Up

4 reps per side of the world's greatest stretch, 5 reps each of inchworm and inverted hamstring stretch, 10 reps of glute bridge

● Featured Exercise

Foam Roller Crush

1. Lie faceup on the floor. The front of your thighs should be facing your chest, and your knees should be bent at 90 degrees.
2. Bend your elbows to 90 degrees, with your upper arms facing the front of your thighs. Place a foam roller between your elbows and your thighs.
3. Drive your elbows and thighs into the foam roller, contracting your abs as tightly as possible.
4. Hold for time and repeat for reps.

Complete Workout

A. Single-side kettlebell squat (#254)
- 3 sets × 8 reps/side
- 90 seconds of rest

B1. Foam roller crush
- 4 sets × 20 seconds per set
- 45 seconds of rest

B2. Hanging leg raise (#217)
- 4 sets × 10 reps
- 45 seconds of rest

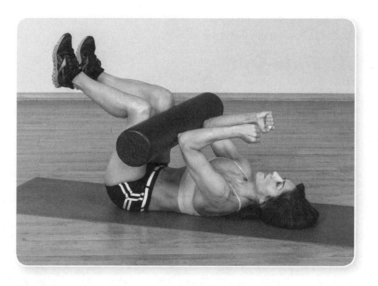

OPTIONS

Easy Option   Perform 3 sets of the foam roller crush and hanging leg raise.

Step It Up   Increase the foam roller crush to 30 seconds per set.

Cool-Down   Double lat stretch, hamstring stretch, calf stretch.

Slideshow

There are many different sects of training: bodybuilding, powerlifting, sports performance, CrossFit, group fitness, spinning—the list goes on and on. Naturally you will gravitate toward one or two of these forms and stick with them. But don't be afraid to step out of your comfort zone and try one of these different modalities from time to time. You may learn to appreciate something you are not familiar with or actually learn something you can bring into your own training. Don't be closed-minded when it comes to a different style of training that's not your own.

Warm-Up

5 reps of inchworm, 6 reps per side of quadruped T-spine rotation, 10 reps of cat–cow

Featured Exercise

Ab Slide-Out

1. Start in a push-up position with your hands on Valslides, paper plates, or gym towels directly under your shoulders (a), and lower yourself to the floor.

2. Keeping your torso braced and not allowing your hips to sag, extend one hand forward, keeping your arm straight (b).

3. Once you have reached maximal extension, brace your abs and slide your hands back to the original position. Repeat with the other hand (c).

Complete Workout

A1. Barbell front squat (#44)
- 4 sets × 6 reps
- 75 seconds of rest

A2. Dumbbell step-up (#121)
- 4 sets × 6 reps/side
- 75 seconds of rest

B1. Medicine ball bridge (#215)
- 3 sets × 10 reps
- 60 seconds of rest

B2. Ab slide-out
- 3 sets × 10 reps
- 60 seconds of rest

OPTIONS

Easy Option Perform 3 sets of the barbell front squat and dumbbell step-up.

Step It Up Add 2 reps to each exercise.

Cool-Down Double lat stretch, cross-body stretch, hamstring stretch.

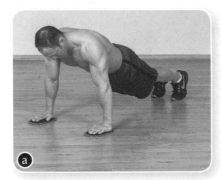
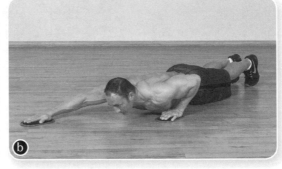
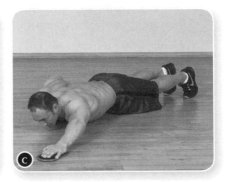

The Hip Dip

The external oblique muscles, found on the sides of your abdomen, have several functions including aiding in pulling your chest down toward your ribs (as with a crunch) and allowing for bracing of your entire midsection during the Valsalva maneuver (taking a big inhale and holding your breath in order to create more stability in your trunk). However, just as important, the obliques limit the amount of flexion and rotation you can achieve in your spinal column, which helps keep you safe from back injury when moving dynamically. Needless to say, oblique training should be a priority, and the side plank with hip touch in this workout is designed to ensure your obliques stay strong.

Warm-Up

6 reps of squat to stand, 6 reps per side of quadruped T-spine rotation, 8 reps of glute bridge, 10 reps of cat–cow

● Featured Exercise

Side Plank With Hip Touch

1. Lie on the ground on your right side.
2. Place your elbow directly under your shoulder and your left foot in front of your right (your left heel should be touching or just in front of your right toes).

3. Press yourself up so you are creating a straight line from head to heels, with only your elbow, forearm, and feet touching the ground (a).
4. Allow your hip to dip down toward the ground and make contact with the floor (b). Once your hip touches, bring it back to the starting position. Complete all reps on one side before switching.

Complete Workout

This workout uses a wave-loading scheme. As the number of reps decreases for the barbell overhead press, increase the load used. The second time through the wave (sets 4, 5, and 6), attempt more weight than you used for the corresponding number of reps on sets 1, 2, and 3. For example, your second set of 6 reps (set 5) should be heavier than your first set of 6 (set 2).

A. Barbell overhead press (#36)
- 6 sets × 8, 6, 4, 8, 6, 4 reps
- 75 seconds of rest

B1. Side plank with hip touch
- 3 sets × 12 reps/side
- 60 seconds of rest

B2. Hanging leg raise (#217)
- 3 sets × 12 reps
- 60 seconds of rest

OPTIONS

Easy Option Reduce the number of reps of the side plank with hip touch and hanging leg raise to 8 per set.

Step It Up Increase the number of reps of the side plank with hip touch and hanging leg raise to 15 per set.

Cool-Down Standing quad stretch, 90-degree stretch, double lat stretch.

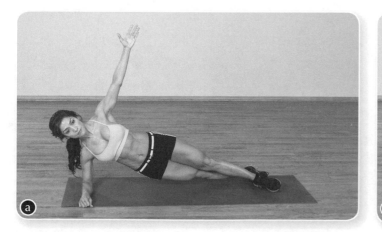

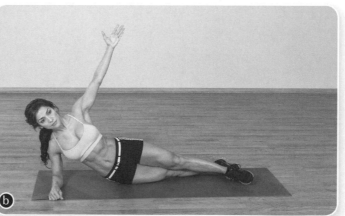

V Is for Victory

Although your rectus abdominis, more commonly known as your six-pack, is only one muscle (tendons that traverse the muscle give it that blocky look), it's still advantageous to train it from multiple angles. The V-up, which is featured in this workout, has the benefit of including flexion from the top down (bringing your rib cage toward your hips) and the bottom up (bringing your hips toward your sternum). If this movement is too advanced, you can always break it down into separate parts by performing standard crunches followed by a set of reverse crunches.

Warm-Up

5 reps of inchworm, 6 reps per side of quadruped T-spine rotation, 10 reps of cat–cow

Featured Exercise

V-Up

1. Lie faceup on the floor, with your legs and arms straight and your arms directly overhead (a).

2. In one motion, lift your legs and torso off the floor and reach to touch your toes. Only your butt should be on the floor (your body should look like a V) (b). Keep your spine as neutral as possible, and keep your head in line with your body.

3. Lower back down to the floor and repeat for reps.

Complete Workout

A. Sumo deadlift (#82)
- 4 sets × 5 reps
- 90 seconds of rest

B1. Hanging leg raise (#217)
- 2 sets × 10 reps
- 30 seconds of rest

B2. Negative sit-up (#227)
- 2 sets × 10 reps
- 30 seconds of rest

B3. V-up
- 2 sets × 10 reps
- 30 seconds of rest

B4. Side plank (#175)
- 2 sets × 30 seconds/side
- 30 seconds of rest

OPTIONS

Easy Option   Eliminate 2 sets of the sumo deadlift.

Step It Up   Add one set to each of the B exercises.

Cool-Down   Double lat stretch, cross-body stretch, hamstring stretch.

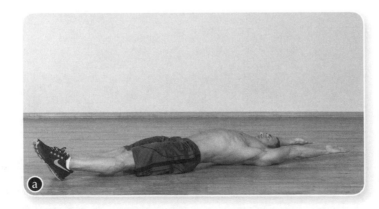

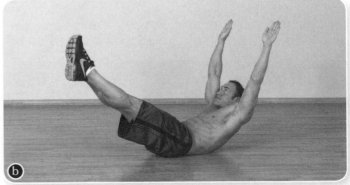

Pike's Peak

Occasionally your gym will not have a piece of equipment that you want for a specific exercise. If this is something like an Olympic lifting platform, a Prowler, or a 600 lb tractor tire, you're probably out of luck. But if your gym does not have a pair of sliders (which are utilized in the featured exercise of this workout), you can easily use a pair of Valslides, furniture sliders, or even paper plates or face towels on a hardwood floor to get the desired training effect. As long as your equipment substitutions are safe and effective, there's no reason to break the bank picking up the highest-priced solutions.

Warm-Up

6 reps of squat to stand, 6 reps per side of quadruped T-spine rotation, 8 reps of glute bridge, 10 reps of cat–cow

● Featured Exercise

Slider Pike

1. Assume a push-up position, with your feet on a pair of sliders (a). Make sure you are keeping a neutral spine and a slight external rotation of your shoulders.

2. Keeping your legs straight, slide your feet toward your hands by raising your butt in the air and bringing your head down between your arms (b).

3. Drive the pike as high as possible. When you reach the top of your range of motion, reverse until you return to the push-up plank position. Repeat for reps.

Complete Workout

A. Barbell back squat (#63)
   - 3 sets × 10 reps
   - 60 seconds of rest

B1. Toes to bar (#28)
   - 3 sets × 10 reps
   - 45 seconds of rest

B2. Slider pike
   - 3 sets × 10 reps
   - 45 seconds of rest

B3. Burpee (#7)
   - 3 sets × 10 reps
   - 45 seconds of rest

OPTIONS

Easy Option   Perform 8 reps of all exercises.

Step It Up   Add an additional set to each exercise.

Cool-Down   Standing quad stretch, 90-degree stretch, double lat stretch.

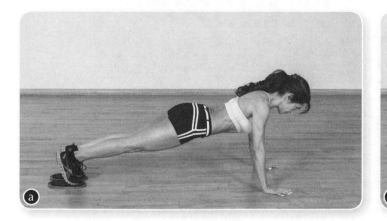
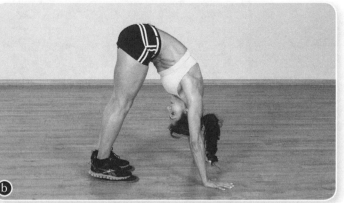

Eight-Pack

Although there are benefits to varying the speed at which you lower and lift weights, and some exercises demand more power and explosiveness by their very nature, the concentric (or lifting) phase of nearly every exercise should be done with the intent of moving the bar or your body as quickly as possible. This intention will not only allow you to lift the largest amount of weight but also set you up to be faster and more dynamic on the track, field, or court.

Warm-Up

5 reps of inchworm, 6 reps per side of quadruped T-spine rotation, 10 reps of cat–cow

● Featured Exercise

Kneeling Cable Crunch

1. Grab a rope handle set at a high pulley of a cable station. Kneel facing the weight stack, with your elbows bent and the ends of the rope at your collarbones (a).

2. Begin with a flat back, and crunch your rib cage toward your pelvis. Contract your abs hard at the end position (b).

3. Under control, return to the starting position. Repeat for reps.

Complete Workout

Standing lateral cable rope chop (#219)
- 4 sets × 10 reps/side
- 30 seconds of rest

Toes to bar (#28)
- 4 sets × 12 reps
- 30 seconds of rest

Kneeling cable crunch
- 4 sets × 12 reps
- 30 seconds of rest

Plank (figure 1.8)
- 4 sets × 60 seconds
- 30 seconds of rest

OPTIONS

Easy Option Reduce the number of sets to 3 per movement.

Step It Up Add 2 reps per set of the standing lateral cable rope chop, toes to bar, and kneeling cable crunch, and add 30 seconds to the plank.

Cool-Down Double lat stretch, cross-body stretch, hamstring stretch.

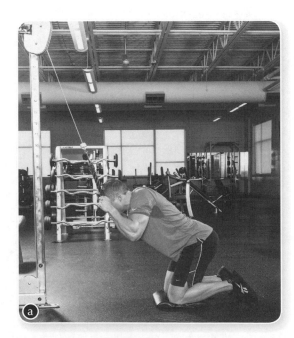
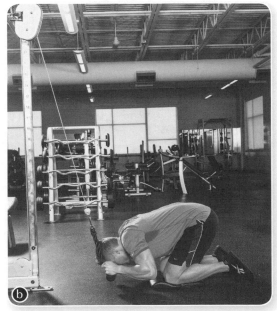

To a T

In strength training there is a tendency to overemphasize certain planes of motion, specifically the sagittal plane, which incorporates the majority of pushing, pulling, and squatting movements. This workout places a greater priority on rotational movements, which help develop structural balance and athleticism. The takeaway: Don't make your training one-dimensional.

Warm-Up

6 reps of squat to stand, 6 reps per side of quadruped T-spine rotation, 8 reps of glute bridge, 10 reps of cat–cow

● Featured Exercise

T Push-Up

1. Assume a push-up position, with your hands directly under your shoulders and your body forming a straight line from your head to your heels (*a*).

2. Unlock your elbows and lower yourself toward the floor, keeping your elbows tucked toward your rib cage.

3. After reaching the bottom range of motion (*b*), forcefully drive your hands into the ground to lift yourself back toward the starting position.

4. As you approach the top, lift your left hand off the floor, rotate your torso, and reach your left hand toward the ceiling (your body should look like the letter T lying on its side) (*c*).

5. Rotate your torso back to the plank position, placing your left hand on the floor. Repeat the push-up, but this time lift your right hand toward the ceiling at the top. Continue to alternate until you've completed all reps.

Complete Workout

Complete 5 rounds of the following circuit.

T push-up
- 8 reps/side
- 30 seconds of rest

Standing lateral cable rope chop (#219)
- 8 reps/side
- 30 seconds of rest

Barbell rollout (#228)
- 15 reps
- 60 seconds of rest

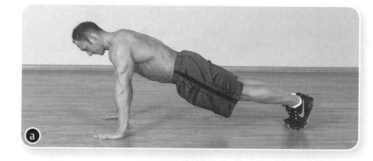

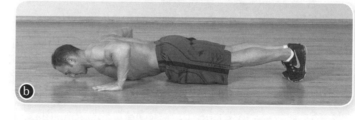

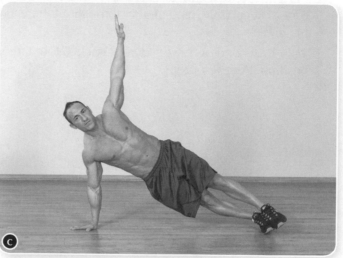

OPTIONS

Easy Option Reduce the number of total circuits to 4.

Step It Up Increase to 12 reps per side of the standing lateral cable rope chop and barbell rollout.

Cool-Down Standing quad stretch, 90-degree stretch, double lat stretch.

Negative Reinforcement

Once you gain a bit of experience in the iron game, you'll realize how much of your success and progress is dependent on your state of mind. If you don't believe you can add one more pound, perform one more rep, or shave one second off your time, you probably won't be able to. And although it's true that we all have different genetics, all humans have many more similarities than differences. So keep in mind that there are many, many people out there who are outlifting or outperforming you based on sheer will and dedication alone. Your goal should be to believe you can close this gap and do and be more than you ever thought you could.

Warm-Up

4 reps per side of the world's greatest stretch, 6 reps per side of hip rocker and inverted hamstring stretch, 8 reps per side of shoulder sweeps

● Featured Exercise

Negative Sit-Up

1. Sit with your feet flat on the floor, knees bent, and hands across your chest (a).
2. Raise your torso up to a seated position, making sure to keep your spine neutral throughout the entire movement (b).
3. Take 10 seconds to lower yourself back to the starting position. Repeat for reps.

Complete Workout

Complete 4 rounds of the following circuit, resting as little as needed between exercises and rounds.

Toes to bar (#28)
- 12 reps

Barbell rollout (#228)
- 12 reps

Negative sit-up
- 12 reps

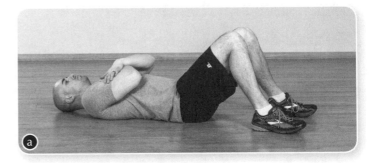

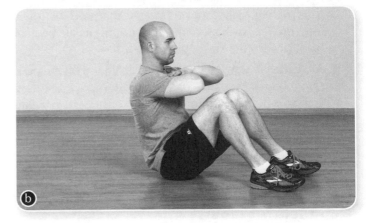

OPTIONS

Easy Option   Perform 3 rounds of the circuit.

Step It Up   Increase the reps of all three exercises to 15 per round.

Cool-Down   Standing quad stretch, 90-degree stretch, double lat stretch.

Washboard

One of the most common mistakes we make when training the abdominals is the overreliance on crunches and sit-ups. The core benefits from being trained in multiple planes of movement, including top-to-bottom flexion (crunches), bottom-to-top flexion (leg raises), antirotation (cable holds), and rotation (chops) as well as isometrics (planks).

Warm-Up

4 reps per side of the world's greatest stretch, 6 reps per side of hip rocker and inverted hamstring stretch, 8 reps per side of shoulder sweeps

● Featured Exercise

Barbell Rollout

1. Add round weights to each end of a barbell. Kneel down (you may need a pad for under your knees), and grab the barbell with an overhand grip (a).

2. Keeping your arms fully extended and maintaining a straight line from your shoulders to your knees, roll the bar away from you, extending as far as possible (b). Do not allow your hips or trunk to sag.

3. When you reach maximum extension, reverse the motion, pulling the barbell back toward your knees. Repeat for reps.

Complete Workout

Perform 4 rounds of the following circuit.

Hanging leg raise (#217)
- 8 reps
- 30 seconds of rest

Barbell rollout
- 10 reps
- 30 seconds of rest

Foam roller crush (#220)
- 30 seconds
- 30 seconds of rest

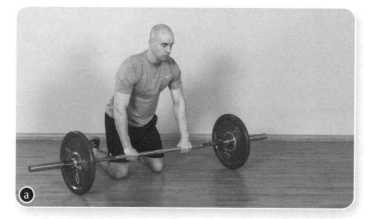

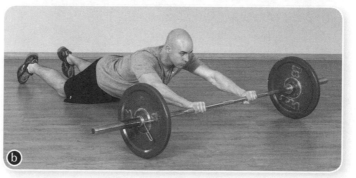

OPTIONS

Easy Option Perform 3 rounds of the circuit.

Step It Up Add 2 reps to the hanging leg raise and barbell rollout.

Cool-Down Hamstring stretch, calf stretch, pec stretch.

On a Roll

Although targeted abdominal training should be part of your overall training program, keep in mind that many compound movements such as squats, deadlifts, and even overhead presses and push-ups also train your core muscles. So, just because a crunch, rotation, or plank isn't part of a particular workout, don't be fooled into thinking your core isn't being trained.

Warm-Up

6 reps of squat to stand, 6 reps per side of quadruped T-spine rotation, 8 reps of glute bridge, 10 reps of cat–cow

● Featured Exercise

Foam Roller Reverse Crunch

1. Lie faceup on the floor. Place a foam roller securely between the back of your ankles and hamstrings. Extend your arms overhead, and grab a heavy dumbbell, kettlebell, or medicine ball (*a*).

2. Bring your knees in toward your chest, being sure to keep the foam roller in position (*b*).

3. Contract your abs at the top, and lower to the starting position. Repeat for reps.

Complete Workout

A. Barbell front squat (#44)
- 5 sets × 4 reps
- 90 seconds of rest

B1. Foam roller reverse crunch
- 4 sets × 10 reps
- 45 seconds of rest

B2. Barbell rollout (#228)
- 4 sets × 10 reps
- 45 seconds of rest

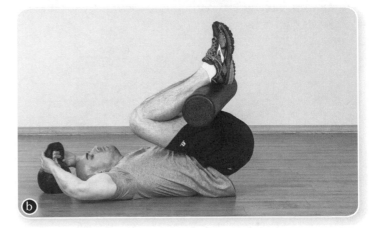

OPTIONS

Easy Option   Perform 3 sets of the foam roller reverse crunch and barbell rollout.

Step It Up   Reduce rest on the foam roller reverse crunch and barbell rollout to 30 seconds.

Cool-Down   Standing quad stretch, 90-degree stretch, double lat stretch.

CHAPTER 22

Let's Push! Let's Pull!

This chapter focuses on workouts that feature noncompeting supersets, a fancy way of saying exercises performed back-to-back that utilize completely different muscle groups. By training in this manner, you are allowing one group of muscles to rest while the other group is working, which allows for a very efficient workout without a lot of downtime. Alternating pushing and pulling movements (e.g., a squat with a hamstring curl or a chin-up with an overhead press) is a very common way of organizing this type of training because pulling exercises and pushing exercises most often do not utilize the same primary muscles. This method can be used to gain strength and put on size, while the minimal rest required can contribute to fat loss as well.

Sleeve Stretcher

For every unilateral (single arm or single leg) exercise in this book, it's recommended that you begin with your right side. However, it's a great idea to start any unilateral movements with the weaker arm or leg. This will allow you to train your weaker side while you are fresher and have more energy as well as match the number of reps you performed on your weaker side with your stronger side, preventing you from creating even greater strength imbalances.

Warm-Up

5 reps of inchworm, 6 reps per side of quadruped T-spine rotation, 10 reps of cat–cow

● Featured Exercise

Alternating Dumbbell Hammer Curl

1. Grab a pair of dumbbells. Allow your arms to hang straight down at your sides, with your palms facing each other (a).
2. Keeping an upright torso and your abs braced, curl the right dumbbell up until it is just in front of your right shoulder. Hold your upper arm next to your rib cage, and keep your elbow from driving forward as you curl (b).
3. Return the dumbbell to the starting position, and repeat the movement on the left side.
4. Continue to alternate in this manner until all reps have been completed.

Complete Workout

A1. Barbell floor press (#166)
- 5 sets × 4 reps
- 90 seconds of rest

A2. Weighted chin-up (#160)
- 5 sets × 4 reps
- 90 seconds of rest

B1. Alternating dumbbell hammer curl
- 4 sets × 8 reps/side
- 45 seconds of rest

B2. Decline EZ-bar triceps extension (#145)
- 4 sets × 10 reps
- 45 seconds of rest

OPTIONS

Easy Option   Perform 3 sets of the alternating dumbbell hammer curl and decline EZ-bar triceps extension.

Step It Up   Reduce rest on the alternating dumbbell hammer curl and decline EZ-bar triceps extension to 30 seconds.

Cool-Down   Double lat stretch, cross-body stretch, hamstring stretch.

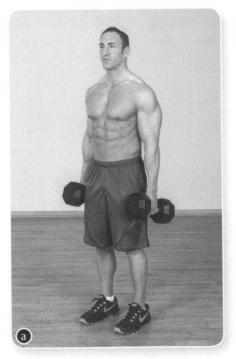
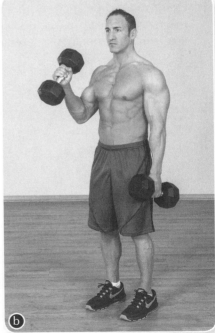

Push–Pull Tabata

The term *Tabata* stems from research performed in Japan by a scientist and researcher named Izumi Tabata. Tabata conducted tests on two groups of athletes, comparing moderate high-intensity training with high-intensity interval training. His famous protocol required that athletes perform intervals with an all-out effort for 20 seconds while recovering for 10 seconds, repeated 8 times (for a total workout of 4 minutes). He proved that training in this manner could increase both aerobic and anaerobic conditioning in these athletes. Any interval-type training that uses this 20 on, 10 off protocol has become synonymous with his name.

Warm-Up

5 reps of inchworm, 6 reps per side of quadruped T-spine rotation, 10 reps of cat–cow

Complete Workout

Complete as many reps as possible of the following two exercises for 20 seconds, followed by 10 seconds of rest, for 8 sets (4 minutes total).

Pull-up
- 8 sets × 20 seconds
- 10 seconds of rest
- 4 minutes of rest

Push-up (#12)
- 8 sets × 20 seconds
- 10 seconds of rest

● Featured Exercise

Pull-Up

1. Begin by grabbing a pull-up bar with an overhand grip just outside shoulder width.
2. Every rep should begin with your arms fully extended (*a*). Depress your shoulder blades, and use your back and arms to pull yourself toward the bar.
3. Complete the rep by touching your chest to the bar (*b*). Lower back to the starting position.
4. Do not utilize momentum or bring your knees up or legs forward during each rep.

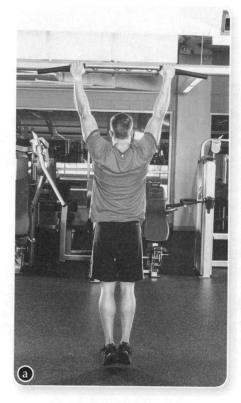

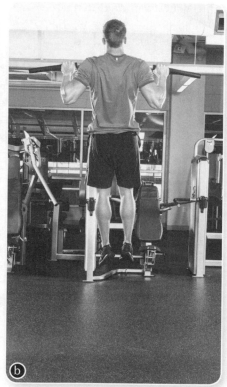

OPTIONS

Easy Option   Perform a half Tabata by completing 4 rounds of each movement.

Step It Up   Perform each Tabata twice, for a total of 16 rounds of each exercise (resting 4 minutes between each set of 8 intervals).

Cool-Down   Double lat stretch, cross-body stretch, hamstring stretch.

Half Squat

A half squat is not usually recommended for optimal training. However, in this workout, we are going to use a partial range of motion squat to help you get stronger. The partial will allow you to use more weight than you would on a full ROM lift and should carry over to more strength when you return to the full ROM movement.

Warm-Up

5 reps of squat to stand; 6 reps per side of kneeling adductor stretch, hip rocker, and quadruped T-spine rotation

● Featured Exercise

Partial Squat

1. Unrack the barbell (*a*), and initiate a squat by bringing your hips back and bending your knees.

2. Lower the bar down to a partial squat (*b*), being sure to keep your abs braced.

3. Return to the starting position and repeat for reps.

Complete Workout

Perform all sets of the partial squat using 90 to 110 percent of your usual 3-5RM squat weight. Complete all sets of the partial squat before moving on to the superset of the dumbbell split squat and barbell Romanian deadlift.

A1. Partial squat
- 4 sets × 3 to 5 reps
- 2 minutes of rest

B1. Barbell front-foot elevated split squat (#140)
- 4 sets × 6 to 8 reps
- Proceed to next exercise without rest

B2. Barbell Romanian deadlift (#295)
- 4 sets × 6 to 8 reps
- 75 seconds of rest

OPTIONS

Easy Option Use 80 to 95 percent of your 3-5RM squat weight for the partial squat.

Step It Up Work up to 130 percent of your 3-5RM squat weight for the partial squat.

Cool-Down Standing quad stretch, 90-degree stretch, cross-body stretch.

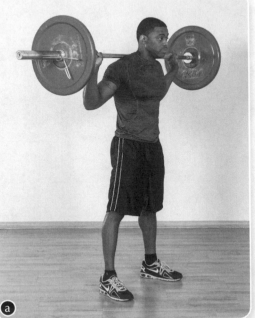
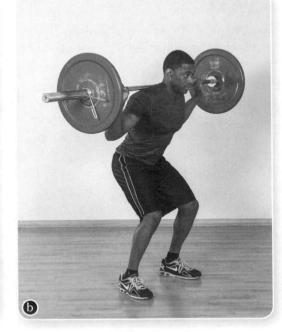

Chairman of the Board

For years, powerlifters have used board presses (a bench press variation in which you place a wooden board on your chest to limit the range of motion of the bar) to improve triceps development and lockout. However, most gyms do not offer boards, which are obviously critical for this exercise. Enter the towel press (featured in this workout). By placing towels, instead of boards, on your sternum to limit the range of motion, you can get similar benefits without the need for extra equipment.

Warm-Up

4 reps per side of the world's greatest stretch, 5 reps of inchworm, 8 reps per side of shoulder sweeps

● Featured Exercise

Towel Press

1. Set up in a flat bench press station with your head, upper back, and glutes on the bench. Keep both feet flat on the floor and your eyes directly under the bar. Place a folded towel on your sternum (you can use one folded towel or stack up several based on how much you want to limit the range of motion) (*a*).
2. Unrack the bar. Keeping your elbows close to your rib cage, lower the bar until it touches the towel (*b*).
3. Forcefully drive the bar back up until you reach lockout. Repeat for reps.

Complete Workout

A. Towel press
- 6 sets × 4 reps
- 90 seconds of rest

A2. Chin-up (#73)
- 6 sets × 4 reps
- 90 seconds of rest

B1. TRX face pull (#270)
- 2 sets × 8 reps
- 60 seconds of rest

B2. Standing underhand rear lateral raise (#125)
- 2 sets × 8 reps
- 60 seconds of rest

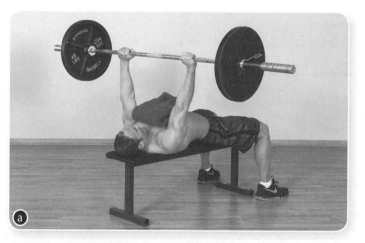

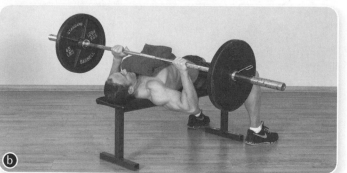

OPTIONS

Easy Option Perform 4 sets of the towel press and chin-up. Replace the chin-up with the kneeling lat pull-down (#120).

Step It Up Use a narrow grip on the towel press, and add weight to the chin-up.

Cool-Down Pec stretch, double lat stretch, 90-degree stretch.

Bound for Glory

Bounding is simply the act of repeatedly jumping forward (think about those broad jumps you did during the physical fitness tests as a kid; now put a few of them in a sequence). They can be done on one leg (jump forward off your right leg, land on your left, jump off your left, land on your right, repeat) or on both legs, as in the following workout. Bounding is one of those very simple, effective, yet demanding plyometric movements that truly allow you to express power. Improve your capabilities in your bounding exercises, and watch your cleans, snatches, and squats improve.

Warm-Up

4 reps per side of the world's greatest stretch, 5 reps each of inchworm and inverted hamstring stretch, 10 reps of glute bridge

● Featured Exercise

Double-Leg Bound

1. Begin with your feet hip-width apart. Flex your knees and bring your arms directly behind you (*a*).

2. Drive your forefoot into the ground, swing your arms forward, and explosively propel yourself as far forward as possible (*b*).

3. Land on your full foot with flexed knees (*c*).

4. Reset and repeat for reps (as you get more advanced, you can complete the bounds in a continuous series).

Complete Workout

A. Double-leg bound
   - 4 sets × 6 reps
   - 60 seconds of rest

B1. Trap bar deadlift (#8)
   - 3 sets × 4 to 6 reps
   - 75 seconds of rest

B2. Barbell walking lunge (#112)
   - 3 sets × 6 to 8 reps/leg
   - 75 seconds of rest

B3. Seated calf raise (#154)
   - 3 sets × 8 to 10 reps
   - 75 seconds of rest

OPTIONS

Easy Option   Perform 2 sets of the trap bar deadlift, barbell walking lunge, and seated calf raise.

Step It Up   Perform 5 sets of the trap bar deadlift, barbell walking lunge, and seated calf raise.

Cool-Down   Double lat stretch, hamstring stretch, calf stretch.

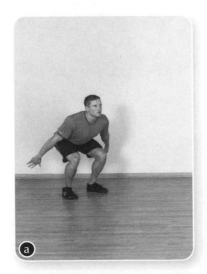
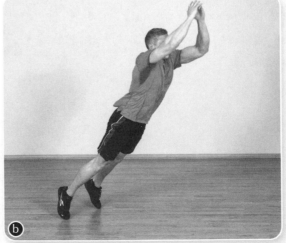
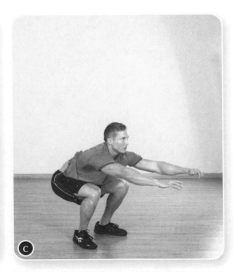

Arm-ageddon

Compound lifts set the stage for an anabolic hormonal environment. If you want to produce the hormones that stimulate muscle growth, you should be including big lifts such as the squat, deadlift, and chin-up in your program. However, if you want bigger biceps or calves, you are going to have to train those muscle groups directly as well. You're not going to get giant triceps if you never perform any triceps-focused movements.

Warm-Up

4 reps per side of the world's greatest stretch, 5 reps of inchworm, 8 reps per side of shoulder sweeps

● Featured Exercise

Reverse-Grip Biceps Curl

1. With an overhand grip (palms facing down), begin with a barbell in front of your thighs (*a*).
2. Keeping your arms tight to your sides, curl the bar up to your shoulders. Do not bring your elbows forward as you reach the top of the movement (*b*).
3. Lower to the starting position and repeat for reps.

Complete Workout

A1. Close-grip bench press (#131)
- 2 sets × 8 reps
- 60 seconds of rest

A2. Decline EZ-bar triceps extension (#145)
- 2 sets × 10 reps
- 30 seconds of rest

A3. Triceps rope press-down (#64)
- 2 sets × 12 reps
- 60 seconds of rest

B1. Chin-up (#73)
- 2 sets × 8 reps
- 60 seconds of rest

B2. Offset-grip incline dumbbell biceps curl (#243)
- 2 sets × 10 reps
- 30 seconds of rest

B3. Reverse-grip biceps curl
- 2 sets × 12 reps
- 60 seconds of rest

OPTIONS

Easy Option Replace the chin-up with the kneeling lat pull-down (#120).

Step It Up Add 1 set to each of the exercises.

Cool-Down Pec stretch, double lat stretch, 90-degree stretch.

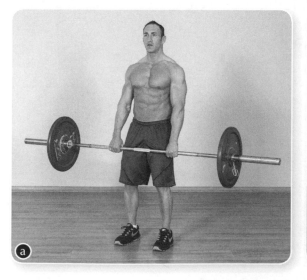

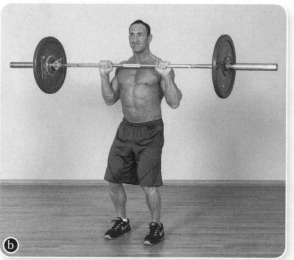

Broadway

Plyometrics, such as the broad jump in this workout, are a great way of developing explosive power, particularly in the lower body. However, plyos are also extremely demanding, placing a high amount of stress on your joints and structures. When including these types of movements in your training, respect the demand they place on your body, and limit the number of repetitions you perform in each workout.

Warm-Up

4 reps per side of the world's greatest stretch, 5 reps each of inchworm and inverted hamstring stretch, 10 reps of glute bridge

● Featured Exercise

Broad Jump

1. Begin in a standing position, feet at hip width and facing forward.

2. Bend your knees, bringing your hips back and your arms straight behind you (a).

3. Explosively leap forward as far as possible (b), landing on both feet with knees slightly bent to absorb the impact (c).

4. Reset to the starting position and repeat for reps.

Complete Workout

Broad jump
- 6 sets × 3 reps
- 30 seconds of rest

Barbell Romanian deadlift (#295)
- 6 sets × 8 reps
- 2 minutes of rest

OPTIONS

Easy Option Reduce the number of reps of the barbell Romanian deadlift to 6 per set.

Step It Up Increase the number of broad jumps to 5 per set.

Cool-Down Double lat stretch, hamstring stretch, calf stretch.

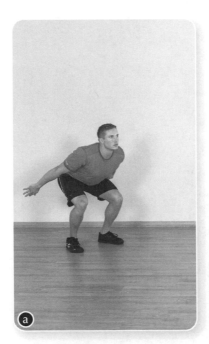
(a)

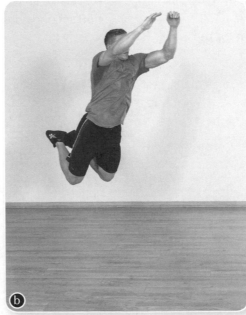
(b)

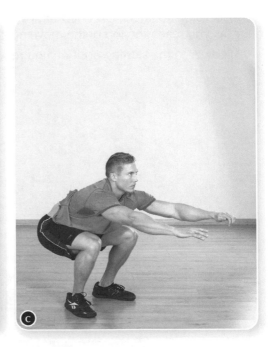
(c)

Crisscross

It's difficult to think of a more effective upper body pulling exercise than the pull-up (and its variations). By utilizing the muscles in the upper back, lats, forearms, and biceps, you are truly getting a lot of bang for your buck out of this movement. There is a reason it's remained a standard in fitness tests ranging from grade school through the military—it's just a tough exercise to beat for functionality, strength, and building muscle. In this workout, you'll be utilizing the pull-up along with its equally great counterpart, the push-up, in a crisscross pattern, increasing the reps per set of one exercise while decreasing the reps per set of the other.

Warm-Up

5 reps of inchworm, 6 reps per side of quadruped T-spine rotation, 10 reps of cat–cow

Complete Workout

This workout is performed as an ascending/descending ladder. In the first set, complete 10 repetitions of the neutral-grip pull-up and 1 repetition of the push-up. In the second set, complete 9 repetitions of the neutral-grip pull-up and 2 repetitions of the push-up. Keep decreasing the reps in the pull-up by one each set while increasing the reps of the push-up by one each set until, in the 10th set, you are completing 1 pull-up and 10 push-ups.

Neutral-grip pull-up
- 10 sets × 10, 9, 8, 7, 6, 5, 4, 3, 2, 1 reps

Push-up (#12)
- 10 sets × 1, 2, 3, 4, 5, 6, 7, 8, 9, 10 reps

● Featured Exercise

Neutral-Grip Pull-Up

1. Begin by grabbing a pull-up bar with a neutral grip (palms facing each other).
2. Every rep should begin with your arms fully extended (a). Depress your shoulder blades, and use your back and arms to pull yourself toward the bar. Do not utilize momentum or bring your knees up or legs forward.
3. Complete the rep by touching your chest to the bar (b). Lower back to the starting position and repeat for reps.

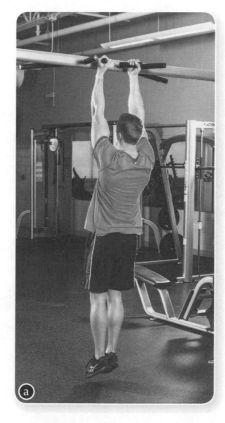
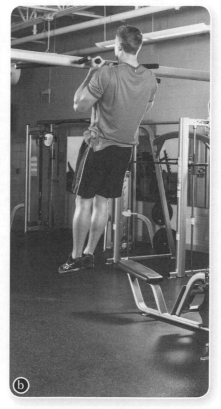

Paused Reps: Romanian Deadlift

Although an excellent strength exercise in its own right, the Romanian deadlift can be used as a great teaching tool to improve technique on the traditional deadlift. Because the lift begins in the top position, it eliminates many of the mobility issues associated with getting into the proper position to lift a barbell off the floor. And the fact that the initial movement pattern is the hip hinge really drives home this critical position. So if you are having a hard time mastering the deadlift, try starting with the RDL—it could be the missing piece of the puzzle.

Warm-Up

4 reps per side of the world's greatest stretch, 5 reps each of inchworm and inverted hamstring stretch, 10 reps of glute bridge

● Featured Exercise

Paused Barbell Romanian Deadlift

1. Begin with a barbell directly in front of your thighs. Feet should be hip width, hands grasping the bar with a pronated grip at shoulder width (a).

2. Keeping a neutral spine and the bar close to your legs throughout the entire movement, unlock your knees slightly and hinge at your hips.

3. Keep your chin tucked and drive your butt back, creating tension in your hamstrings (for more on proper squat technique, see chapter 1, Ramping Up).

4. You've reached the bottom of your range of motion when you can no longer drive your hips back without increasing the bend in your knees or bending from your lower back (b).

5. Pause for 3 seconds in the bottom position before reversing the motion by driving your hips forward. Repeat for reps.

Complete Workout

A. Paused barbell Romanian deadlift
- 4 sets × 8 reps
- 2 minutes of rest

B1. Lying hamstring curl (#168)
- 3 sets × 12 reps
- 60 seconds of rest

B2. Goblet squat (#2)
- 3 sets × 12 reps
- 60 seconds of rest

OPTIONS

Easy Option   Reduce the length of the pause on the paused barbell Romanian deadlift to 2 seconds.

Step It Up   Increase the length of the pause on the paused barbell Romanian deadlift to 4 seconds.

Cool-Down   Double lat stretch, hamstring stretch, calf stretch.

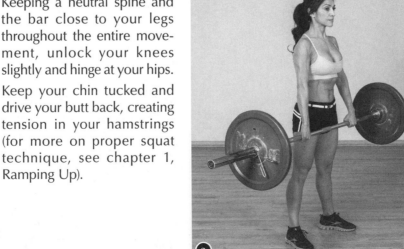

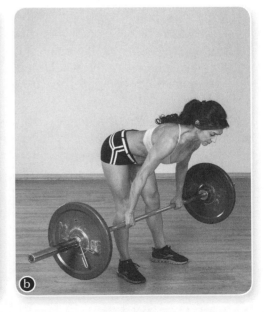

Moon Shot

In 1969, man first set foot on the moon. And if you survive this gravity-defying workout, you'll probably feel as if you are on cloud nine. This workout starts with a power exercise, moves on to a pair of unilateral (single limb) movements, and then ends with a 25-rep killer. Prepare for blastoff.

Warm-Up

6 reps of squat to stand, 6 reps per side of quadruped T-spine rotation, 8 reps of glute bridge, 10 reps of cat–cow

● Featured Exercise

Single-Arm Dumbbell Snatch

1. Begin with a shoulder-width stance and a dumbbell directly between your feet.
2. Reach down and grab the handle of the dumbbell with your right hand by bringing your hips back and keeping your chest tall (a).

3. In one explosive motion, keeping the dumbbell close to your body, drive your hips forward, shrug your right shoulder, and drive the dumbbell overhead (b-c).
4. Return the weight to the starting position, and repeat all the reps for one side before switching to the other.

Complete Workout

A. Single-arm dumbbell snatch
- 4 sets × 3 reps/side
- 60 seconds of rest

B1. Alternating step-back lunge (#24)
- 3 sets × 8 reps/side
- 60 seconds of rest

B2. Alternating dumbbell row (#246)
- 3 sets × 8 reps/side
- 60 seconds of rest

C. Push-up (#12)
- 1 set × 25 reps

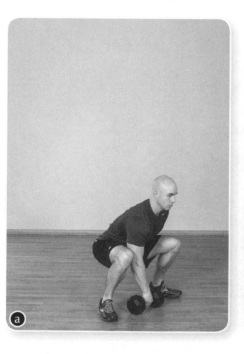
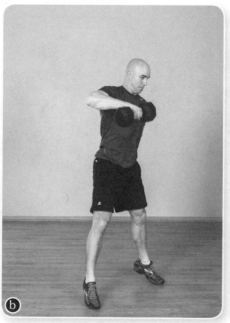
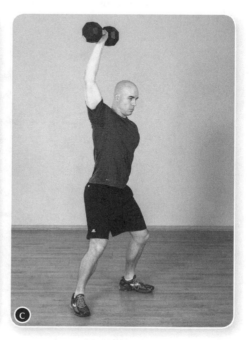

OPTIONS

Easy Option Reduce the number of push-ups to 15 reps.

Step It Up Increase the number of push-ups to 35 reps.

Cool-Down Hamstring stretch, calf stretch, pec stretch.

Im-Pressed

When it comes to overhead pressing with a barbell, the most challenging portion of the movement is usually the bottom—getting the bar from the collarbones to the forehead. The workout uses a partial that emphasizes the strongest part of the movement, from the forehead to lockout, allowing you to use more weight and develop more pressing strength.

Warm-Up

4 reps per side of the world's greatest stretch, 5 reps of inchworm, 8 reps per side of shoulder sweeps

Featured Exercise

Partial Press

1. Set the safety bars in a power rack so that a barbell is at forehead height when sitting on a bench.
2. Sit tall on the bench (feel free to use one with back support) and grab the bar with a double-overhead grip just outside shoulder-width (*a*).
3. Keeping your heels on the floor and torso tight, press the bar overhead until you reach lockout (*b*).
4. Return to the starting position and repeat for desired reps.

Complete Workout

Perform all sets of the partial press using 90 to 110 percent of your usual bench press weight. Complete all sets of the partial press before moving on to the superset of the seated dumbbell overhead press and reverse cable fly.

A. Partial press
- 4 sets × 3 to 5 reps
- 2 minutes of rest

B1. Seated dumbbell shoulder press (#209)
- 4 sets × 6 to 8 reps

B2. Face pull (#127)
- 4 sets × 6 to 8 reps
- 75 seconds of rest

OPTIONS

Easy Option Use 80 to 95 percent of your 3-5RM shoulder press weight for the partial press.

Step It Up Work up to 130 percent+ of your 3-5RM shoulder press weight for the partial press.

Cool-Down Pec stretch, double lat stretch, 90-degree stretch.

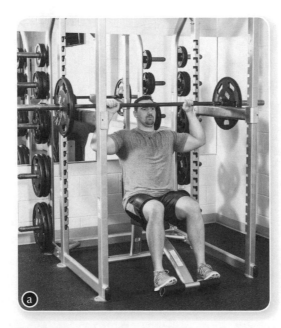
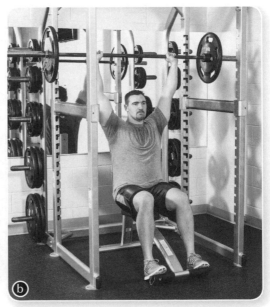

Breaking Point

If you are struggling with performing a full pistol, or single-leg squat (#245), the single-leg box squat (featured in this workout) is a great tool to start improving strength and range of motion. As you progress, be sure to use lower boxes. After a few weeks, you should have the ankle and hip mobility as well as leg and core strength to get your butt down to your heels and back up. This will also carry over to your bilateral squats, lunges, and Olympic lifts—so it's definitely worth the time and energy.

Warm-Up

4 reps per side of the world's greatest stretch, 5 reps each of inchworm and inverted hamstring stretch, 10 reps of glute bridge

Complete Workout

A. Sumo deadlift (#82)
- 4 sets × 6 reps
- 90 seconds of rest

B1. Single-leg box squat
- 3 sets × 8 reps/leg
- 45 seconds of rest

B2. Barbell walking lunge (#112)
- 3 sets × 8 reps/leg
- 45 seconds of rest

● Featured Exercise

Single-Leg Box Squat

1. Sit tall on a box with a neutral spine. Hold your arms straight in front of you and stand up (this will determine how far away from the box you should stand).
2. Raise your right foot off the floor (a), reach your hips back, and sit on the box (b).
3. Maintaining that same upright posture, drive your right foot into the floor to come back to standing. Repeat all reps for one side before switching to the other.

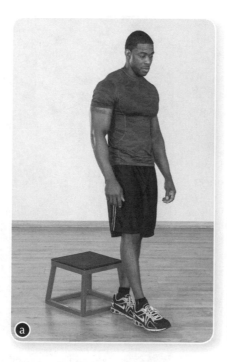

(a)

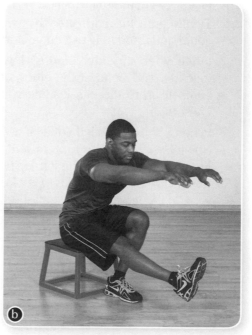

(b)

OPTIONS

Easy Option Perform 3 sets of the sumo deadlift and 2 sets of the single-leg box squat and barbell walking lunge.

Step It Up Replace the single-leg box squat with a single-leg squat (#245).

Cool-Down Double lat stretch, cross-body stretch, hamstring stretch.

Hanging On

The body is incredibly adaptable and will get very efficient at skills you practice and repeat. This allows us to not have to think when performing a movement we've done hundreds of times. However, sometimes it's good to throw your system a movement curveball in order to challenge your body in a way it has not been tested before. By changing your grip, using a different apparatus (e.g., kettlebells instead of dumbbells), or even performing an exercise at a different tempo, you'll stimulate your central nervous system and force your body into an even greater state of adaptation.

Warm-Up

5 reps of inchworm, 6 reps per side of quadruped T-spine rotation, 10 reps of cat–cow

● Featured Exercise

Towel-Grip Chin-Up

1. Hang two gym towels over a pull-up bar. Tightly grab the end of each towel with your hands, and fully extend your arms (a).
2. Drive your shoulder blades down and together, and bend at the elbows to pull yourself up to the bar, leading with your chest (b).
3. When you have pulled yourself as high as possible, reverse the motion and slowly lower yourself back to the starting position. Repeat for reps. The goal is to not lose your grip on the towels for the entire set.

Complete Workout

A1. Towel-grip chin-up
- 3 sets × 6 reps
- 60 seconds of rest

A2. Incline barbell bench press (#179)
- 3 sets × 6 reps
- 60 seconds of rest

B1. Seated cable row with hip flexion (#174)
- 3 sets × 10 reps
- 45 seconds of rest

B2. Flat dumbbell bench press (#109)
- 3 sets × 10 reps
- 45 seconds of rest

OPTIONS

Easy Option Perform 4 reps per set of the towel-grip chin-up.

Step It Up Increase the number of reps of the towel-grip chin-up and incline barbell bench press to 8 per set.

Cool-Down Double lat stretch, cross-body stretch, hamstring stretch.

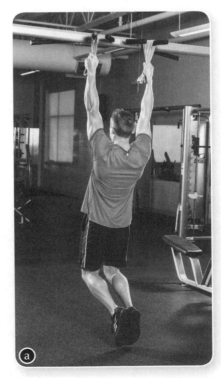
(a)

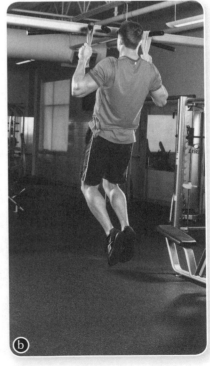
(b)

In Arms' Way

You would think that gripping a dumbbell would be simple, right? Just grab the handle and go. However, where you place your hand on the handle actually makes a difference. Take the incline dumbbell biceps curl, for example. If you use an offset grip in which your thumb rests against one of the weight plates, you'll be targeting more of the short head of the biceps. Slide your hand the other way so your pinkie is against the weight plate, and you'll instantly feel the curl get much more challenging. Don't be afraid to play around with different hand placements from time to time to vary training stimulus—just don't do it when you are about to max out on weight.

Warm-Up

5 reps of inchworm, 6 reps per side of quadruped T-spine rotation, 10 reps of cat–cow

● Featured Exercise

Offset-Grip Incline Dumbbell Biceps Curl

1. Set an adjustable bench to a 45-degree angle. Grab a pair of dumbbells with an offset grip (your thumb against the weight plate) (a), and sit on the bench with your upper back resting against the pad.

2. Begin with your arms hanging directly down from your shoulder (b).

3. Without allowing your elbow to come forward, curl up the dumbbells (c).

4. Contract your biceps hard at the top of the movement, and return the dumbbells back to the starting position. Repeat for reps.

Complete Workout

Perform 4 rounds of the following circuit.

Three-position EZ-bar curl (#151)
- 8 reps
- 30 seconds of rest

Decline EZ-bar triceps extension (#145)
- 8 reps
- 30 seconds of rest

Offset-grip incline dumbbell biceps curl
- 12 reps
- 30 seconds of rest

Triceps rope press-down (#64)
- 12 reps
- 30 seconds of rest

OPTIONS

Easy Option   Perform 3 rounds of the circuit.

Step It Up   Perform 5 rounds of the circuit.

Cool-Down   Double lat stretch, cross-body stretch, hamstring stretch.

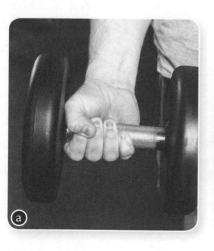

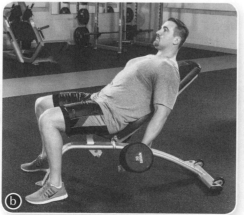

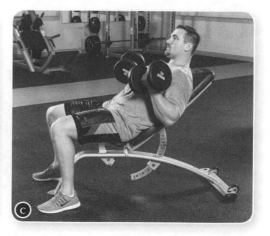

Combo Platter

Combination exercises (taking two movements that are often performed separately and combining them into one continuous movement) are not always great for building strength because you are limited to using a weight that allows you to complete the weakest part of the movement. For example, in the curl to overhead press, you are likely able to overhead press more than you can curl, but you have to use the weight you can curl for the entire movement. However, because you are using a lot of muscle mass and the reps usually involve a longer time under tension (total length of the rep), combo exercises are a great choice for workouts that have a metabolic focus.

Warm-Up

4 reps per side of the world's greatest stretch, 6 reps per side of hip rocker and inverted hamstring stretch, 8 reps per side of shoulder sweeps

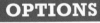 **Featured Exercise**

Lying Dumbbell Pullover to Extension

1. Grab a pair of dumbbells, and lie faceup on a flat bench. Press the dumbbells up directly over your shoulders, with your palms facing each other (a).

2. Without moving your upper arms, flex at the elbows to lower the dumbbells until your forearms are parallel to the floor (b).

3. Lower the dumbbells back beyond your head. You should feel a stretch in your lats (c).

4. Reverse the entire movement until you are back to the starting position. Repeat for reps.

Complete Workout

A. Barbell thruster (#6)
- 4 sets × 8 reps
- 90 seconds of rest

B1. Alternating dumbbell hammer curl (#230)
- 3 sets × 10 reps
- 30 seconds of rest

B2. Lying dumbbell pullover to extension
- 3 sets × 10 reps
- 30 seconds of rest

OPTIONS

Easy Option Perform 2 sets of the alternating dumbbell hammer curl and lying dumbbell pullover to extension.

Step It Up Add 2 reps to each set of the alternating dumbbell hammer curl and lying dumbbell pullover to extension.

Cool-Down Standing quad stretch, 90-degree stretch, double lat stretch.

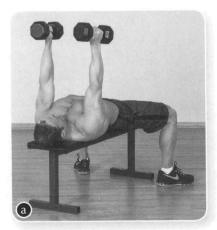
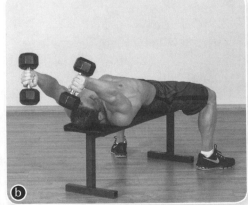
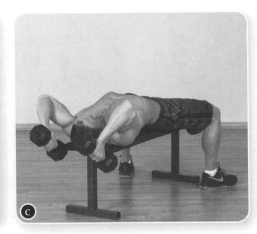

The Pistol

Performing a single-leg squat (aka pistol squat) not only demands strength but also requires proper core stability, mobility in the ankle and hip, and great thoracic extension. There is certainly a larger learning curve to the single-leg squat than many other exercises, so feel free to begin by holding onto a squat rack or a TRX, or lower yourself down to a high box in order to work on the movement pattern and develop the other physical requirements before attempting the free-standing version of this impressive exercise.

Warm-Up

4 reps per side of the world's greatest stretch, 5 reps each of inchworm and inverted hamstring stretch, 10 reps of glute bridge

● Featured Exercise

Single-Leg Squat

1. Begin with your feet hip-width apart. Lift your right foot off the floor, and place the heel directly in line with your left toes (*a*).

2. Keeping your back flat and chest tall, begin bending the knee on your left leg while keeping your right leg straight and off the floor. As you descend, bring both arms directly out in front of your torso as counterbalance.

3. Continue to descend until your butt reaches your left heel (*b*). Press your left foot into the ground to reverse the movement until you are back at the standing position. Complete all reps for one side before switching.

Complete Workout

A. Conventional deadlift (#5)
- 4 sets × 6 reps
- 90 seconds of rest

B1. Overhead squat (#167)
- 2 sets × 12 reps
- 60 seconds of rest

B2. Single-leg squat
- 2 sets × 6 reps/side
- 60 seconds of rest

B3. Leg press calf raise (#136)
- 2 sets × 12 reps
- 60 seconds of rest

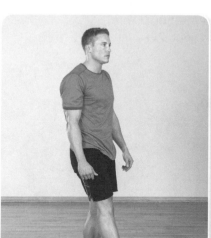
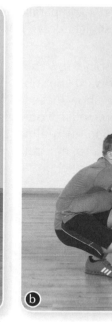

OPTIONS

Easy Option   Perform 4 reps per side of the single-leg squat.

Step It Up   Add an extra set to the barbell overhead squat, single-leg squat, and leg press calf raise.

Cool-Down   Double lat stretch, hamstring stretch, calf stretch.

Invincible

As much as you may like looking at yourself in the mirror, it's best to avoid doing so when performing exercises that require you to bend over. By lifting your chin and keeping your head up when your chest is facing the floor, you are, at best, decreasing the amount of neurological signaling that you can send to your muscles (similar to putting a kink in a hose) and making yourself weaker. At worst, you are risking a neck or back injury. So limit the mirror-gazing to checking yourself out after the workout.

Warm-Up

5 reps of inchworm, 6 reps per side of quadruped T-spine rotation, 10 reps of cat–cow

● **Featured Exercise**

Alternating Dumbbell Row

1. Grab a pair of dumbbells, bend at the hips, and lower your torso until it's nearly parallel to the floor. Your arms should hang straight down from your shoulders (*a*).

2. Keeping a neutral spine, row the left dumbbell up toward your rib cage, keeping your elbow tucked in. As you row up, rotate your hand from a supinated (palm facing your thighs) to neutral (palm facing your rib cage) position (*b*).

3. After reaching the top of your range of motion, lower the dumbbell back to the starting position and repeat for the left side. Be sure your right arm is locked out before rowing with the left. Continue to alternate until all reps are complete.

Complete Workout

A1. Neutral-grip pull-up (#237)
- 4 sets × 10 reps
- 60 seconds of rest

A2. Wide-hands push-up (#191)
- 4 sets × 10 reps
- 60 seconds of rest

B1. Alternating dumbbell row
- 3 sets × 12 reps/side
- 60 seconds of rest

B2. Incline dumbbell chest press (#210)
- 3 sets × 12 reps/side
- 60 seconds of rest

OPTIONS

Easy Option Reduce the number of sets of the neutral-grip pull-up and wide-hands push-up to 3.

Step It Up Add weight to the neutral grip pull-up.

Cool-Down Double lat stretch, cross-body stretch, hamstring stretch.

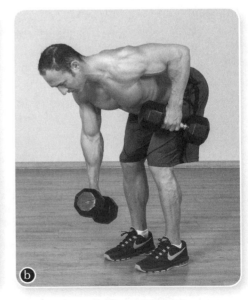

Bolder Shoulders

The shoulder is one of the most complex joints in the body. A ball-and-socket joint, the shoulder is capable of a wide range of movements, but this makes it rather susceptible to injury as well. So although it's highly recommended to use a variety of movements and angles to train shoulders and help them reach their full aesthetic and strength potential, it's always important to do so in a safe manner. Make sure you are using loads you can handle as well as performing the proper mobility work (outlined in the warm-up) in order to make sure your shoulders remain bulletproof.

Warm-Up

5 reps of inchworm, 6 reps per side of quadruped T-spine rotation, 10 reps of cat–cow

Featured Exercise

Seated Barbell Shoulder Press

1. Grab a barbell with an overhand grip just outside shoulder width, and sit at the end of a bench, your torso upright (try not to use a back-supported bench) (a).

2. Keeping your abs braced and feet flat on the floor, press the barbell overhead until your arms are locked out and the bar is directly over your shoulders (b).

3. Return the bar to the starting position in front of your collarbones and repeat for reps.

Complete Workout

A1. Seated barbell shoulder press
- 4 sets × 6 reps
- 60 seconds of rest

A2. Wide-grip pull-up (#117)
- 4 sets × 6 reps
- 60 seconds of rest

B1. Cable diagonal raise (#137)
- 2 sets × 10 reps
- 60 seconds of rest

B2. TRX face pull (#270)
- 2 sets × 10 reps
- 60 seconds of rest

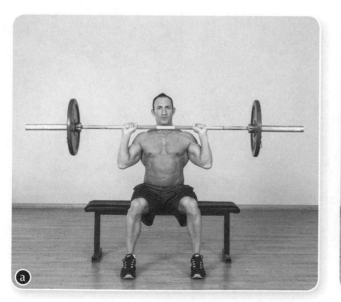

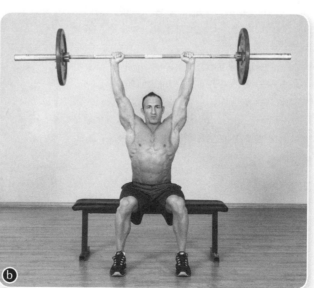

OPTIONS

Easy Option Replace the wide-grip pull-up with a kneeling lat pull-down (#120).

Step It Up Add weight to the wide-grip pull-up. Replace the TRX face pull with a heavier face pull (#127).

Cool-Down Double lat stretch, cross-body stretch, hamstring stretch.

Total Recall

As a general rule of thumb, total-body routines that use larger muscle groups (quads, lats, pecs) are better for fat loss than body-part splits that focus more on isolation movements using smaller muscle groups (biceps, triceps, calves). These splits tend to be of greater value in mass-building phases. However, most people would be well served to utilize both total-body and split routines in their year-long workout plans. And, of course, both goals of fat loss and mass building are very dependent on an appropriate nutrition plan.

Warm-Up

5 reps of inchworm, 6 reps per side of quadruped T-spine rotation, 10 reps of cat–cow

● Featured Exercise

Trap Bar Romanian Deadlift

1. Step into a trap bar with your feet just outside shoulder width and your hands grasping the center of the handles.
2. Stand up with the trap bar. Maintaining a neutral spine, reach your hips back, keeping a slight (10 degree) bend in your knees (a).
3. Without bending your knees farther, continue to reach your hips back until you've reached maximum range of motion (b).
4. Drive your hips forward to return to a standing position. Repeat for reps.

Complete Workout

A1. Trap bar Romanian deadlift
  • 4 sets × 8 reps
  • 60 seconds of rest

A2. Incline dumbbell chest press (#210)
  • 4 sets × 8 reps
  • 60 seconds of rest

B1. Barbell front-foot elevated split squat (#140)
  • 3 sets × 8 reps/side
  • 60 seconds of rest

B2. Alternating dumbbell row (#246)
  • 3 sets × 8 reps/side
  • 60 seconds of rest

OPTIONS

Easy Option   Perform 3 sets of the trap bar Romanian deadlift and incline dumbbell chest press.

Step It Up   Add 2 reps to each set of the barbell front-foot elevated split squat and alternating dumbbell row.

Cool-Down   Double lat stretch, cross-body stretch, hamstring stretch.

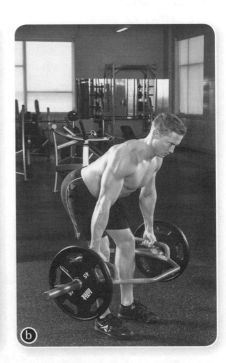

Paused Reps: Front Squat

Whenever you use specialized techniques that cause a mechanical disadvantage such as pauses, fat grips, or altered stances, it is critical that you adjust the weight accordingly to compensate for that disadvantage. The last thing you want to do is drive up the degree of difficulty on an exercise and then perform the lift with bad form. Leave your ego at the gym door, and back off the amount of weight you use.

Warm-Up

6 reps of squat to stand, 6 reps per side of quadruped T-spine rotation, 8 reps of glute bridge, 10 reps of cat–cow

● Featured Exercise

Paused Front Squat

1. Set up a barbell just below collarbone height in a squat rack.
2. Grab the bar in a rack position—hands grasping the bar just outside shoulder width, upper arms parallel to the floor, bar resting across the front deltoids (*a*).

3. Tighten up your upper body, unlock your hips, bend your knees, and lower your body toward the ground, trying to sit as low as possible while keeping the bar over the center of your foot (for more on proper squat technique, see chapter 1, Ramping Up) (*b*).
4. Once you reach the bottom of your range, pause for 3 seconds and drive the weight back up to the starting position. Repeat for reps, pausing at the bottom each time.

Complete Workout

A. Paused front squat
- 4 sets × 8 reps
- 2 minutes of rest

B1. Leg press (#114)
- 3 sets × 12 reps
- 60 seconds of rest

B2. Dumbbell Romanian deadlift (#267)
- 3 sets × 12 reps
- 60 seconds of rest

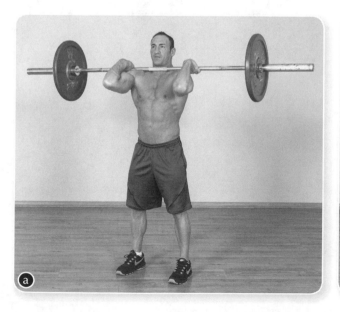

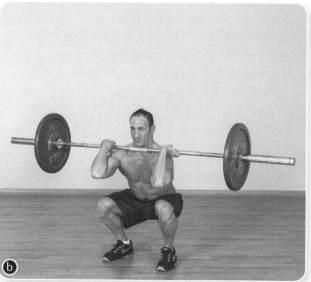

OPTIONS

Easy Option   Reduce the length of the pause on the paused front squat to 2 seconds.

Step It Up   Increase the length of the pause on the paused front squat to 4 seconds.

Cool-Down   Standing quad stretch, 90-degree stretch, double lat stretch.

Up, Up, and Away

One of the most maligned exercises in recent history is the sit-up. After being a staple in the exercise vernacular for decades, the sit-up has now been tagged as a worthless exercise at best and a movement that will destroy your spinal discs at worst. The truth is, spinal flexion (which is what happens when you perform a sit-up) is a normal and valid part of everyday movement demands. The trouble occurs when sit-ups are done incorrectly or are the exclusive core movement performed in a program. Avoid both mistakes by keeping a relatively neutral spine throughout all reps and by not pulling on your head with your arms as you lift. Balance out your program with exercises that incorporate extension, rotational, and antirotational movements as well and you will have a well-developed core without risking neck and back pain.

Warm-Up

5 reps of inchworm, 6 reps per side of quadruped T-spine rotation, 10 reps of cat–cow

● Featured Exercise

Sit-Up

1. Sit with your feet flat on the floor, knees bent, and hands behind your ears (do not pull on your neck) (a).

2. Raise your torso up to a seated position, keeping your spine neutral throughout the entire movement (b).

3. Lower yourself under control to the starting position. Repeat for reps.

Complete Workout

A. Barbell overhead press (#36)
- 4 sets × 6 reps
- 75 seconds of rest

B1. Wide-hands push-up (#191)
- 2 sets × 12 reps
- 45 seconds of rest

B2. Wide-grip pull-up (#117)
- 2 sets × 12 reps
- 45 seconds of rest

B3. Sit-up
- 2 sets × 25 reps
- 45 seconds of rest

OPTIONS

Easy Option   Perform 3 sets of the barbell overhead press.

Step It Up   Add 1 set to the wide-grip push-up, wide-grip pull-up, and sit-up.

Cool-Down   Double lat stretch, cross-body stretch, hamstring stretch.

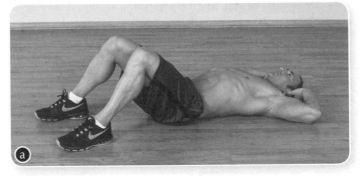

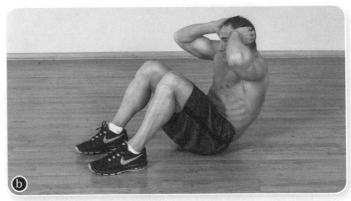

Face the Pain

When it comes to training, you should always prioritize perfecting technique before adding speed and resistance. This will ensure you stay safe and develop solid movement patterns. Think about it this way: You wouldn't enter a high-speed car race before you learned how to drive.

Warm-Up

5 reps of inchworm, 6 reps per side of quadruped T-spine rotation, 10 reps of cat–cow

● **Featured Exercise**

Seated Cable Face Pull

1. Set up a box or bench in front of a cable station. Attach a rope to the pulley, and set it at eye level (when seated on the bench).

2. Grab the rope with a neutral grip (as if you were shaking hands with the rope), keeping your shoulders down and your arms straight (*a*).

3. Pull the rope toward your ear lobes, keeping your upper arms parallel to the floor. Your thumbs should be facing behind you at the end range of the movement (*b*).

4. Return the rope to the starting position and repeat for reps.

Complete Workout

A1. Incline barbell bench press (#179)
 • 3 sets × 8 reps
 • 60 seconds of rest

A2. Seated cable face pull
 • 3 sets × 8 reps
 • 60 seconds of rest

B1. Kneeling lat pull-down (#120)
 • 3 sets × 10 reps
 • 45 seconds of rest

B2. Seated dumbbell shoulder press (#209)
 • 3 sets × 10 reps
 • 45 seconds of rest

OPTIONS

Easy Option Perform 2 sets of all the B exercises.

Step It Up Add 2 reps to each set of the B exercises.

Cool-Down Double lat stretch, cross-body stretch, hamstring stretch.

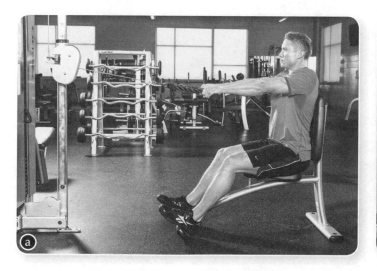

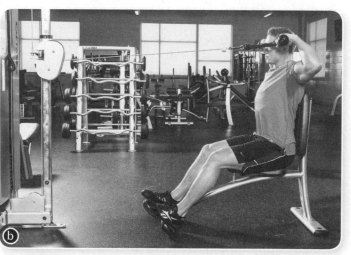

The Luger

Although the Olympic lifts (snatch, clean and jerk) are the most technically demanding movements in the gym, they can be broken down into smaller parts—making them much easier to learn while still delivering much of the benefit. The snatch-grip jump shrug (featured in this workout) will improve grip, upper back, and hamstring strength as well as explosive jumping power—all without having to receive the bar and completing the overhead squat as required in the full snatch. Of course the snatch still has huge benefits (total body mobility and stability), but movements such as the snatch-grip jump shrug will help you start grooving these movement patterns without having to hoist a bar over your head.

Warm-Up

5 reps of inchworm, 6 reps per side of quadruped T-spine rotation, 10 reps of cat–cow

Complete Workout

A. Snatch-grip jump shrug
- 5 sets × 3 reps
- 90 seconds of rest

B1. Barbell overhead press (#36)
- 2 sets × 8 reps
- 30 seconds of rest

B2. Goblet squat (#2)
- 2 sets × 10 reps
- 30 seconds of rest

B3. Kneeling lat pull-down (#120)
- 2 sets × 12 reps
- 30 seconds of rest

● **Featured Exercise**

OPTIONS

Easy Option Reduce the number of sets of the snatch-grip jump shrug to 4.

Step It Up Add 1 set to the barbell overhead press, goblet squat, and kneeling lat pull-down.

Cool-Down Double lat stretch, cross-body stretch, hamstring stretch.

Snatch-Grip Jump Shrug

1. Grab a barbell with a double overhand grip at approximately twice shoulder width (or your usual snatch grip).
2. Keeping your back flat and tight, bend your hips and knees until your shoulders are in line with the bar (a).
3. Drive your knees back to slowly pull the bar off the floor.
4. Once the bar is above your midthighs, explosively extend your hips, knees, and ankles (as you would in a vertical jump), sending the bar upward (b).
5. Once your heels return to the floor, place the bar in the starting position and repeat for reps.

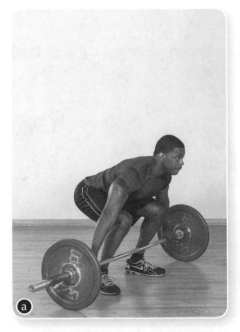

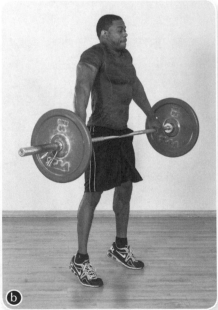

Pullover

The pullover has long been considered an exercise that works the lats. However, it can also be an effective chest and triceps builder because both these muscle groups get involved in this movement, as well. When designing a chest and back workout, such as the one featured here, the pullover becomes a great bang-for-your-buck exercise that allows you to hit these two muscle groups at once.

Warm-Up

5 reps of inchworm, 6 reps per side of quadruped T-spine rotation, 10 reps of cat–cow

● Featured Exercise

EZ-Bar Pullover

1. Grab an EZ bar with a shoulder-width grip, and lie down on a flat bench. Press the EZ bar so it is directly over your chin. This is your starting position (a).

2. Keeping your arms straight, lower the bar back and overhead until your arms are approximately parallel to the floor (b).

3. Contract your lats and bring the bar back to the starting position. Repeat for reps.

Complete Workout

A1. Barbell bench press (#54)
  • 4 sets × 6 reps
  • 60 seconds of rest

A2. Neutral grip pull-up (#237)
  • 4 sets × 6 reps
  • 60 seconds of rest

B1. Cable chest fly (#181)
  • 3 sets × 8 to 10 reps
  • 60 seconds of rest

B2. EZ-bar pullover
  • 3 sets × 8 to 10 reps
  • 60 seconds of rest

OPTIONS

Easy Option   Perform 3 sets of the barbell bench press and neutral-grip pull-up.

Step It Up   Add weight to the neutral-grip pull-up.

Cool-Down   Double lat stretch, cross-body stretch, hamstring stretch.

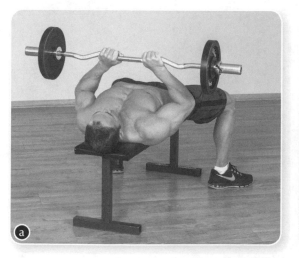

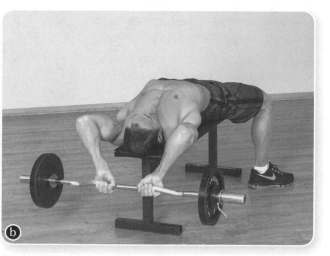

Tree Trunks

Understanding movement patterns and what exercises utilize which muscles is key to both designing a good program and being able to substitute exercises according to equipment availability or preference. So, instead of mindlessly going through your workout, give some thought as to what muscle groups are being activated, and consider what alternatives would be appropriate when needed.

Warm-Up

6 reps of squat to stand, 6 reps per side of quadruped T-spine rotation, 8 reps of glute bridge, 10 reps of cat–cow

● Featured Exercise

Single-Side Kettlebell Squat

1. Begin with a kettlebell in the rack position on your right side. Your wrist should be straight and in line with your forearm, and your elbow should be tucked next to your rib cage. Your feet should be at or just outside shoulder width (*a*).

2. Keeping your chest tall and a neutral spine, bring your hips back and bend at your knees to lower into a full squat (*b*). Resist the urge to lean to one side in order to compensate for the weight.

3. Once you reach the bottom position, straighten your knees while driving your hips forward until you have returned to the starting position. Complete all reps on one side before switching.

Complete Workout

A1. Trap bar deadlift (#8)
- 4 sets × 8 reps
- 60 seconds of rest

A2. Single-side kettlebell squat
- 4 sets × 8 reps/side
- 60 seconds of rest

B1. Lying hamstring curl (#168)
- 3 sets × 10 reps
- 45 seconds of rest

B2. Dumbbell step-up (#121)
- 3 sets × 10 reps
- 45 seconds of rest

OPTIONS

Easy Option   Perform 3 sets of the trap bar deadlift and single-side kettlebell squat.

Step It Up   Add 1 set to the lying hamstring curl and dumbbell step-up.

Cool-Down   Standing quad stretch, 90-degree stretch, double lat stretch.

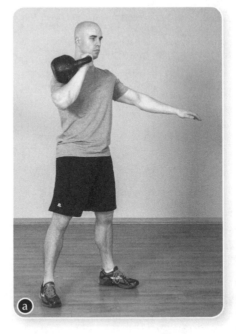
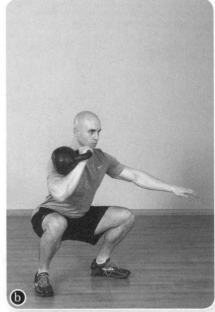

Paused Reps: Bench Press

Pausing for 3 seconds at the bottom of a bench press (as you will do in this workout) does several things. The pause eliminates the stretch reflex that is created when you simply touch the bar to your chest and immediately drive the weight back up, as you would in a standard bench press. This develops more strength from the dead-stop position, which could be the key to breaking a bench press plateau. This pause makes the exercise more demanding by eliminating the use of momentum, so you will have to adjust your weight selection accordingly.

Warm-Up

4 reps per side of the world's greatest stretch, 5 reps of inchworm, 8 reps per side of shoulder sweeps

● Featured Exercise

Paused Barbell Bench Press

1. Begin by lying back on the bench at a bench press station. Your feet should be on the floor, and your butt, the area between your shoulder blades, and your head should all be on the bench. Your eyes should be directly under the bar

2. Grab the bar with a slightly wider than shoulder-width grip. Unrack the bar so it is directly over the center of your chest (a).

3. Keep your elbows tucked toward your rib cage as you lower the bar down to your chest (b).

4. Once the bar reaches the bottom position, pause for 3 seconds before driving up the weight to lockout. Repeat for reps.

Complete Workout

A. Paused barbell bench press
- 4 sets × 8 reps
- 2 minutes of rest

B1. Face pull (#127)
- 3 sets × 12 reps
- 60 seconds of rest

B2. Incline dumbbell chest press (#210)
- 3 sets × 12 reps
- 60 seconds of rest

OPTIONS

Easy Option   Reduce the length of the pause on the paused barbell bench press to 2 seconds.

Step It Up   Increase the length of the pause on the paused barbell bench press to 4 seconds.

Cool-Down   Pec stretch, double lat stretch, 90-degree stretch.

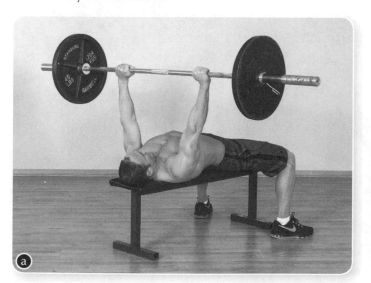

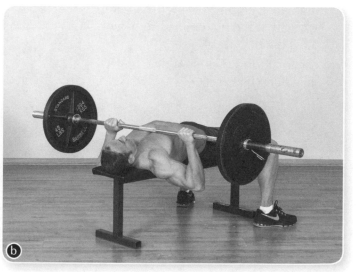

Mix and Match

The mixed-grip chin-up, featured in this workout, is an underutilized but extremely effective exercise. You get not only all the back- and biceps-building benefits you would achieve in a standard chin-up or pull-up but also additional shoulder and core activation because you need to prevent your torso from rotating as you pull up to the bar. So ignore the curious stares of other gym-goers, and get this rarely used movement into your program.

Warm-Up

6 reps of squat to stand, 6 reps per side of quadruped T-spine rotation, 8 reps of glute bridge, 10 reps of cat–cow

Complete Workout

A. Mixed-grip chin-up
- 4 sets × 10 reps
- 90 seconds of rest

B1. Incline barbell bench press (#179)
- 3 sets × 10 reps
- 60 seconds of rest

B2. Seated cable row with hip flexion (#174)
- 3 sets × 10 reps
- 45 seconds of rest

● Featured Exercise

Mixed-Grip Chin-Up

1. Grab a chin-up bar with a mixed grip (one overhand, one underhand) just outside shoulder width (*a*).
2. Depress your shoulder blades and bend your elbows, pulling your chest up to the bar (*b*).
3. Lower yourself to the starting position, making sure your arms are full straight at the bottom before beginning the next rep.
4. Alternate the overhand and underhand grip each set.

OPTIONS

Easy Option   Perform 2 sets of the incline barbell bench press and seated cable row.

Step It Up   Perform as many reps as possible on each set of the mixed-grip chin-up.

Cool-Down   Standing quad stretch, 90-degree stretch, double lat stretch.

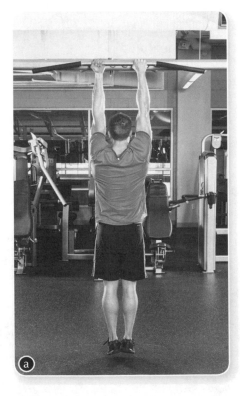

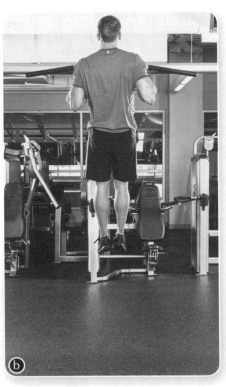

Daggers

The serratus anterior (a thin, flat muscle that sits atop your rib cage) is to the front of your body what the muscles around your scapulae (shoulder blades) are to the back of your body. The serratus plays a big role in maintaining good posture, particularly when you are pressing overhead. And just as the scapular retraction (#258) is a great movement to promote strength around the shoulder blades, the serratus shrug (featured in this workout) is an ideal way to strengthen this often-overlooked muscle.

Warm-Up

4 reps per side of the world's greatest stretch, 5 reps of inchworm, 8 reps per side of shoulder sweeps

Featured Exercise

Serratus Shrug

1. Grab the bars at a dip station, keeping your arms locked out, chest tall, and head forward.

2. Without bending your arms, actively press your shoulders away from your ears to lift your body up.

3. Hold this position for 3 to 5 seconds before returning to the starting position. Repeat for reps.

Complete Workout

A. Push jerk (#81)
- 5 sets × 4 reps
- 90 seconds of rest

B1. Incline dumbbell chest press (#210)
- 3 sets × 8 reps
- 45 seconds of rest

B2. Serratus shrug
- 3 sets × 10 reps
- 45 seconds of rest

B3. Cable diagonal raise (#137)
- 3 sets × 12 reps
- 45 seconds of rest

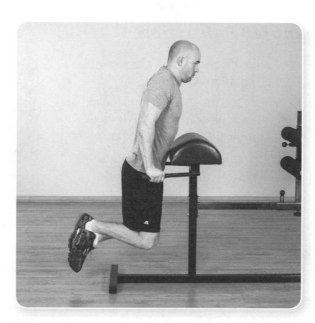

OPTIONS

Easy Option   Perform 2 sets of the incline dumbbell chest press, serratus shrug, and cable diagonal raise.

Step It Up   Reduce the rest on the incline dumbbell chest press, serratus shrug, and cable diagonal raise to 30 seconds.

Cool-Down   Pec stretch, double lat stretch, 90-degree stretch.

Blades of Glory

If you are relying on as much biceps power as possible to initiate the beginning of your pull-up, you are missing out on using some of the biggest and most effective muscles in your body—those of your upper back. Instead, try initiating the pull by driving your scapulae (shoulder blades) downward. This will lift your chest toward the bar before your arms even bend. The scapular retraction hold featured in this workout will begin to train your scaps to do more of the work for you. If you find yourself unable to hold the retraction for at least 10 seconds, you should focus more of your training time on strengthening your upper back.

Warm-Up

5 reps of inchworm, 6 reps per side of quadruped T-spine rotation, 10 reps of cat–cow

● Featured Exercise

Scapular Retraction

1. Grab a pull-up bar with an overhand, outside shoulder-width grip (a).
2. Keeping your arms straight and locked out, pull your shoulder blades downward. Your chest should rise toward the bar without your arms bending (b).
3. Hold this position for 30 seconds.

Complete Workout

A. Incline barbell bench press (#179)
- 5 sets × 4 reps
- 90 seconds of rest

B1. Seated cable row with hip flexion (#174)
- 3 sets × 8 reps
- 30 seconds of rest

B2. Seated dumbbell shoulder press (#209)
- 3 sets × 10 reps
- 30 seconds of rest

B3. Scapular retraction
- 3 sets × 30 seconds
- 30 seconds of rest

OPTIONS

Easy Option Perform 2 sets of all the B exercises.

Step It Up Add 2 reps to each set of the B exercises.

Cool-Down Double lat stretch, cross-body stretch, hamstring stretch.

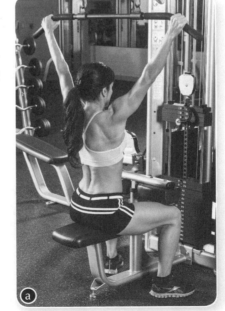
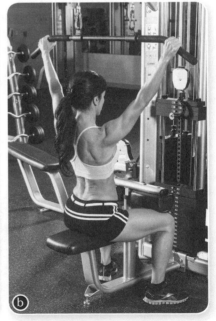

Unbreakable

Your hamstrings have two jobs: to bend your knees, as in a lying hamstring curl (#168), and to extend your hips, as in a Romanian deadlift (#267). The stability ball hip raise and leg curl (featured in this workout) trains both of these functions of the hamstrings in one integrated movement, allowing for greater muscle recruitment and exercise efficiency.

Warm-Up

4 reps per side of the world's greatest stretch, 5 reps each of inchworm and inverted hamstring stretch, 10 reps of glute bridge

● Featured Exercise

Stability Ball Hip Raise and Leg Curl

1. Lie faceup on the floor with your heels on a stability ball. Place your arms out to the sides with your palms facing the ceiling (a).
2. Push your hips up until your body forms a straight line from head to heels (b).
3. Press your heels into the ball and roll the ball toward you, getting it as close to your butt as possible. Keep your hips extended the entire time (c).
4. Reverse the motion by rolling the ball away from you until your legs are straight and then lowering your butt to the floor. Repeat for reps.

Complete Workout

A1. Sumo deadlift (#82)
- 4 sets × 10 reps
- 60 seconds of rest

A2. Heel-elevated back squat (#96)
- 4 sets × 10 reps
- 60 seconds of rest

B1. Stability ball hip raise and leg curl
- 3 sets × 12 reps
- 60 seconds of rest

B2. Negative sit-up (#227)
- 3 sets × 12 reps
- 60 seconds of rest

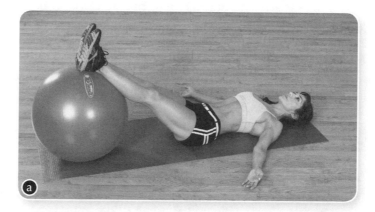

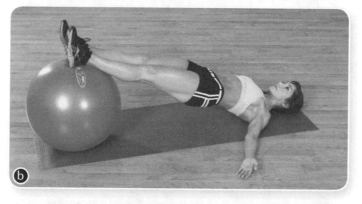

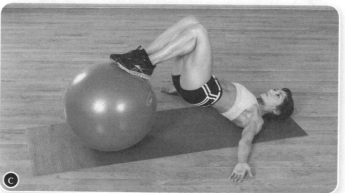

OPTIONS

Easy Option Reduce the number of sets of the sumo deadlift and heel-elevated back squat to 3.

Step It Up Replace the negative sit-up with an overhead squat (#167).

Cool-Down Double lat stretch, hamstring stretch, calf stretch.

Singles Club

If gaining strength is one of your main goals, it's good practice to test your 1RM (1-repetition maximum) every 4 to 8 weeks. Since many strength programs are based on using a specific percentage of that 1RM, testing will not only give you a sense of what your max weights are but also help you more accurately pick your loads when performing a strength-focused training protocol.

Warm-Up

4 reps per side of the world's greatest stretch, 5 reps of inchworm, 8 reps per side of shoulder sweeps

● Featured Exercise

Half-Kneeling Single-Arm Cable Row

1. Begin facing a cable station, with a D handle set at just above knee height.
2. Take a half-kneeling stance (this should look like the bottom of a lunge, with your left leg behind you, knee off the ground, and right leg in front of you at a 90-degree angle, foot flat on the floor). Grab the handle with your left hand (a).
3. Keeping your chest tall, drive your left elbow behind you until your left hand is adjacent to your rib cage (b).
4. Straighten your left arm, and repeat for all reps on one side before switching to the other.

Complete Workout

Increase the weight used on each set of the barbell bench press until you reach your maximum weight on the final set.

A. Barbell bench press (#54)
   - 5 sets × 5, 3, 1, 1, 1 reps
   - 90 seconds of rest

B1. Seated dumbbell shoulder press (#209)
   - 2 sets × 10 reps
   - 60 seconds of rest

B2. Half-kneeling single-arm cable row
   - 2 sets × 10 reps (5 per leg)
   - 60 seconds of rest

B3. Standing Zottman curl (#149)
   - 2 sets × 10 reps
   - 60 seconds of rest

OPTIONS

Easy Option   Eliminate the final single from the barbell bench press.

Step It Up   Add two more singles with your max weight for the barbell bench press (7 sets total).

Cool-Down   Pec stretch, double lat stretch, 90-degree stretch.

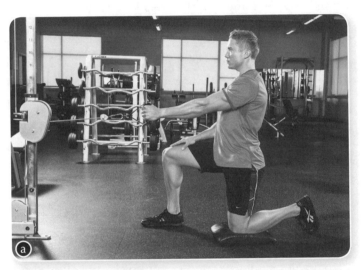

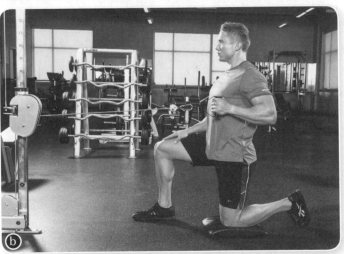

CHAPTER 8

40 Toughest Workouts

You've learned the movement patterns, built up strength, worked on conditioning, and improved lagging body parts. Now it's time to put it all together and see what you can do with all the work you've put in. These 40 workouts combine aspects from all the training you've done up to this point for the ultimate expression of performance. These workouts are tough and certainly not for beginners. So lace up your sneakers and get that postworkout recovery shake ready because, as the saying goes, only the strong will survive.

AMRAP: Back Squat

AMRAP stands for *as many reps as possible*, where you are trying to maximize the number of reps you can perform in a specific amount of time. However, AMRAP workouts are not a place to use anything less than safe and proper form. You are much better off sacrificing a few reps in order to stay injury free than getting hurt and knocking yourself out of training for days or weeks. So although you want to push the pace and your limits, it's important to do so in a way that is safe.

Warm-Up

5 reps of squat to stand; 6 reps per side of kneeling adductor stretch, hip rocker, and quadruped T-spine rotation

● Featured Exercise

Barbell Back Squat

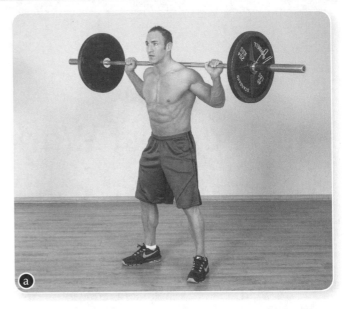

1. Utilizing a shoulder-width stance, step under a bar in a squat rack, with the barbell resting on your upper traps. Take one step back with each foot (*a*).

2. Maintaining a neutral or slightly arched lower back, unlock your hips and begin bringing them back. Almost instantaneously, bend at your knees.

3. Keeping your feet on the ground, continue to lower yourself to as deep a level as possible (you want your hip crease to be at least below your knees) (*b*).

4. When you reach your full range of motion, forcefully drive your feet into the ground and stand up, returning to the starting position. Repeat for reps.

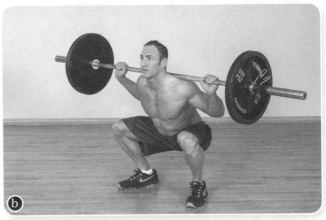

Complete Workout

Perform as many reps as possible of the barbell back squat in 12 minutes using 65 percent of your 1RM. Be sure to use proper technique on each rep. Rest between reps as needed.

Barbell back squat
- 12 minutes × as many reps as possible

OPTIONS

Easy Option   Use 60 percent of your 1RM, and perform as many reps as possible in 9 minutes.

Step It Up   Use 70 percent of your 1RM.

Cool-Down   Standing quad stretch, 90-degree stretch, cross-body stretch.

Body-Weight Blitz

The great thing about challenge workouts is that they give you a time or number of reps to utilize as a benchmark for progress. Therefore, you would be wise to record the results of these workouts and come back to them from time to time to measure progress. Just as a 1RM is a key metric for strength, timed workouts can be extremely useful in monitoring work capacity.

Warm-Up

4 reps per side of the world's greatest stretch, 6 reps per side of hip rocker and inverted hamstring stretch, 8 reps per side of shoulder sweeps

● Featured Exercise

Chin-Up

1. Grab a pull-up bar with a supinated grip (palms facing you) at shoulder width.
2. Start in a dead hang (your arms should be straight) (a), and begin the movement by depressing your shoulder blades.
3. Drive your elbows down and behind you, bending at the elbows in order to pull your chest up toward the bar (b).
4. Once your chin clears the bar, return to the starting position under control. Repeat for reps.

Complete Workout

Complete 4 rounds of the following circuit as quickly as possible. Load the equivalent of your body weight on the barbell bench press and trap bar deadlift.

Barbell bench press (#54)
* 5 reps

Chin-up
* 10 reps

Trap bar deadlift (#8)
* 15 reps

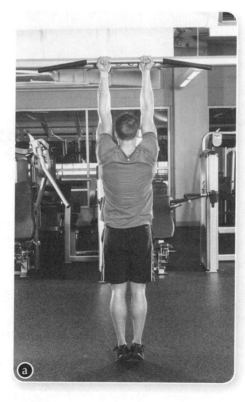
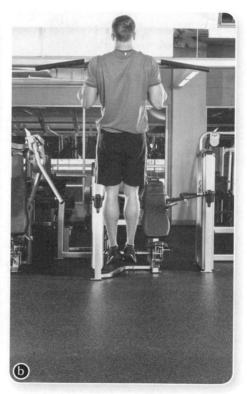

OPTIONS

Easy Option   Use 50 percent body weight on the barbell bench press and trap bar deadlift. Substitute a kneeling lat pull-down (#120) for the chin-up, using 50 percent body weight.

Step It Up   Use 125 percent body weight on the barbell bench press and trap bar deadlift.

Cool-Down   Hamstring stretch, calf stretch, pec stretch.

Hyperdrive

The reverse hyper featured in this workout was developed by one of the all-time great powerlifting coaches, Louie Simmons, who owns and still operates the legendary Westside Barbell club in Ohio. If you have never heard of Simmons, he is certainly worth seeking out because he is a fountain of knowledge on program design for developing maximal strength. The reverse hyper is an excellent exercise for strengthening the posterior chain of the lower body, specifically the glutes and hamstrings, while keeping the lower back stable and supported, eliminating much of the lower back overactivity that people can experience with movements such as Romanian deadlifts and back extensions.

Warm-Up

4 reps per side of the world's greatest stretch, 5 reps each of inchworm and inverted hamstring stretch, 10 reps of glute bridge

● Featured Exercise

Reverse Hyperextension

1. Lie across a reverse hyper bench, with your hips at one edge and grabbing the handles at the other end (a). If you do not have a reverse hyper bench, lie across a stability ball, and grab a bench or squat rack with your arms fully extended for support.

2. Without using momentum, raise your legs up and slightly out until they are parallel to the ground (b). Squeeze your glutes at the top in order to relieve stress on your lower back.

3. Return your legs to the starting position and repeat for reps.

Complete Workout

Perform 4 circuits of the following four exercises, resting as little as possible.

Box jump (#198)
- 8 reps

Barbell thruster (#6)
- 10 reps

Reverse hyperextension
- 12 reps

200-yard (200 m) sprint (#41)

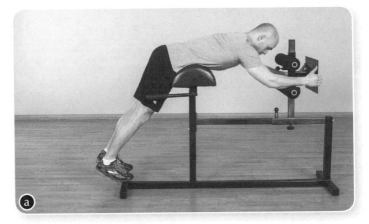

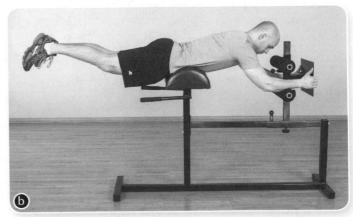

OPTIONS

Easy Option   Complete 2 circuits total.

Step It Up   Complete 6 circuits total.

Cool-Down   Double lat stretch, hamstring stretch, calf stretch.

One-Exercise Challenge: Chin-Up

Want a nice, thick back? Dream of rippling biceps? Nothing will help you achieve these goals more efficiently than the chin-up. The chin-up is one of the few upper body movements that require you to move your body through space (as opposed to pushing weights away from you or pulling weights toward you). This makes for a high strength carryover to everyday movements as well as leads to fantastic muscle gain.

Warm-Up

5 reps of inchworm, 6 reps per side of quadruped T-spine rotation, 10 reps of cat–cow

Complete Workout

Complete as many sets of 8 of the chin-up as you can, resting as little as needed. The goal is to complete as many sets (and total reps) as possible in the time allotted (25 minutes). Rest as little as needed between sets.

Chin-up

- Max sets × 8 reps × 25 minutes

● Featured Exercise

Chin-Up

1. Begin by grabbing a pull-up bar with an underhand grip (palms facing you) at shoulder width.

2. Every rep should begin with your arms fully extended (a). Depress your shoulder blades, and use your back and arms to pull yourself toward the bar. Do not utilize momentum or bring your knees up or legs forward.

3. Complete the rep by touching your chest to the bar (b). Lower back to the starting position and repeat for reps.

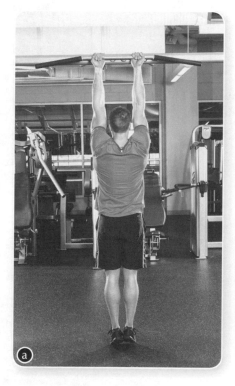
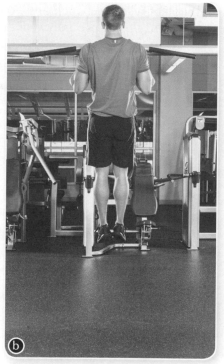

OPTIONS

Easy Option Reduce the total length of the workout to 15 minutes.

Step It Up Attempt to complete at least 1 set every 90 seconds for the entire 25 minutes.

Cool-Down Double lat stretch, cross-body stretch, hamstring stretch.

The Descent

The goal of your training should be to take one more step. Whether that be one more step during a heavy farmer's walk, one more step in that mile run at the end of the workout, or simply one more step toward your goals. The point is not to get overwhelmed by thinking about what you need to accomplish 3 months from now or 5 miles down the road. Just focus on taking one more step today.

Warm-Up

5 reps of inchworm, 6 reps per side of quadruped T-spine rotation, 10 reps of cat–cow

● Featured Exercise

Barbell Bench Press

1. Lie back so your head, upper back, and glutes are in contact with the bench and your feet are flat on the floor. Begin with your eyes directly under the bar.
2. Grab the barbell with a double overhand grip just outside shoulder width (*a*).
3. Keeping your elbows tucked toward your rib cage, lower the bar until it makes contact with your mid-chest (*b*).
4. Drive the bar off your chest until you reach lockout.

OPTIONS

Easy Option   Use 50 percent of your body weight (or less) for the barbell bench press.

Step It Up   Use 1 × body weight for the barbell bench press.

Cool-Down   Double lat stretch, cross-body stretch, hamstring stretch.

Complete Workout

Crisscross the following two exercises, starting with 10 reps per set of the barbell bench press and working down to 1 rep and starting at 1 rep of the barbell front squat and working up to 10 reps. Use 75 percent body weight for the barbell bench press and 50 percent body weight for barbell front squat.

Barbell bench press
- 10 sets × 10, 9, 8, 7, 6, 5, 4, 3, 2, 1 reps

Barbell front squat (#44)
- 10 sets × 1, 2, 3, 4, 5, 6, 7, 8, 9, 10 reps

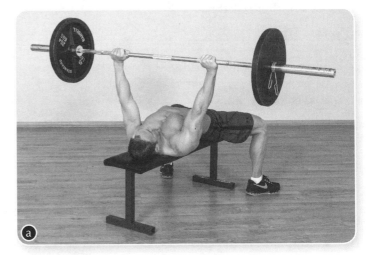

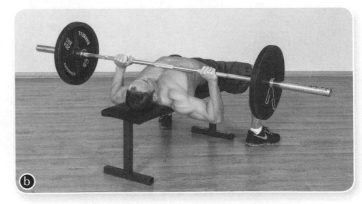

Front Squat Tabata

Front squats vary from back squats in several key areas. First, front squats place more emphasis on the quadriceps muscles because of the positioning of the barbell. They also put you in a more upright posture and require more stability through the upper back and posterior (rear) deltoids. Front squats are often more mechanically effective for taller lifters given that the placement of the weights allows for more extension through the upper back. All these factors allow for a very effective lift that thoroughly challenges the upper body, legs, and core.

Warm-Up

5 reps of squat to stand; 6 reps per side of kneeling adductor stretch, hip rocker, and quadruped T-spine rotation

● Featured Exercise

Barbell Front Squat

1. In a squat rack, begin by placing a barbell across the front of your deltoids, your hands gripping the bar just outside shoulder width, elbows up and upper arms parallel to the floor (*a*).
2. Keeping your chest tall, bring your hips back and bend at the knees to descend into a deep squat position (*b*).
3. Keep your chest tall and maintain a neutral spine throughout the entire movement.
4. Once you reach the bottom position, return to standing and repeat for reps.

Complete Workout

Perform as many reps as possible of the front squat for 20 seconds, followed by 10 seconds of rest, for 8 sets (4 minutes total).

Barbell front squat
- 8 sets × 20 seconds
- 10 seconds of rest

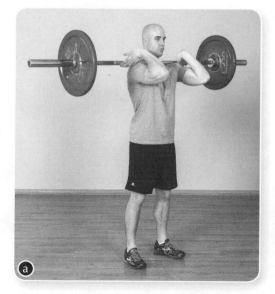

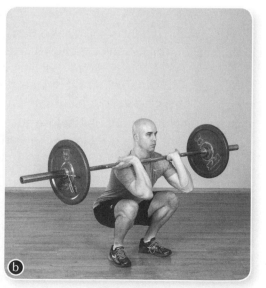

OPTIONS

Easy Option   Perform a half Tabata by completing 4 rounds of the movement.

Step It Up   Perform this Tabata twice, for a total of 16 rounds of the movement, resting 4 minutes between rounds.

Cool-Down   Standing quad stretch, 90-degree stretch, cross-body stretch.

267

Death Circuit

As the name implies, this is not for those of you who scare easily. The death circuit doesn't look so bad on paper, but actually surviving it is another matter altogether. This workout alternates between big upper body and lower body movements, driving up metabolic demands as well as challenging strength.

Warm-Up

6 reps of squat to stand, 6 reps per side of quadruped T-spine rotation, 8 reps of glute bridge, 10 reps of cat–cow

● Featured Exercise

Dumbbell Romanian Deadlift

1. Choose a set of dumbbells. Begin standing straight, arms hanging straight down, palms facing you, with the dumbbells right in front of your thighs (*a*).

2. Keeping your back in a neutral position, unlock your knees and lower the dumbbells along your thighs by bringing your hips back behind you. Do not bend your knees as you lower the weight.

3. Lower the dumbbells as far down as possible only by moving your hips backward (do not get lower by simply pitching your chest forward) (*b*). You should feel a significant stretch in your hamstrings.

4. Keeping the dumbbells close to your legs, stand up and return to the starting position. Repeat for reps.

Complete Workout

Complete 4 rounds of the circuit as quickly as possible, using as little rest as needed between exercises and rounds. Utilize a weight on all exercises that would allow you to complete 15 perfect repetitions.

Barbell back squat (#63)
- 12 reps

Chin-up (#73)
- 12 reps

Dumbbell Romanian deadlift
- 12 reps

Seated dumbbell shoulder press (#209)
- 12 reps

OPTIONS

Easy Option Reduce the reps to 8 per exercise.

Step It Up Complete 5 rounds of the circuit.

Cool-Down Hamstring stretch, calf stretch, pec stretch.

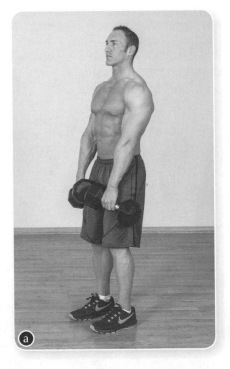
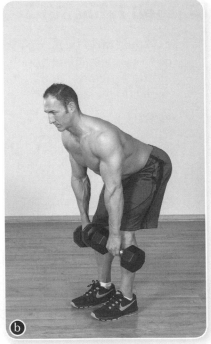

Glenn's Ladder

This workout includes an exercise called the Pendlay row (named after Olympic lifting coach Glenn Pendlay), which is a modified version of the bent-over barbell row that requires you to bring your torso parallel to the ground and perform each row off the floor. Although this version eliminates much of the cheating that occurs with standard bent-over rows (people tend to stand more and more upright as the weight gets challenging), it also requires good hamstring flexibility as well as the ability to keep a neutral lower back. If you cannot keep this position, utilize standard bent-over rows instead. Your lower back will thank you for this decision later.

Warm-Up

4 reps per side of the world's greatest stretch, 6 reps per side of hip rocker and inverted hamstring stretch, 8 reps per side of shoulder sweeps

● Featured Exercise

Pendlay Row

1. Begin with a loaded barbell on the floor. Bend forward at the hips so your torso is parallel to the ground, knees slightly bent. Grab the bar slightly wider than you would for a traditional bent-over barbell row (*a*).
2. Maintaining this posture, explosively row the barbell to your upper abs/lower chest (*b*).
3. Return the barbell to the floor and repeat for reps.

Complete Workout

Perform the following circuit for as many rounds as possible in 12 minutes. Note that you are increasing the reps by 1 rep per set for the push press, 2 reps per set for the Pendlay row, and 3 reps per set for the prisoner squat. Rest as needed, but keep in mind that the goal is to get as many reps as possible in the 12 minutes.

Push press (#16)
- Begin with 1 rep and then increase by 1 rep each set (1, 2, 3, 4, etc.)

Pendlay row
- Begin with 2 reps and then increase by 2 reps each set (2, 4, 6, 8, etc.)

Prisoner squat (#188)
- Begin with 3 reps and then increase by 3 reps each set (3, 6, 9, 12, etc.)

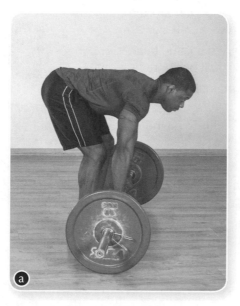

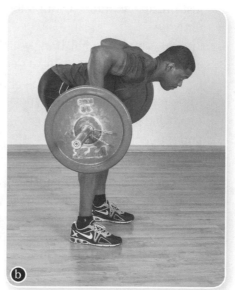

OPTIONS

Easy Option   Perform as many reps as possible for 8 minutes.

Step It Up   Perform as many reps as possible for 15 minutes.

Cool-Down   Standing quad stretch, 90-degree stretch, double lat stretch.

One-Exercise Challenge: Barbell Back Squat

Performing one exercise for 25 minutes can be as mentally challenging as it is physically grueling. I challenge you to stay focused and determined and make every rep in this workout a high-quality rep. When you are done your legs will burn, your mind will be mush, your resolve will be broken. But as you feel the rush of exhaustion, you will feel more accomplished than you may ever have before in a squat rack.

Warm-Up

5 reps of squat to stand; 6 reps per side of kneeling adductor stretch, hip rocker, and quadruped T-spine rotation

● **Featured Exercise**

Barbell Back Squat

1. In a squat rack, begin by placing a barbell across the back of your upper traps, your hands gripping the bar just outside shoulder width, elbows tight toward the body (a).
2. Keeping your chest tall, bring your hips back and bend at the knees to descend into a deep squat position (b).
3. Be sure to keep your chest tall and maintain a neutral spine throughout the entire movement.
4. Once you reach the bottom position, return to standing and repeat for reps.

Complete Workout

Complete as many sets of 8 of the barbell back squat as you can, resting as little as needed. The goal is to complete as many sets (and total reps) as possible in the time allotted (25 minutes).

Barbell back squat
  • Max sets × 8 reps × 25 minutes

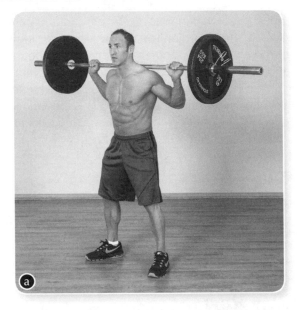

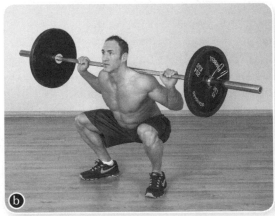

OPTIONS

Easy Option   Reduce the total length of the workout to 15 minutes.

Step It Up   Attempt to complete at least one set every 90 seconds for the entire 25 minutes.

Cool-Down   Standing quad stretch, 90-degree stretch, cross-body stretch.

The Ranger

The Rangers are members of the U.S. Army elite infantry and are known for being highly trained and incredibly skilled. And although you do not need to go to Ranger school to survive this workout, you will need more toughness, focus, and endurance than nearly anyone else in your gym to make it through. Save the Ranger for a day when you can't wait to get in the gym and give it everything you've got—because that is what it will take to make it to the end of this workout.

Warm-Up

4 reps per side of the world's greatest stretch, 5 reps each of inchworm and inverted hamstring stretch, 10 reps of glute bridge

● Featured Exercise

TRX Face Pull

1. Grab a set of TRX handles, with your palms facing the floor. Walk your feet toward the anchor point to create an angle with your body that is anywhere between 45 and 75 degrees (a).

2. Keeping your arms high and perpendicular to your torso, bend at the elbows and pull your hands toward your jawline (b).

3. Squeeze your upper back and shoulder blades at the top position and then return, under control, to the starting position. Repeat for reps.

Complete Workout

Perform the sprint every minute on the minute (start at the top of the minute, perform the exercise, rest the remainder of the minute, begin the next set at the top of the next minute, repeat until all sets are complete). Rest 3 minutes. Complete 3 circuits of the remaining exercises, resting as little as possible between movements and between circuits.

Sprint (#41)
  - 20 yards (20 m)
  - Every minute on the minute for 10 minutes

Neutral-grip pull-up (#237)
  - 10 reps

Barbell thruster (#6)
  - 15 reps

TRX face pull
  - 20 reps

Burpee (#7)
  - 25 reps

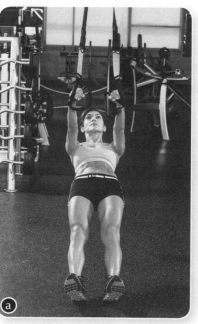

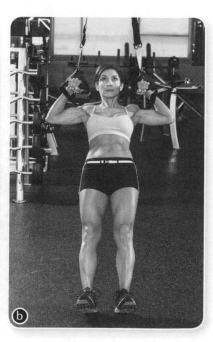

OPTIONS

Easy Option   Perform 2 rounds of the circuit after you've finished the sprints.

Step It Up   Perform the sprints every minute on the minute for 15 minutes.

Cool-Down   Double lat stretch, hamstring stretch, calf stretch.

The 10 Spot

Although a caloric deficit is helpful for losing body fat, there is diminishing returns in setting your caloric intake too low. First, you won't have energy to train appropriately, nor will you have enough nutrients available for protein synthesis and muscle repair. Your body will also become efficient at using fewer calories, hurting your metabolism. If you are eating high-quality foods and feel the need to reduce portions in order to support body-fat reduction, start by simply reducing calories by 10 percent. This should be enough to kickstart results while still keeping your system running smooth.

Warm-Up

5 reps of inchworm, 6 reps per side of quadruped T-spine rotation, 10 reps of cat–cow

● Featured Exercise

Trap Bar Deadlift

1. Step into a loaded trap bar, with your feet at shoulder width.
2. Grab the handles at their center, bend your knees, pull your hips down, and retract your shoulder blades (a).
3. Lift the bar by simultaneously extending your knees and driving your hips forward.

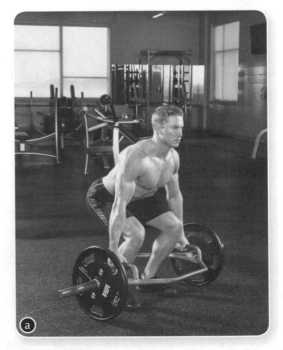
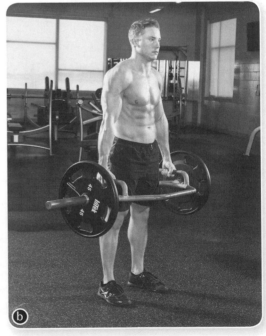

4. Complete the movement by fully locking out your hips at the top (b).
5. Reverse the motion by bringing your hips back and flexing the knees. Maintain a tall chest and neutral spine in all phases of the movement. Repeat for reps.

Complete Workout

Perform the following circuit in as little time as possible, resting only as needed. Place your body weight on the bar for the trap bar deadlift.

Trap bar deadlift
- 10 sets × 10, 9, 8, 7, 6, 5, 4, 3, 2, 1 reps

Chin-up (#73)
- 10 sets × 10, 9, 8, 7, 6, 5, 4, 3, 2, 1 reps

Frog sit-up (#27)
- 10 sets × 10, 9, 8, 7, 6, 5, 4, 3, 2, 1 reps

OPTIONS

Easy Option   Perform 7 sets total, starting with 7 reps per set and working down to 1 rep.

Step It Up   Use 1.25 × body weight for the trap bar deadlift.

Cool-Down   Double lat stretch, cross-body stretch, hamstring stretch.

AMRAP: Deadlift

The most unexpected tool you can use to help you reach your fitness goals may just be the calendar. Scheduling a photo shoot, working toward fitting into a dress for a wedding, aiming for a performance goal by a specific date, or prepping to look great at your high school reunion will all give you the focus and drive you'll need in order to get motivated and make things happen.

Warm-Up

4 reps per side of the world's greatest stretch, 5 reps each of inchworm and inverted hamstring stretch, 10 reps of glute bridge

● Featured Exercise

Conventional Deadlift

1. Approach a barbell set up on the floor by placing your feet under the bar so it is 2 to 3 inches (5 to 8 cm) in front of your shins. Your stance should be approximately hip width.
2. Bend down and grab the bar just outside your legs, with either a double overhand or mixed grip.
3. Pull your hips down and bring your shins in contact with the bar. Keep your chest tall, and maintain a neutral spine (a).

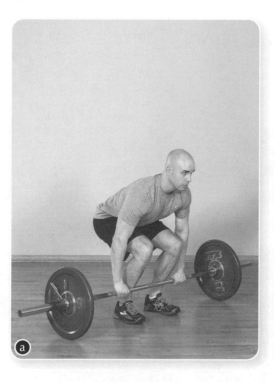

4. Stand up by rising simultaneously at your hips and shoulders, driving your hips forward until you reach lockout (b). Repeat for reps.

Complete Workout

Perform as many reps as possible of the conventional deadlift in 12 minutes, using 65 percent of your 1RM. Be sure to use proper technique on each rep. Rest between reps as needed.

Conventional deadlift
- 12 minutes × as many reps as possible

Warning: The deadlift is a very demanding exercise that can put you at risk for injury if done with bad form. End each set when you can no longer perform the reps with correct technique.

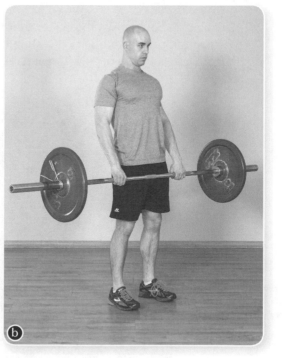

OPTIONS

Easy Option Use 60 percent of your 1RM, and perform as many reps as possible in 9 minutes.

Step It Up Use 70 percent of your 1RM.

Cool-Down Double lat stretch, hamstring stretch, calf stretch.

Back Squat Plus

Although flexibility is valuable for improving range of motion and reducing the risk of injury, it is possible to have too much of a good thing. Too much mobility can come at the expense of stability and strength, which, at best, will leave you weak in the basic movement patterns and, at worst, will open you up for injuries at your joints. Finding the proper balance between flexibility and stability in the gym, on the field, and in day-to-day life is what you should be after.

Warm-Up

5 reps of squat to stand; 6 reps per side of kneeling adductor stretch, hip rocker, and quadruped T-spine rotation

● Featured Exercise

Barbell Back Squat

1. Utilizing a shoulder-width stance, step under a bar in a squat rack, with the barbell resting on your upper traps. Take one step back with each foot (*a*).

2. Maintaining a neutral or slightly arched lower back, unlock your hips and begin bringing them back. Almost instantaneously, bend at your knees.

3. Keeping your feet on the ground, continue to lower yourself to as deep a level as possible (you want your hip crease to be at least below your knees) (*b*).

4. When you reach your full range of motion, forcefully drive your feet into the ground and stand up, returning to the starting position. Repeat for reps.

Complete Workout

Load 50 percent of your 1RM for the back squat onto a barbell. Perform 2 reps every minute on the minute (start at the top of each minute, and rest whatever remains of that minute after your set is complete). Increase the weight on the bar by 10 lb (4.5 kg) every minute. Continue until you hit a weight where you can no longer complete 2 reps.

Barbell back squat
- As many sets as possible, as described

OPTIONS

Easy Option Increase the weight by 5 lb (2.5 kg) every set.

Step It Up Perform 3 reps per set.

Cool-Down Standing quad stretch, 90-degree stretch, cross-body stretch.

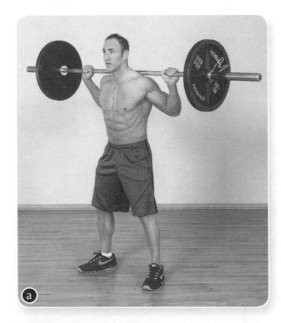

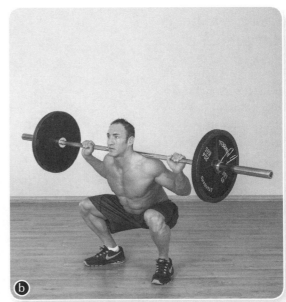

One-Exercise Challenge:
Barbell Bench Press

So, you love to bench press? Well, how do you feel about 25 minutes of nonstop benching? Your chest will ache. Your triceps will burn. And you may have a hard time pushing the door open when it's time to leave the gym. You've been warned: After this workout, you may never feel the same way about bench pressing again.

Warm-Up

4 reps per side of the world's greatest stretch, 5 reps of inchworm, 8 reps per side of shoulder sweeps

● Featured Exercise

Barbell Bench Press

1. At a barbell bench press station, grab the bar just outside shoulder width, and unrack it from the barbell catches.

2. Keeping a slight natural arch in your lower back (a), lower the bar until it touches your torso at midchest level (about nipple height) (b). Keep your elbows tucked toward your sides as you lower the bar; and keep your head, upper back, and butt on the bench at all times.

3. Forcefully drive the weight back up until you achieve lockout of your elbows. Repeat for reps.

Complete Workout

Complete as many sets of 8 of the barbell bench press as you can, resting as little as needed. The goal is to complete as many sets (and total reps) as possible in the time allotted (25 minutes).

Barbell bench press
- Max sets × 8 reps × 25 minutes

 Warning: Always perform difficult bench presses with a spotter.

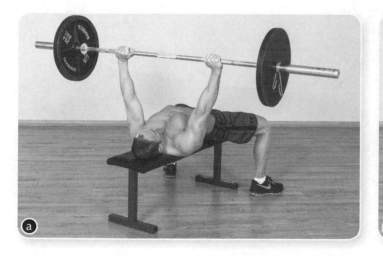

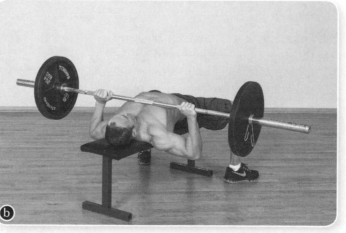

OPTIONS

Easy Option   Reduce the total length of the workout to 15 minutes.

Step It Up   Attempt to complete at least 1 set every 90 seconds for the entire 25 minutes.

Cool-Down   Pec stretch, double lat stretch, 90-degree stretch.

El Diablo

Body-weight exercises are not always easier to perform than weighted movements that work the same muscle groups. The handstand push-up, featured in this workout, is a great example of an extremely challenging body-weight movement that requires not only shoulder strength but shoulder and core stability as well.

Warm-Up

4 reps per side of the world's greatest stretch, 6 reps per side of hip rocker and inverted hamstring stretch, 8 reps per side of shoulder sweeps

● Featured Exercise

Handstand Push-Up

1. Place your hands at wider than shoulder width on the floor, a few inches (about 10 cm) away from a wall.

2. Kick both feet up so you are in a handstand position, with your heels supported on the wall (*a*).

3. Lower yourself under control until the top of your head touches the floor (*b*).

4. Forcefully press yourself back up to the starting position and repeat for reps. If you cannot achieve full range of motion, feel free to place a pad on the floor and bring your head to the pad.

Complete Workout

Complete as many rounds of the following circuit in 15 minutes, resting only as needed. Use a load equivalent to your body weight for the conventional deadlift.

Handstand push-up
- 5 reps × as many sets as possible

Conventional deadlift (#5)
- 5 reps × as many sets as possible

OPTIONS

Easy Option Substitute standard push-ups (#12) for the handstand push-ups.

Step It Up Use 1.5 × body weight for the conventional deadlift.

Cool-Down Hamstring stretch, calf stretch, pec stretch.

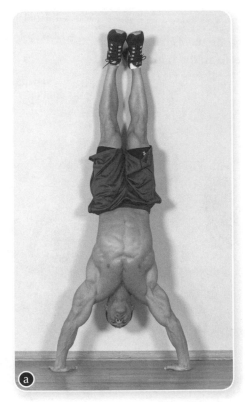
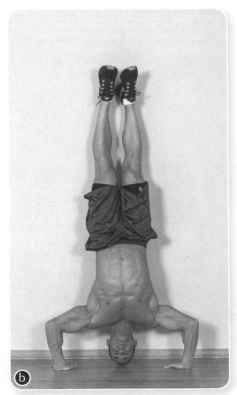

Intensity

Whether or not to take a preworkout supplement is completely up to you. Caffeine, beta-alanine, citrulline malate, and carnitine as well as many other compounds have proven to increase exercise drive and stave off muscle fatigue in many trainees. Some people react very well to preworkout supplementation, while others can get overstimulated or agitated. If you do plan on experimenting with a supplement, start with a minimal dose and number of ingredients. If you find it's working for you, you can always choose to increase the serving from there.

Warm-Up

6 reps of squat to stand, 6 reps per side of quadruped T-spine rotation, 8 reps of glute bridge, 10 reps of cat–cow

● Featured Exercise

Barbell Thruster

1. Rack a barbell on your shoulders with a double overhand grip. Your elbows should be forward of the bar.

2. Unlock your hips and squat down toward the floor, keeping your chest tall and eyes forward throughout the entire movement (a).

3. Once you've reached the bottom of your range of motion (your upper legs should be at or below parallel to the floor) (a), reverse your motion, driving your hips forward (b).

4. As you return to the standing position, drive the barbell overhead until reaching full lockout (c).

5. Rerack the barbell at your shoulders and repeat for reps.

Complete Workout

Perform the following four exercises within 5 minutes. Continue to add additional rounds until you can no longer complete all the exercises as prescribed within the 5-minute time frame. If you finish before the 5-minute mark, use the additional time as rest.

Barbell thruster
- 8 reps × 50 percent body weight

Pull-up (#231)
- 10 reps

Push-up (#12)
- 20 reps

Sprint (#41)
- 200 yards (200 m)

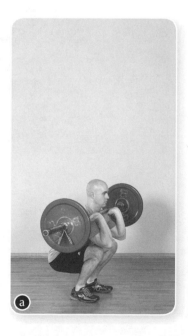

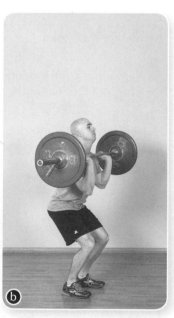

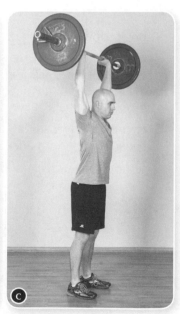

OPTIONS

Easy Option Reduce the number of pull-ups to 8 reps and number of push-ups to 15 reps.

Step It Up Perform the entire circuit in 4 minutes.

Cool-Down Standing quad stretch, 90-degree stretch, double lat stretch.

Running Rebel

Although running is considered by many to be a basic movement pattern and is possibly the most common form of exercise, running mechanics are actually extremely complicated. Running is a form of plyometric exercise that involves the coordination of the entire body along with significant impact on the ankle, knee, and hip joints. Add in that many of us spend too many hours in a sitting posture during the day, putting our muscular system in a compromised state, and the demands of running become that much greater. If you are serious about adding running and sprinting to your routine, you'd be well served to seek out a good running coach who can analyze your form and make improvements.

Warm-Up

4 reps per side of the world's greatest stretch, 5 reps each of inchworm and inverted hamstring stretch, 10 reps of glute bridge

● Featured Exercise

Sprinting

1. Begin slowly running on a treadmill or a track.
2. Accumulate speed by striking your forefoot on the ground or treadmill and actively pulling your foot up toward your glutes (avoid striking your heel on the ground).
3. Prioritize longer strides and faster turnover to improve speed and performance during sprints.

Complete Workout

400-yard (400 m) sprint
- 4 minutes of rest

300-yard (300 m) sprint
- 3 minutes of rest

200-yard (200 m) sprint
- 2 minutes of rest

100-yard (100 m) sprint

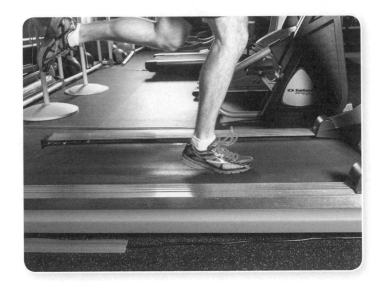

OPTIONS

Easy Option   Cut all the sprint distances in half (200, 150, 100, 50).

Step It Up   Reduce the rest between sprint by 1 minute each.

Cool-Down   Double lat stretch, hamstring stretch, calf stretch.

One-Exercise Challenge: Barbell Overhead Press

Three reasons why the barbell overhead press is superior to the bench press: (1) With an overhead press, there is no bench to support you, requiring much more stability through your entire body. (2) Getting stronger on the overhead press has proven to increase your bench press strength; the reverse has not been proven. (3) Although the bench press utilizes the often-overworked anterior deltoids and pecs as their prime movers, the overhead demands more work from your posterior delts, lats, upper back, and core.

Warm-Up

4 reps per side of the world's greatest stretch, 5 reps of inchworm, 8 reps per side of shoulder sweeps

3. As the bar passes the crown of your head, drive your head slightly forward so that your upper arms are in line with your ears.

4. Finish by locking out your elbows with the bar directly over the top of your head (b). Bring the bar down to the starting position and repeat for reps.

Complete Workout

Complete as many sets of 8 of the barbell overhead press as you can, resting as little as needed. The goal is to complete as many sets (and total reps) as possible in the time allotted (25 minutes).

Barbell overhead press
- Max sets × 8 reps × 25 minutes

● **Featured Exercise**

Barbell Overhead Press

1. Begin by grabbing a barbell with an overhand grip directly outside shoulder width. The bar should be in front of your collarbones (a).

2. Keeping your body tight and your knees locked, drive the bar directly overhead.

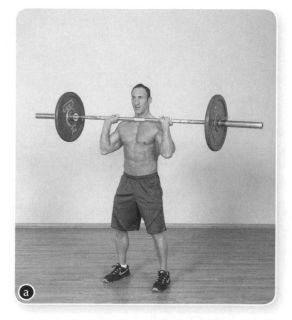

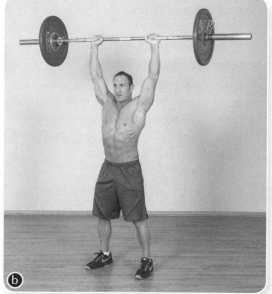

OPTIONS

Easy Option Reduce the total length of the workout to 15 minutes.

Step It Up Attempt to complete at least one set every 90 seconds for the entire 25 minutes.

Cool-Down Pec stretch, double lat stretch, 90-degree stretch.

Milo's Ladder

This workout is named after the mythic Milo of Croton, a champion Olympic wrestler in the 6th century BC, who set out to be the world's strongest man. In his most famous tale, Milo began carrying a calf from his farm to the town square on his daily trips to gather supplies. Every day the calf got bigger, so Milo had to get stronger. Ultimately, the mighty Milo got so strong that he was able to carry the now full-grown bull on his shoulders. Milo's story relates well to one of the most basic principles of weight training, called progressive overload, which states that, to get stronger, you have to lift progressively heavier weights.

Warm-Up

4 reps per side of the world's greatest stretch, 6 reps per side of hip rocker and inverted hamstring stretch, 8 reps per side of shoulder sweeps

● Featured Exercise

Double Kettlebell Swing

1. Begin with a kettlebell in each hand at your sides and your feet at hip-width apart.
2. Swing the kettlebells behind you by hinging at your hips (*a*).
3. Drive your hips forward, allowing the power you've generated to swing the kettlebells forward and up. Keep your arms straight at all times. The kettlebells should rise to anywhere between navel and shoulder height (*b*).
4. Once the kettlebells reach their apex, pull them down and behind you, once again hinging at the hips. Repeat for reps.

Complete Workout

Perform the following circuit for as many rounds as possible in 12 minutes. Note that you are increasing the reps by 1 rep per set for the hang power snatch, 2 reps per set for the chin-up, and 3 reps per set for the double kettlebell swing. Rest as needed, but keep in mind that the goal is to get as many reps as possible in the 12 minutes.

Hang power clean (#93)
  - Begin with 1 rep and then increase by 1 rep each set (1, 2, 3, 4, etc.)

Chin-up (#73)
  - Begin with 2 reps and then increase by 2 reps each set (2, 4, 6, 8, etc.)

Double kettlebell swing
  - Begin with 3 reps and then increase by 3 reps each set (3, 6, 9, 12, etc.)

OPTIONS

Easy Option   Perform as many reps as possible for 8 minutes.

Step It Up   Perform as many reps as possible for 15 minutes.

Cool-Down   Standing quad stretch, 90-degree stretch, double lat stretch.

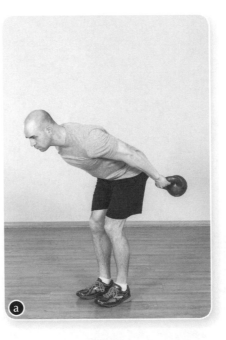
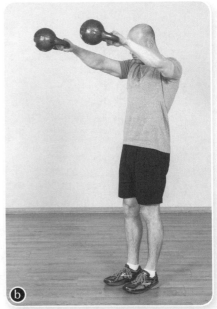

Basic Training

You can never go wrong focusing on basic exercise movements and equipment. Squats, deadlifts, presses, pull-ups, and lunges with dumbbells, barbells, kettlebells, and medicine balls have been getting people stronger, more powerful, and fitter for years. These are all tried and true exercises that make up the foundation of human movement and as such should be the foundation of your training program. Does that mean you can never get creative and try something new? Of course not. Experimenting can lead to great discoveries and alleviate boredom. But don't just blindly follow fitness fads and trends. Find your way back to the basics, and you will always make progress.

Warm-Up

6 reps of squat to stand, 6 reps per side of quadruped T-spine rotation, 8 reps of glute bridge, 10 reps of cat–cow

Complete Workout

Complete 4 rounds of the following circuit. You can rest as much as needed between exercises and between rounds. The goal is to use as much weight as possible (while maintaining good form) for each exercise.

Barbell back squat (#63)
- 6 reps

Barbell push press
- 8 reps

Trap bar deadlift (#8)
- 10 reps

Wide-grip pull-up (#117)
- As many reps as possible

⬤ Featured Exercise

Barbell Push Press

1. Begin with a barbell in the rack position, sitting across your anterior (front) deltoids, your hands in a clean grip and your upper arms parallel to the ground.
2. Keeping your back straight, bend your knees until you have reached a quarter-squat position (*a*).
3. In one explosive motion, straighten your legs and drive the bar overhead (*b*).
4. Return the barbell to the starting position and repeat for reps.

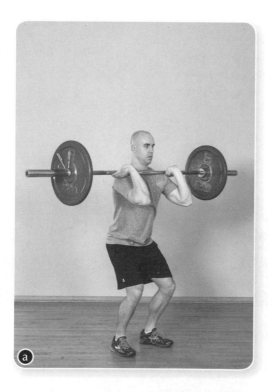

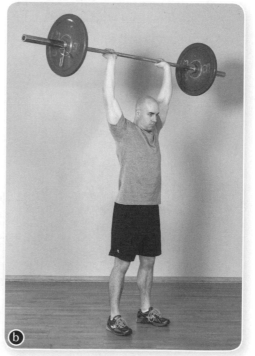

OPTIONS

Easy Option   Perform 3 rounds of the circuit.

Step It Up   Perform 5 rounds of the circuit.

Cool-Down   Standing quad stretch, 90-degree stretch, double lat stretch.

The Quadruple Century

Some days you walk into the gym, realize what challenges face you, get yourself psyched up, train hard, and walk out feeling accomplished. Then there are other days when the workout is so daunting you are not sure how you are going to survive it. The quadruple century falls into this latter category. It will test not only your endurance in several key body-weight exercises but your will and mental toughness as well. It's up to you to get your mind right and make it to the end of this challenge.

Warm-Up

6 reps of squat to stand, 6 reps per side of quadruped T-spine rotation, 8 reps of glute bridge, 10 reps of cat–cow

● Featured Exercise

Single-Contact Mountain Climber

1. Begin in a push-up position, with your hands slightly outside shoulder width and your body forming a straight line from your head to your heels (a).
2. Keeping your left foot on the floor, lift your right foot and bring your knee in toward your chest. Do not let your right foot touch the floor (hence the name *single contact*) (b).

3. Bring your right foot back to the starting position by straightening your leg. As your right foot touches the ground, simultaneously bring your left foot into your chest (c).
4. Continue to alternate in this manner until all reps are complete.

Complete Workout

Perform 100 reps of each exercise before moving on to the next. Rest as needed during and between sets.

Prisoner squat (#188)
- 100 reps

Chin-up (#73)
- 100 reps

Push-up (#12)
- 100 reps

Single-contact mountain climber
- 100 reps

OPTIONS

Easy Option   Perform 50 reps of the prisoner's squat, push-up, and single-contact mountain climber and 25 reps of the chin-up.

Step It Up   Perform 200 reps of the single-contact mountain climber.

Cool-Down   Standing quad stretch, 90-degree stretch, double lat stretch.

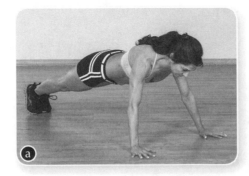
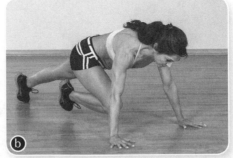
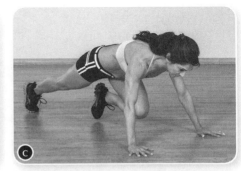

5, 4, 3, 2, 1

Using body weight as a standard for choosing loads is a great way to scale exercises to body size. If you are training with a partner or a group, it instantly levels the playing field. It also gives you different standards and benchmarks to try to shoot for as your training progresses. Can you perform a deadlift for reps using twice your body weight? How about 10 front squats with your body weight on the bar? Slowly try working up to certain rep and set schemes using your body weight as a marker. It's great motivation and a surefire way to ensure your strength levels are progressing.

Warm-Up

6 reps of squat to stand, 6 reps per side of quadruped T-spine rotation, 8 reps of glute bridge, 10 reps of cat–cow

● **Featured Exercise**

Behind-the-Neck Push Press

1. Begin with a barbell sitting across your traps, your hands in a clean grip just outside shoulder width.

2. Keeping your back straight, bend your knees until you have reached a quarter-squat position (a).

3. In one explosive motion, straighten your legs and drive the bar overhead (b).

4. Return the barbell to the behind-the-neck position and repeat for reps.

Complete Workout

Perform 5 rounds of the following circuit, starting with 5 reps of each the first round and reducing by 1 rep each set. Use 1 × body weight for the barbell front squat, 50 percent body weight for the behind-the-neck push press, and 1.5 × body weight on the trap bar deadlift. Complete the circuit in as little time as possible, being sure to use good form on each rep.

Barbell front squat (#44)
- 5 sets × 5, 4, 3, 2, 1 reps

Behind-the-neck push press
- 5 sets × 5, 4, 3, 2, 1 reps

Trap bar deadlift (#8)
- 5 sets × 5, 4, 3, 2, 1 reps

 Warning: The behind-the-neck push press requires adequate shoulder mobility. If you cannot perform a press from this position, utilize the standard push press as an alternative.

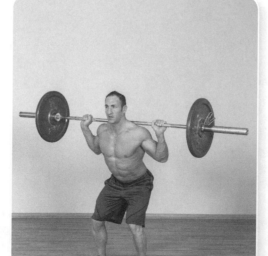

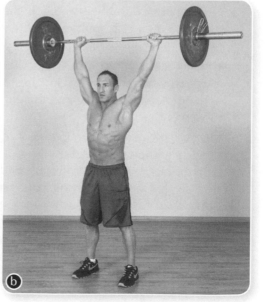

OPTIONS

Easy Option Use 75 percent of your body weight (or less) for the barbell front squat and 1 × body weight for the trap bar deadlift.

Step It Up Use 1.25 × body weight for the barbell front squat and 2 × body weight for the trap bar deadlift.

Cool-Down Standing quad stretch, 90-degree stretch, double lat stretch.

Multi-Tabata

The term *Tabata training* gets thrown around a lot these days. And although the true protocol that Izumi Tabata used with high-level athletes in Japan is almost impossible for even more advanced trainees to replicate, it's safe to say that most people these days refer to any high-intensity, negative-rest (meaning the rest period is shorter than the work period) interval training as Tabata. This terminology isn't 100 percent accurate, but let's not throw out the baby with the bathwater. Performing intervals in this manner is a great way to test your work capacity and stimulate fat loss. So call it Tabata, high-intensity interval training, or anything else you'd like—as long as you put everything you have into those work intervals, you are going to see some serious results.

Warm-Up

4 reps per side of the world's greatest stretch, 6 reps per side of hip rocker and inverted hamstring stretch, 8 reps per side of shoulder sweeps

● **Featured Exercise**

OPTIONS

Easy Option Cut the number of intervals in half, performing 4 rounds for each exercise.

Step It Up Rest 3 minutes between exercises.

Cool-Down Hamstring stretch, calf stretch, pec stretch.

Complete Workout

Perform 8 rounds (4 minutes) of intervals for each of the following exercises. You should be working as hard as possible for 20 seconds and resting completely for 10 seconds. Once you complete all 8 rounds, rest for 5 minutes and then repeat for the remaining exercises.

Dumbbell thruster
- 8 rounds of 20 seconds × as many reps as possible followed by 10 seconds of rest
- 5 minutes of rest

Push-up (#12)
- 8 rounds of 20 seconds × as many reps as possible followed by 10 seconds of rest
- 5 minutes of rest

Burpee (#7)
- 8 rounds of 20 seconds × as many reps as possible followed by 10 seconds of rest

Dumbbell Thruster

1. Grab a pair of dumbbells and hold them with a neutral grip (palms facing each other) at your shoulders (*a*).

2. Unlock your hips and squat down toward the floor, keeping your chest tall and eyes forward throughout the entire movement.

3. Once you've reached the bottom of your range of motion (your upper legs should be at or below parallel to the floor) (*b*), reverse the motion, driving your hips forward.

4. As you return to the standing position, drive the dumbbells overhead until they reach lockout (*c*).

5. Bring the dumbbells back to shoulder height and repeat for reps.

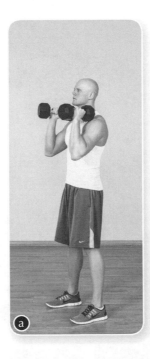
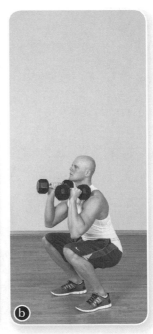
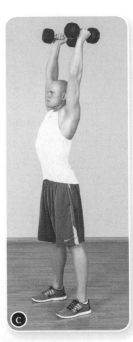

Animal

Everyone wants to look and feel better. And a huge part of accomplishing that goal is paying attention to your nutrition. Although nutrition is very complicated and needs individualized planning, a few principles hold true for anyone looking to improve body composition. Try not to rely on processed foods. Make sure the ingredients you are using are of the highest quality. Eat plenty of vegetables, but make sure you consume adequate protein and healthy fats as well. Don't overdo it on the sugars and processed grains. If you manage to follow those tips while also training hard, your body will have no choice but to look and feel its best.

Warm-Up

6 reps of squat to stand, 6 reps per side of quadruped T-spine rotation, 8 reps of glute bridge, 10 reps of cat–cow

● Featured Exercise

Wall Ball

1. Begin with a medicine ball in front of your torso and your hands on either side of it (*a*).

2. Squat down until your hip creases are below your knees (you can put a medicine ball behind you and touch the ball with your glutes as a reference) (*b*). Keep your chest tall and a neutral spine position as you squat.

3. Once you reach the bottom position, stand up and throw the ball against a target 9 to 12 feet (3 to 4 m) above the floor (*c*). This should be done as one continuous motion.

4. Catch the ball and immediately descend into the squat. Repeat for reps.

Complete Workout

Perform as many rounds as you can of the following workout in 12 minutes, resting as needed.

Chin-up (#73)
- 15 reps

Wall ball
- 25 reps

Burpee (#7)
- 35 reps

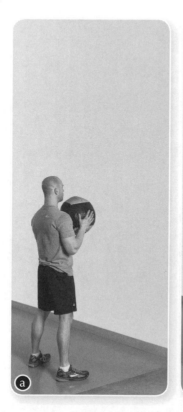
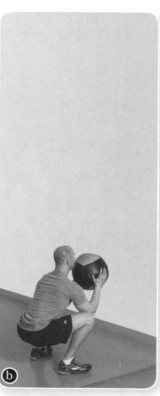
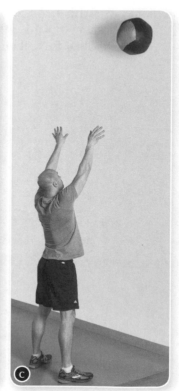

OPTIONS

Easy Option Perform as many rounds as possible in 9 minutes.

Step It Up Increase the number of reps per exercise by 5 (20, 30, 40).

Cool-Down Hamstring stretch, calf stretch, pec stretch.

The Sweet Spot

There is nothing magical about the most popular set and rep scheme on the planet: 3 sets of 10 reps. Although 3 × 10 is effective, particularly for building muscle mass, it should not be the only scheme you follow for indefinite periods of time. Changing the number of reps and sets will help you train different strength qualities, allow you to use varying weights, and force your body to adapt. Don't fall in love with any number of reps, sets, or even exercises. Doing so will certainly get you stuck at a plateau.

Warm-Up

5 reps of inchworm, 6 reps per side of quadruped T-spine rotation, 10 reps of cat–cow

● Featured Exercise

Wide-Hands Push-Up

1. Start with your hands well outside shoulder width and your body in a plank position, creating a straight line from shoulder to heel (a).

2. Keeping your elbows tucked toward your rib cage and maintaining a neutral spine, slowly lower your body until your chest nearly touches the ground (b).

3. Drive your hands into the floor, and reverse the motion until your elbows reach lockout and you have returned to the starting position. Repeat for reps.

Complete Workout

Perform the following circuit in as little time as possible, resting only as needed. Place your body weight on the bar for the barbell back squat.

Barbell back squat (#63)
- 10 sets × 10, 9, 8, 7, 6, 5, 4, 3, 2, 1 reps

Wide-hands push-up
- 10 sets × 10, 9, 8, 7, 6, 5, 4, 3, 2, 1 reps

Hanging leg raise (#217)
- 10 sets × 10, 9, 8, 7, 6, 5, 4, 3, 2, 1 reps

OPTIONS

Easy Option Use 75 percent body weight for the barbell back squat. Perform 7 sets total, starting with 7 reps per set and working down to 1 rep.

Step It Up Use 1.25 × body weight for the barbell back squat.

Cool-Down Double lat stretch, cross-body stretch, hamstring stretch.

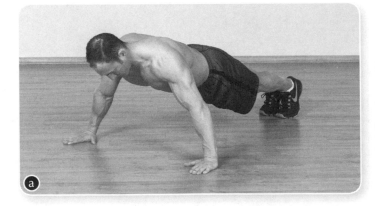
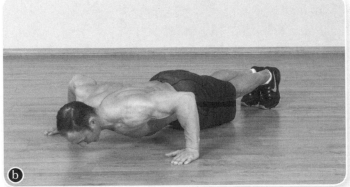

Awful

When performing exercises or a circuit for time, a number of strategies—such as how to best utilize rest in order to maximize performance—come into play. One thing you may want to avoid is redlining—getting your heart rate up over 90 percent. By backing off before spiking your heart rate to that level, you will likely have a bit more stamina over the long haul than if you simply tried to get as many reps as possible as fast as possible. So when your heart is almost to that point when it feels as if it's going to explode out of your chest, take a couple of seconds to recover before your next rep. It may save you in the long run.

Warm-Up

4 reps per side of the world's greatest stretch, 6 reps per side of hip rocker and inverted hamstring stretch, 8 reps per side of shoulder sweeps

● Featured Exercise

Barbell Bench Press

1. Lie back so your head, upper back, and glutes are in contact with the bench and your feet are flat on the floor. Begin with your eyes directly under the bar.

2. Grab the barbell with a double overhand grip just outside shoulder width (*a*).

3. Keeping your elbows tucked toward your rib cage, lower the bar until it makes contact with your mid-chest (*b*).

4. Drive the bar off your chest until you reach lockout. Repeat for reps.

Complete Workout

Perform the following four exercises within 5 minutes. Continue to add additional rounds until you can no longer complete all the exercises as prescribed within the 5-minute time frame. If you finish before the 5-minute mark, use the additional time as rest.

Conventional deadlift (#5)
- 5 reps × body weight

Barbell bench press
- 8 reps × body weight

Pull-up (#231)
- 10 reps

Rower (#212)
- 500 meters

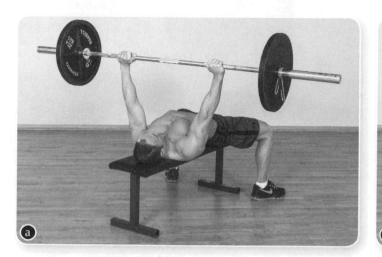

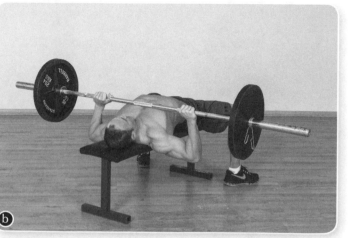

OPTIONS

Easy Option Use 75 percent body weight on the conventional deadlift and barbell bench press, and reduce the number of pull-ups to 8 reps.

Step It Up Complete the circuit in 4 minutes.

Cool-Down Standing quad stretch, 90-degree stretch, double lat stretch.

AMRAP: Overhead Press

Although it's easy to find plenty of nutrition strategies that work for fat loss, the one component that is critical to all of them yet rarely discussed is the need for a change of behaviors. How you schedule your meals and make time to prepare for your needs can be just as important to your success as what you are eating. So take time to look at the habits you have formed around eating, and determine what needs to change in your approach to ensure success.

Warm-Up

4 reps per side of the world's greatest stretch, 5 reps of inchworm, 8 reps per side of shoulder sweeps

● Featured Exercise

Barbell Overhead Press

1. Grab a loaded bar just outside shoulder width at collarbone height. The bar should be resting on top of your anterior deltoids (front of your shoulders) (*a*).

2. Take a deep breath in, brace your core, and begin driving the bar overhead.

3. As the bar passes over the top of your head, drive your body slightly forward so the bar is over the center of your foot (do not, however, jut your chin out or extend your neck).

4. Continue to press the bar overhead until you have achieved full lockout (*b*). Return the bar to the starting position and repeat for reps.

Complete Workout

Perform as many reps as possible of the barbell overhead press in 12 minutes, using 65 percent of your 1RM. Be sure to use proper technique on each rep. Rest between reps as needed.

Barbell overhead press
- 12 minutes × as many reps as possible

OPTIONS

Easy Option   Use 60 percent of your 1RM, and perform as many reps as possible in 9 minutes.

Step It Up   Use 70 percent of your 1RM.

Cool-Down   Pec stretch, double lat stretch, 90-degree stretch.

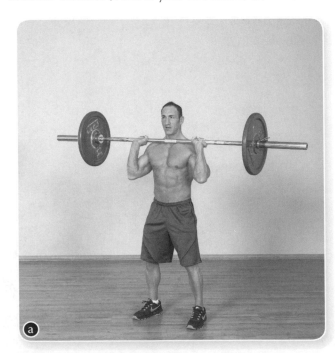

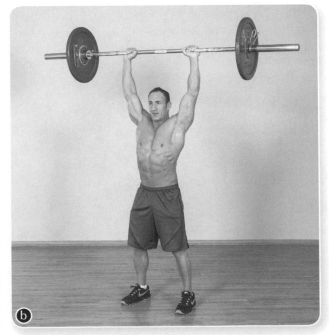

10-20-30-40

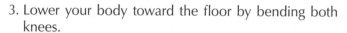

Some workouts push your limits by using a high number of repetitions to test muscular endurance and lactic threshold. Others combine challenging exercises with minimal rest periods in order to drive metabolic demand sky-high. This workout uses both these methods to produce one of the most difficult workouts you'll do all year. Complete this workout and give yourself a well-deserved pat on the back—if you can still lift your arms once it's over.

Warm-Up

6 reps of squat to stand, 6 reps per side of quadruped T-spine rotation, 8 reps of glute bridge, 10 reps of cat–cow

● **Featured Exercise**

Barbell Walking Lunge

1. Place a barbell across your upper back as you would for a barbell back squat (a).
2. Take a long step forward with your right leg.

3. Lower your body toward the floor by bending both knees.
4. Once the back knee touches the floor (b), press your front foot into the floor and bring both feet together.
5. Repeat the sequence by stepping forward with your left leg (c). Continue to alternate in this manner until all reps are complete.

Complete Workout

Complete 3 rounds of the following circuit, resting as little as possible between exercises and rounds.

Barbell walking lunge
- 10 reps/side

Chin-up (#73)
- 20 reps

Push-up (#12)
- 30 reps

Double-arm kettlebell swing (#13)
- 40 reps

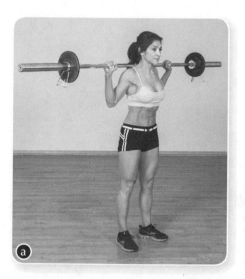

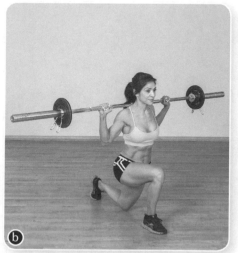

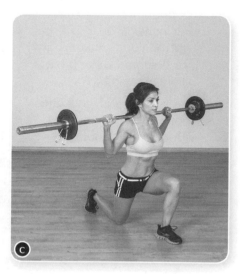

OPTIONS

Easy Option Cut all reps in half (5 per side on the barbell walking lunge, 10 chin-ups, 15 push-ups, and 20 kettlebell swings).

Step It Up Perform 4 rounds of the entire circuit.

Cool-Down Standing quad stretch, 90-degree stretch, double lat stretch.

Deadlift Plus

One of the worst things you can do for your body is something you probably do every day—sitting. Excessive sitting can decrease the amount of power you can produce from your hips and glutes, produces a forward-rounded posture in your upper back and shoulders, reduces coordination between your core and other muscles, and produces neck strain. Although completely eliminating sitting is probably not possible in today's society, do your best to reduce the amount you sit by getting up from your desk or chair for 15 minutes every hour.

Warm-Up

4 reps per side of the world's greatest stretch, 5 reps each of inchworm and inverted hamstring stretch, 10 reps of glute bridge

● Featured Exercise

Conventional Deadlift

1. Approach a barbell set up on the floor by placing your feet under the bar so it is 2 to 3 inches (5 to 8 cm) in front of your shins. Your stance should be approximately hip width.

2. Bend down and grab the bar just outside your legs with either a double overhand or mixed grip.

3. Pull your hips down and bring your shins in contact with the bar (a). Keep your chest tall, and maintain a neutral spine.

4. Stand up by rising simultaneously at your hips and shoulders, driving your hips forward until your reach lockout (b). Repeat for reps.

Complete Workout

Load 50 percent of your 1RM for the conventional deadlift onto a barbell. Perform 2 reps every minute on the minute (start at the top of each minute, and rest whatever remains of that minute after your set is complete). Increase the weight on the bar by 10 lb (4.5 kg) every minute. Continue until you hit a weight where you can no longer complete 2 reps.

Conventional deadlift

- As many sets as possible, as described

OPTIONS

Easy Option Perform 1 rep per set.

Step It Up Perform 3 reps per set.

Cool-Down Double lat stretch, hamstring stretch, calf stretch.

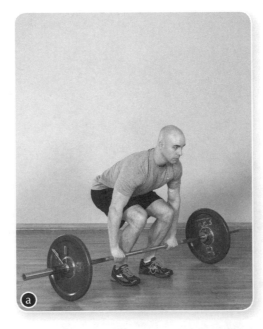
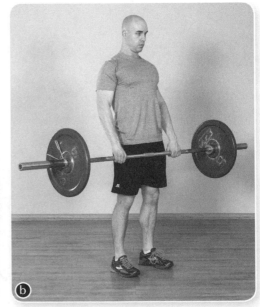

Dirty Dozen

If you are going to get serious about your training, you have to get serious about your recovery—particularly how you treat your body after training sessions. Finding a soft-tissue or licensed massage therapist who can help you with deep tissue massage, trigger point therapy, muscle activation techniques (MAT), active release techniques (ART), and other modalities can prove invaluable in keeping you healthy and performing at your best. Don't shortchange this aspect of your training.

Warm-Up

4 reps per side of the world's greatest stretch, 6 reps per side of hip rocker and inverted hamstring stretch, 8 reps per side of shoulder sweeps

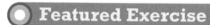
Featured Exercise

Burpee With Push-Up

1. From a tall standing position (a), place your hands on the floor and kick yourself back into a push-up position (b).

2. Perform one push-up (c), keeping your hands just outside shoulder width and your elbows tucked toward your rib cage, your body forming a straight line from head to heels.

3. Kick both feet up toward your chest and quickly stand up, adding in a small jump at the top (d).

4. Land with slightly flexed knees and immediately begin the next rep. Repeat for reps.

Complete Workout

Complete as many rounds of the following circuit as possible in 12 minutes.

Dumbbell push press (#51)
- 12 reps

Burpee with push-up
- 24 reps

Wall ball (#25)
- 36 reps

Single-contact mountain climber (#281)
- 48 reps (per leg)

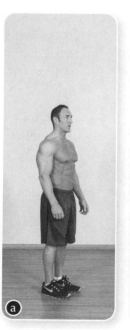

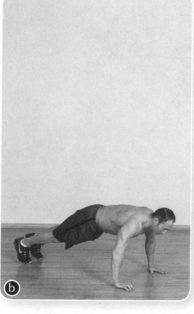

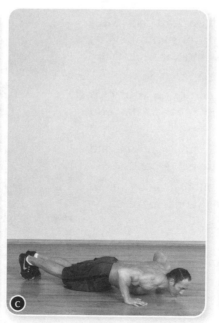

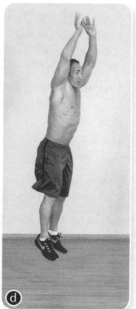

OPTIONS

Easy Option   Perform as many reps as possible in 9 minutes.

Step It Up   Perform as many reps as possible in 15 minutes.

Cool-Down   Standing quad stretch, 90-degree stretch, double lat stretch.

ATG

There is a lot of misinformation floating around regarding squat depth and knee health. Most of this revolves around a faulty older study showing that 90-degree, or parallel, squat depth was the safest and most effective range of motion. Very little could be further from the truth. Your goal should be to squat as deeply as possible, dropping your hips between your heels and attempting to touch your hamstrings to your calves. This not only leads to the best lower body muscle development but also helps keep your knees safe by allowing you to reverse directions when the joint is more stable. In fact the title of this workout stands for "Ass To Grass," or how deep you should be attempting to go (given you have full range of motion).

Warm-Up

5 reps of squat to stand; 6 reps per side of kneeling adductor stretch, hip rocker, and quadruped T-spine rotation

● **Featured Exercise**

Overhead Squat

1. Begin with the barbell on your back, your hands in a snatch-grip position (outside shoulder width). Press the bar straight up, locking out your elbows at the top (a).
2. Keeping your chest tall, bring your hips back and bend at the knees to descend into a squat (b).
3. Keep the bar directly over or slightly behind your head for the entire movement.
4. Once you reach the bottom position, return to a standing position. Repeat for reps.

Complete Workout

For the overhead squat, begin with a weight you can comfortably complete for 3 or 4 reps. Perform 1 rep. Rest 60 seconds, and add weight for set number 2. Continue in this manner (adding weight each set) until you have completed 5 singles. Using the same weights you used for the 5 sets of the overhead squat, perform 6 reps per set of the barbell front squat. When you have completed those 5 sets, use the same weights to complete all 5 sets of 10 reps of the barbell back squat. For example, if you used 135 lb, 155 lb, 165 lb, 175 lb, and 180 lb for the overhead squat singles, use those same weights for the sets of front squat and back squat (but with the increased number of reps).

Overhead squat
- 5 sets × 1, 1, 1, 1, 1 reps
- 60 seconds rest

Barbell front squat (#44)
- 5 sets × 6, 6, 6, 6, 6 reps
- 60 seconds of rest

Barbell back squat (#63)
- 5 sets × 10, 10, 10, 10, 10 reps
- 60 seconds of rest

OPTIONS

Easy Option   Reduce to 3 sets of each exercise.

Step It Up   Add 1 set to each exercise.

Cool-Down   Standing quad stretch, 90-degree stretch, cross-body stretch.

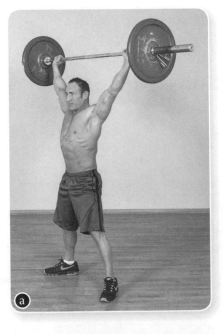
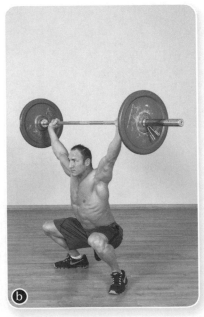

A Taste for Blood

When training at absolute maximum work capacity, some intense physical phenomena will occur—your lungs will burn, sweat will pour into your eyes, and you may get the taste of blood in your mouth. Every fiber in your being will tell you to stop training. It's at this moment that you need to put the pain aside and try to push yourself that much harder. Doing so will improve not only your work capacity but also your character. You'll prove to yourself that you have no limits. And nothing will make you stronger than that belief.

Warm-Up

4 reps per side of the world's greatest stretch, 5 reps each of inchworm and inverted hamstring stretch, 10 reps of glute bridge

Featured Exercise

Farmer's Walk

1. Grab a pair of dumbbells, kettlebells, or farmer's walk handles. Stand tall, with your shoulders down and back.
2. Begin walking forward by taking short, quick steps.
3. When you reach the distance, lower the weight back to the floor.

Complete Workout

Perform the following circuit in as little time as possible, resting only as needed. Load 1 × body weight on the bar for the deadlift and 50 percent body weight per hand on the farmer's walk. Remember, you are alternating between these two movements (8 reps of the deadlift, followed by a farmer's walk, back to the deadlift for 7 reps, and so on)

Conventional deadlift (#5)
- 8 sets × 8, 7, 6, 5, 4, 3, 2, 1 reps

Farmer's walk
- 8 sets × 30 yards (30 m)

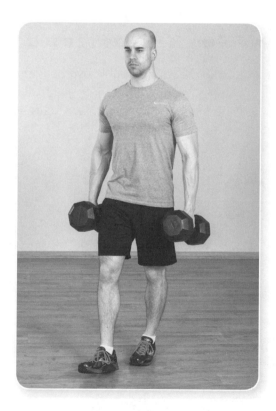

OPTIONS

Easy Option Use 75 percent body weight for the conventional deadlift and 25 percent body weight per hand on the farmer's walk.

Step It Up Use 1.5 × body weight on the deadlift and 75 percent body weight per hand on the farmer's walk.

Cool-Down Double lat stretch, hamstring stretch, calf stretch.

The Ascent

Although there are some theories as to when the perfect time to train may be, in reality there is no perfect time. However, if you are consistent with the time of day you train, your body will adapt and expect to train at that time. With that being said, there may be an advantage to having more meals in your day before training, so if you can get in at least one meal, preferably two, before you hit the gym, you may see an increase in performance.

Warm-Up

5 reps of inchworm, 6 reps per side of quadruped T-spine rotation, 10 reps of cat–cow

Featured Exercise

Double-Arm Kettlebell Swing

1. Grab a kettlebell with a double overhand grip (*a*).
2. Begin gaining momentum by forcefully swinging the kettlebell between your legs, making sure to keep it high (directly below your crotch) (*b*).
3. As the kettlebell is traveling through your legs, perform a hip hinge (described in chapter 1, Ramping Up), keeping your arms straight and chest tall.
4. Reverse the motion by driving your hips forward, keeping your arms straight, and propelling the kettlebell forward. All the power should be generated by your hips—do not use your arms to lift the kettlebell.
5. Once the kettlebell reaches its pinnacle (*c*), reverse the motion and drive it back through your legs. Repeat for reps.

Complete Workout

Alternate the following two exercises as described. Use 1 × body weight for the barbell back squat and a 44, 53, or 70-lb kettlebell for the swing.

Barbell back squat (#63)
- 10 sets × 10, 9, 8, 7, 6, 5, 4, 3, 2, 1 reps

Double-arm kettlebell swing
- 10 sets × 1, 2, 3, 4, 5,6, 7, 8, 9, 10 reps

OPTIONS

Easy Option   Use 75 percent body weight (or less) for the barbell back squat.

Step It Up   Use 1.25 × body weight for the barbell back squat.

Cool-Down   Double lat stretch, cross-body stretch, hamstring stretch.

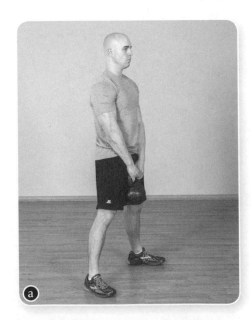

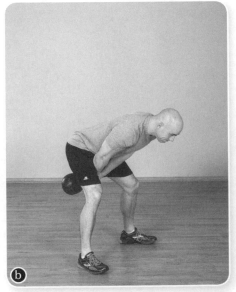

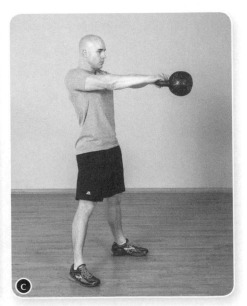

The Seal

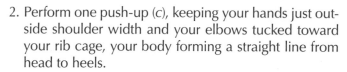

It has been argued that there is no more exclusive group in the U.S. military than the Navy SEALs. SEAL training is notoriously brutal, pushing only the top candidates to their physical, psychological, mental, and emotional limits. And although it is impossible to equate a training session to what it takes to become a member of this elite force, this workout will push both your physical limits and mental focus further than you may have thought possible.

Warm-Up

4 reps per side of the world's greatest stretch, 5 reps each of inchworm and inverted hamstring stretch, 10 reps of glute bridge

● Featured Exercise

Burpee With Push-Up

1. From a tall standing position (*a*), place your hands on the floor and kick yourself back into a push-up position (*b*).

2. Perform one push-up (*c*), keeping your hands just outside shoulder width and your elbows tucked toward your rib cage, your body forming a straight line from head to heels.

3. Kick both feet up toward your chest and quickly stand up, adding in a small jump at the top (*d*).

4. Land with slightly flexed knees and immediately begin the next rep. Repeat for reps.

Complete Workout

Perform 1 round of the following circuit.

Sprint (#41)
- 400 yards (400 m)

Neutral-grip pull-up (#237)
- 100 reps

Burpee with push-up
- 100 reps

Sprint (#41)
- 400 yards (400 m)

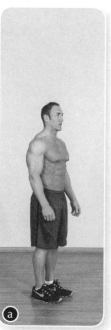

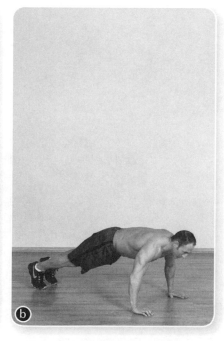

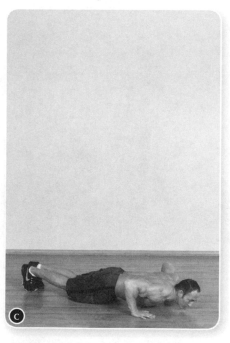

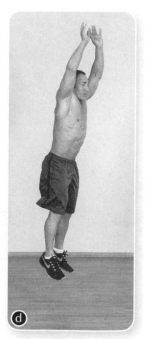

OPTIONS

Easy Option   Perform 25 reps of the pull-up and 50 reps of the burpee.

Step It Up   Wear a weighted vest for the pull-up and the burpee.

Cool-Down   Double lat stretch, hamstring stretch, calf stretch.

Brutal

This workout is so demanding, so challenging, so awful, the only name that seemed suitable was Brutal. By combining full-body pulling, pressing, lower body, upper body, and ballistic exercises, this circuit will challenge your strength, your grip, your work capacity, and your will. Save this one for a day when you walk into the gym feeling as if you can tear the head off a lion—you'll need that kind of enthusiasm to survive it.

Warm-Up

6 reps of squat to stand, 6 reps per side of quadruped T-spine rotation, 8 reps of glute bridge, 10 reps of cat–cow

● Featured Exercise

Barbell Romanian Deadlift

1. Grab a barbell with a double overhand grip just outside shoulder width. Begin with the bar in front of your thighs with your arms straight. Your knees should be unlocked but not bent (a).

2. Lower the barbell by reaching your hips back. Keep your back flat and your chin tucked. Keep the bar very close to your legs, but do not drag it down your thighs.

3. You've reached your end range of motion when you've lost the ability to continue driving your hips back (b). Once you reach this point, reverse the motion by standing with the bar. Repeat for reps.

Complete Workout

Perform 4 rounds of this circuit as quickly as possible, resting as little as needed within sets and between exercises. Perform 18 reps the first round, 15 reps the second round, 10 reps the third round, and 8 reps the fourth round.

Barbell thruster (#6)

Barbell Romanian deadlift

Pull-up (#231)

Double-arm kettlebell swing (#13)

OPTIONS

Easy Option   Perform 12, 9, 6, and 4 reps per round.

Step It Up   Add 2 reps to each round.

Cool-Down   Standing quad stretch, 90-degree stretch, double lat stretch.

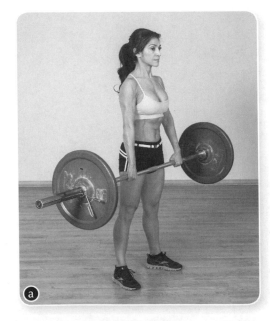
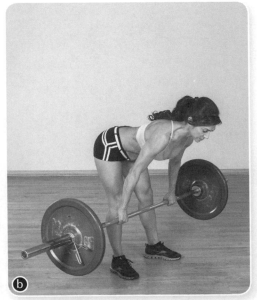

The Savior

Some workouts leave you feeling energized, ready to take on your day. Other workouts may make you feel a bit woozy after pushing yourself really hard. Then there are those workouts that leave you lying on the gym floor, with visions of holy spirits filling your head. You try to catch your breath, you try to recover, but even a couple of hours later you're still feeling it and decide to leave work early, go home, and lie down. This is that workout.

Warm-Up

6 reps of squat to stand, 6 reps per side of quadruped T-spine rotation, 8 reps of glute bridge, 10 reps of cat–cow

● Featured Exercise

Dumbbell Hang Snatch

1. Grab a dumbbell with your right hand, and assume a shoulder-width stance with your feet. Keeping your chest tall, bend at the knees and bring your hips back until the dumbbell is right above knee level (*a*).

2. Explosively drive your hips forward, shrug your right shoulder, and extend at the ankle, driving the dumbbell up and overhead (*b*). Keep the dumbbell close to your body for the entire movement.

3. Catch the dumbbell with your arm fully extended and directly above the same-side shoulder (*c*). Lower the dumbbell back to the starting position. Complete all reps for one side before switching.

Complete Workout

Complete 4 rounds of the following circuit.

Box jump (#198)
- 8 reps

Dumbbell hang snatch
- 4 reps/side

Neutral-grip pull-up (#237)
- 10 reps

Barbell rollout (#228)
- 12 reps

Rower (#212)
- 500 meters
- 2 minutes of rest

OPTIONS

Easy Option Perform the entire circuit 2 times.

Step It Up Add 2 reps to each of the exercises.

Cool-Down Standing quad stretch, 90-degree stretch, double lat stretch.

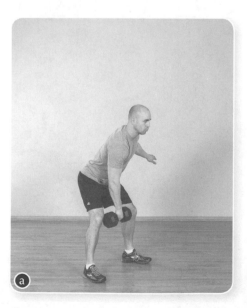

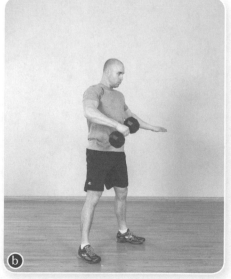

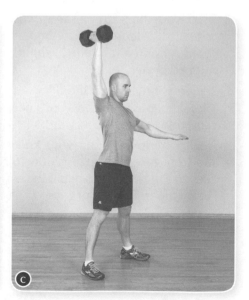

One-Exercise Challenge: Trap Bar Deadlift

Is it a squat? Is it a deadlift? The trap bar deadlift combines the two "kings" of lower body movements into one exercise. By using a more upright posture, the trap bar deadlift utilizes more of the musculature of the anterior (front) thigh than the traditional deadlift. However, the positioning of the bar allows for more of a hip-hinge movement pattern than the squat. You are truly getting the best of both worlds from this tremendous leg builder.

Warm-Up

4 reps per side of the world's greatest stretch, 5 reps each of inchworm and inverted hamstring stretch, 10 reps of glute bridge

Complete Workout

Complete as many sets of 8 of the trap bar deadlift as you can, resting as little as needed. The goal is to complete as many sets (and total reps) as possible in the time allotted (25 minutes).

Trap bar deadlift
- Max sets × 8 reps × 25 minutes

● Featured Exercise

Trap Bar Deadlift

1. Begin by standing inside the trap bar, feet at shoulder-width, grasping the middle of the handles.
2. Pull your hips down, keep your chest tall, depress your shoulder blades, and maintain a slightly arched or neutral spine (a).
3. Drive your feet into the floor, and simultaneously extend your knees and bring your hips forward.
4. Finish by locking out your knees and hips in the top position (b). Reverse the motion to return the bar to the floor. Repeat for reps.

OPTIONS

Easy Option Reduce the total length of the workout to 15 minutes.

Step It Up Attempt to complete at least 1 set every 90 seconds for the entire 25 minutes.

Cool-Down Double lat stretch, hamstring stretch, calf stretch.

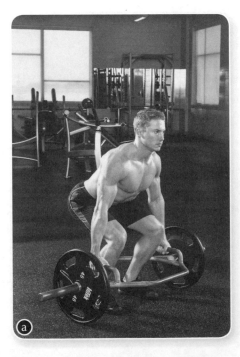

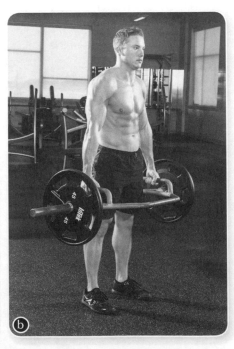

Going Down

As you become more advanced and experienced in your training, working off of specific percentages can be very helpful in determining appropriate loads and making sure you are continuing to gain strength. Keeping an accurate record of your 1RM (as well as your maximums in other rep ranges) on the big lifts such as squat, bench, overhead press, and deadlift will give you a gauge on what loads will be appropriate in future workouts. Of course you can always give yourself the green light to go heavier if you feel great or lighter if you are dragging, but using percentages of maximums is great way to make sure you've got the right weight on the bar.

Warm-Up

5 reps squat to stand, 6 reps per side of kneeling adductor stretch, hip rocker, and quadrupled T-spine rotation.

● Featured Exercise

Kettlebell Shoulder Press

1. Clean a pair of kettlebells up to the rack position. Your hands should be at your collarbones with the kettlebells resting on your forearms (*a*).
2. Keeping your torso tight, drive the kettlebells overhead until your elbows are locked out (*b*). Your palms should be facing away from you in this top position.
3. Return the kettlebells to the rack position and repeat for reps.

Complete Workout

Complete 10 sets of the following circuit in as quickly as possible. This workout features a descending ladder rep scheme, meaning you will perform 10 reps of each exercise in the first set, 9 reps of each in the second set until you perform one rep of each exercise in the last set.

Sumo deadlift (#82)
- 10 × 10, 9,8,7,6,5,4,3,2,1 reps

3-for-1 wall ball (#38)
- 10 × 10, 9,8,7,6,5,4,3,2,1 reps

Kettlebell shoulder press
- 10 × 10, 9,8,7,6,5,4,3,2,1 reps

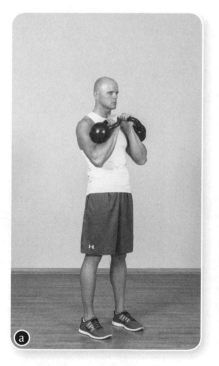

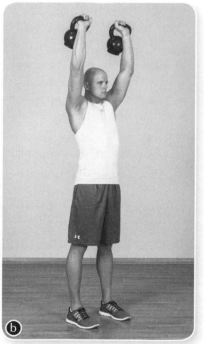

OPTIONS

Easy Option   Perform 7 sets of the circuit beginning with 7 reps in the first set.

Step It Up   Perform 12 sets of the circuit beginning with 12 reps in the first set.

Cool-Down   Standing quad stretch, 90-degree stretch, cross body stretch.

Redemption

Any missed training sessions. Any of this week's cheat meals. Any nights spent staying out late instead of recovering. All of this week's missteps are about to be redeemed with this workout. Redemption involves more dynamic and explosive movements than a typical circuit, driving up metabolic demand and requiring additional focus to execute the movements correctly. The physical and mental challenges will make this one of the toughest circuits you're likely to encounter.

Warm-Up

6 reps of squat to stand, 6 reps per side of quadruped T-spine rotation, 8 reps of glute bridge, 10 reps of cat–cow

Complete Workout

Perform 4 rounds of the following circuit, resting as little as needed.

Box jump (#198)
- 8 reps

Toes to bar (#28)
- 8 reps

Single-arm dumbbell snatch
- 4 reps/side

Farmer's walk (#187)
- 20 yards (20 m)

Featured Exercise

Single-Arm Dumbbell Snatch

1. Begin with a dumbbell on the floor between your feet. Bend down and grab the dumbbell with your right arm, keeping your butt back and chest tall (a).
2. Explosively pull the dumbbell off the floor by driving your hips forward, shrugging your right traps and extending at the ankles (b).
3. Keep the dumbbell close to your body as you drive your elbow high.
4. Allow the dumbbell to continue overhead, and catch it in the top position, with your arm straight and knees slightly bent (c).
5. Bring the dumbbell down to your shoulder and back to the floor. Complete all reps for one side before switching to the other.

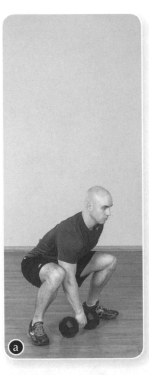
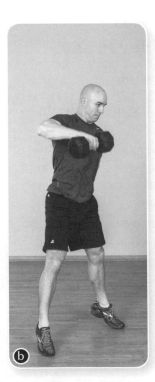
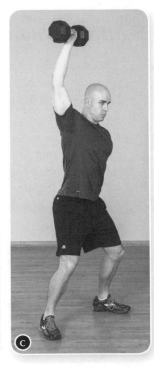

OPTIONS

Easy Option   Perform 3 rounds of the circuit.

Step It Up   Perform 5 rounds of the circuit.

Cool-Down   Standing quad stretch, 90-degree stretch, double lat stretch.

The Century

Four movements, 100 total reps. Seems simple enough. But by combining some of the toughest compound movements you'll find in the gym that alternate from lower body dominant to upper body dominant and back again, you'll have to push past your current limits to finish this intense workout. You will most certainly need to take rest periods during each of these sets. That is absolutely fine; just make sure you take that rest in a safe position (e.g., put the bar down during the trap bar deadlifts, or drop from the chin-up bar so your feet are on the ground).

Warm-Up

4 reps per side of the world's greatest stretch, 6 reps per side of hip rocker and inverted hamstring stretch, 8 reps per side of shoulder sweeps

● **Featured Exercise**

Trap Bar Deadlift

1. Begin by standing inside the trap bar, feet at shoulder-width, grasping the middle of the handles.
2. Pull your hips down, keep your chest tall, depress your shoulder blades, and maintain a slightly arched or neutral spine (a).
3. Drive your feet into the floor, and simultaneously extend your knees and bring your hips forward.
4. Finish by locking out your knees and hips in the top position (b). Reverse the motion to return the bar to the floor. Repeat for reps.

Complete Workout

Perform the following circuit, resting as little as needed within and between sets.

Barbell back squat (#63)
  • 25 reps

Barbell bench press (#54)
  • 25 reps

Trap bar deadlift
  • 25 reps

Chin-up (#73)
  • 25 reps

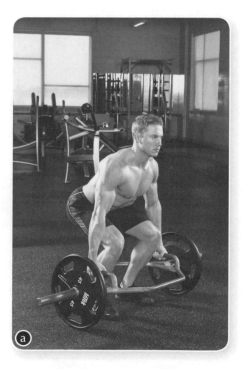
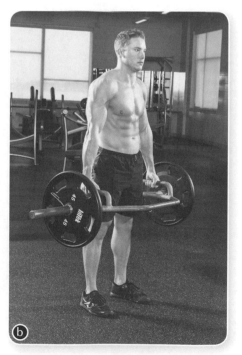

OPTIONS

Easy Option   Complete 15 reps of each exercise.

Step It Up   Go for a double century: Repeat the circuit.

Cool-Down   Standing quad stretch, 90-degree stretch, double lat stretch.

Conclusion

Congratulations! You've made it through a year's worth of tough training, and I guarantee you have a stronger, leaner, and more athletic body to show for all your hard work. Even if you had to stick with the easy options, I have no doubt you've trained hard and made some incredible progress. But you are far from reaching your maximum potential. So go back to the start of the book, add some weight to the bar, and try the Step It Up options. Remember, fitness has no finish line.

Workout Index

Note: The workout number is given after each workout name. The name and page number of the workouts in the "Ramping Up" chapter are indicated in *italics*.

Exercise Index

Note: Each exercise is followed by workout numbers indicating where the exercise is used. The **boldface** workout numbers indicate where to find step-by-step instructions for featured exercises. The name and page number of the fundamental movements and stretches in the "Ramping Up" chapter are indicated in *italics*.

About the Author

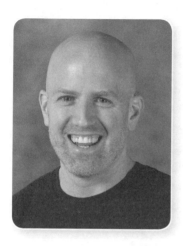

Dan Trink is a certified strength and conditioning specialist (CSCS), the highest level of certification bestowed by the National Strength and Conditioning Association (NSCA), along with being a United States of America Weightlifting Association (USAW) Sports Performance Coach. He also earned a level 3 certification from the Poliquin International Certification Program, an honor reserved for trainers who have coached athletes at the national championship level and have placed in the top 10 percent at their events.

Trink is the director of training operations at Peak Performance in New York City, where he trains a full roster of clients and athletes.

Trink was among the first group to receive the Precision Nutrition sports and exercise nutrition certification and is a BioSignature Modulation practitioner—a nutrition and lifestyle approach designed to optimize hormonal balance within the client or athlete.

Trink has published articles and been cited as a source for leading health and fitness websites and magazines including *Men's Fitness*, *Greatist*, *T Nation*, *Livestrong*, and *Muscle and Fitness*, while his name has appeared in the *Huffington Post* and other general media outlets. He is also a member of the fitness advisory board for Men's Fitness Magazine and a part of the expert panel for greatist.com.

Trink also coaches for the Personal Trainer Development Center (PTDC), an international organization whose mission is to improve the quality of the personal training industry. He has worked with professional athletes at the championship level including developing strength and conditioning programs for boxers preparing for title fights, working with NBA All-Stars as well as countless international-level jiu-jitsu practitioners and mixed martial arts fighters. A featured presenter at both the corporate and international level discussing both nutrition and strength training, Trink has other specialty certifications from TRX (Suspension Training System); FMS (functional movement screen); Dynamax Medicine Balls and many others.

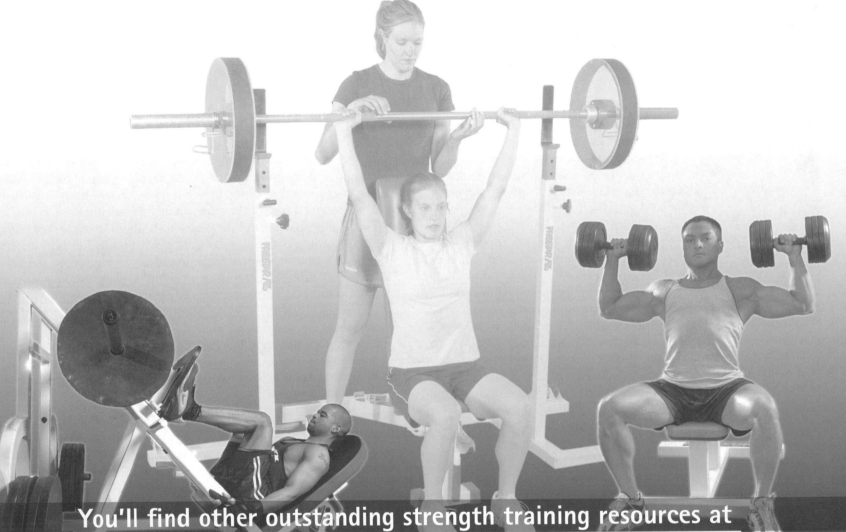

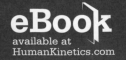